Also by Charles W. Kane

Wild Edible Plants of Texas: A Pocket Guide to the Identification, Collection, Preparation, and Use of 60 Wild Plants of the Lone Star State (2016)

Southern California Food Plants: Wild Edibles of the Valleys, Foothills, Coast, and Beyond (2013)

Sonoran Desert Food Plants: Edible Uses for the Desert's Wild Bounty (2011)

Herbal Medicine: Trends and Traditions (A Comprehensive Sourcebook on the Preparation and Use of Medicinal Plants) (2009)

Medicinal Plants of the American Southwest (2006 & 2011)

MEDICINAL PLANTS

······ of the ······

WESTERN MOUNTAIN STATES

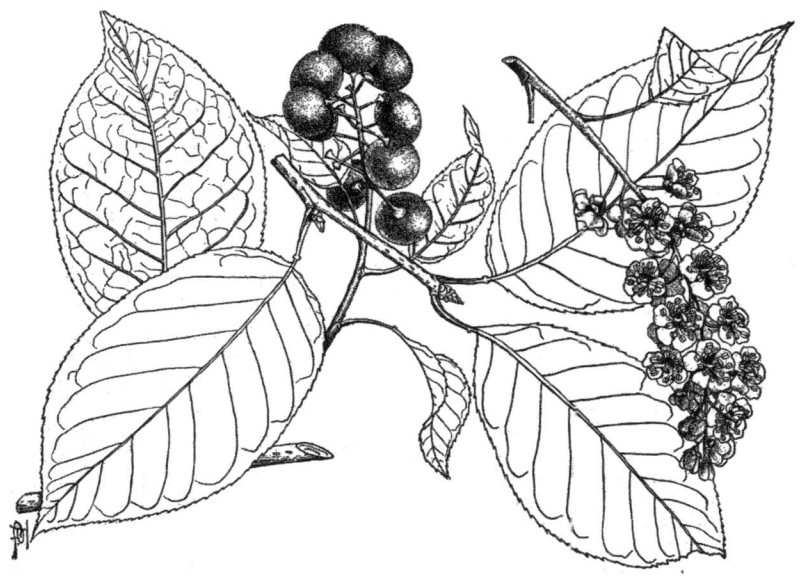

Charles W. Kane

Medicinal Plants of the Western Mountain States
Lincoln Town Press

All rights reserved
Copyright © 2017 by Charles W. Kane
Photo insert © Charles W. Kane

First edition: June 2017

Library of Congress Control Number: 2017904041
ISBN 10: 0–9982871–0–5; ISBN 13: 978–0–9982871–0–2 (Paperback)
ISBN 10: 0–9982871–1–3; ISBN 13: 978–0–9982871–1–9 (Hardcover)

No part of this book may be reproduced or transmitted in any form or by any means, electronic or mechanical, including photocopying, recording, or by any information storage and retrieval system, without written permission from the publisher.

Medicinal Plants of the Western Mountain States is intended solely for educational purposes. The publisher and author disclaim all liability arising from the use of any plant listed in this book.

Printed and bound in the United States of America

CONTENTS

Acknowledgments	12	False Solomon's Seal	133
Introduction	14	Field Mint	135
Format Explanation	18	Figwort	137
Preparations	24	Fir	139
Materia Medica	42	Fireweed	144
Agastache	43	Fragrant Sumac	146
Agrimony	46	Gentian	148
Alfalfa	48	Geranium	151
Alumroot	50	Goldenrod	154
Angelica	52	Green Gentian	156
Apache Plume	55	Grindelia	158
Arnica	57	Hawthorn	161
Asparagus	60	Hedeoma	165
Aspen	62	Henbane	167
Avens	65	Hollyhock	171
Balsam Poplar	67	Hops	173
Balsamroot	72	Hoptree	177
Baneberry	75	Horsetail	180
Barberry	78	Hound's Tongue	182
Bilberry	83	Juniper	183
Birch	85	Larkspur	185
Bistort	88	Ligusticum	188
Bitterbrush	90	Lomatium	191
Bogbean	92	Madrone	195
Buckthorn	94	Marsh Marigold	199
Bugleweed	97	Monarda	203
Checker Mallow	101	Monardella	207
Chicory	103	Mullein	209
Cinquefoil	105	Nettle	211
Cleavers	107	Oak	215
Coral Root	109	Oregongrape	218
Cottonwood	112	Ox–Eye Daisy	221
Cow Parsnip	114	Pedicularis	224
Dandelion	119	Pine	226
Dock	122	Pipsissewa	233
Dogbane	124	Plantain	236
Elder	127	Pulsatilla	238
Evening Primrose	131	Pussytoes	242

Pyrola	244
Rattlesnake Plantain	246
Red Osier Dogwood	247
Red Raspberry	250
Red Root	252
Ribes	256
Sagebrush	258
Scarlet Pimpernel	261
Self Heal	263
Shepherd's Purse	265
Silk Tassel	267
Skullcap	269
Sneezeweed	272
Spearmint	274
Spruce	275
Squawroot	280
St. John's Wort	283
Stachys	286
Sweet Cicely	288
Sweet Clover	290
Toadflax	292
Usnea	295
Uva-Ursi	298
Valerian	301
Verbena	305
Western Mugwort	307
Wild Cherry	310
Wild Iris	313
Wild Rose	316
Wild Strawberry	320
Wild Violet	322
Willow	324
Yarrow	326
Yellow Pond Lily	329
Therapeutic Index	334
Glossary	342
Bibliography	368
Index	394

PHOTOGRAPHS

1. Agastache (Agastache pallidiflora); 2. Agrimony (Agrimonia striata); 3. Alfalfa (Medicago sativa); 4. Alumroot (Heuchera sanguinea); 5. Alumroot (Heuchera sanguinea); 6. Angelica (Angelica pinnata); 7. Angelica (Angelica pinnata); 8. Angelica (Angelica pinnata); 9. Apache plume (Fallugia paradoxa); 10. Arnica (Arnica cordifolia); 11. Asparagus (Asparagus officinalis); 12. Aspen (Populus tremuloides); 13. Aspen (Populus tremuloides); 14. Avens (Geum macrophyllum var. perincisum); 15. Balsam poplar (Populus balsamifera); 16. Balsam poplar (Populus balsamifera); 17. Balsamroot (Balsamorhiza sagittata); 18. Balsamroot (Balsamorhiza sagittata); 19. Baneberry (Actaea rubra); 20. Baneberry (Actaea rubra); 21. Barberry (Berberis fendleri); 22. Barberry (Berberis fendleri); 23. Barberry (Berberis fendleri); 24. Bilberry (Vaccinium myrtillus); 25. Birch (Betula occidentalis); 26. Birch (Betula occidentalis); 27. Birch (Betula occidentalis); 28. Bistort (Bistorta bistortoides); 29. Bistort (Bistorta bistortoides); 30. Bitterbrush (Purshia tridentata); 31. Bogbean (Menyanthes trifoliata); 32. Bogbean (Menyanthes trifoliata); 33. Buckthorn (Rhamnus betulifolia); 34. Buckthorn (Rhamnus californica); 35. Bugleweed (Lycopus americanus); 36. Checker mallow (Sidalcea neomexicana); 37. Checker mallow (Sidalcea neomexicana); 38. Chicory (Cichorium intybus); 39. Cinquefoil (Potentilla fruticosa); 40. Cinquefoil (Potentilla thurberi); 41. Cleavers (Galium aparine); 42. Coral root (Corallorhiza maculata) 43. Cottonwood (Populus angustifolia); 44. Cottonwood (Populus angustifolia); 45. Cow parsnip (Heracleum maximum); 46. Cow parsnip (Heracleum maximum); 47. Cow parsnip (Heracleum maximum); 48. Dandelion (Taraxacum officinale); 49. Dock (Rumex obtusifolius); 50. Dock (Rumex crispus); 51. Dogbane (Apocynum cannabinum); 52. Dogbane (Apocynum cannabinum); 53. Elder (Sambucus cerulea); 54. Elder (Sambucus microbotrys); 55. Evening primrose (Oenothera elata); 56. False Solomon's seal (Maianthemum racemosum); 57. False Solomon's seal (Maianthemum racemosum); 58. Field mint (Mentha arvensis); 59. Figwort (Scrophularia californica); 60. Figwort (Scrophularia parviflora); 61. Fir (Abies concolor); 62. Fireweed (Chamerion angustifolium); 63. Fireweed (Chamerion angustifolium); 64. Fragrant sumac (Rhus aromatica); 65. Gentian (Gentiana affinis); 66. Gentian (Gentiana parryi); 67. Geranium (Geranium richardsonii); 68. Goldenrod (Solidago altissima); 69. Goldenrod (Solidago velutina); 70. Green gentian (Frasera speciosa); 71. Green gentian (Frasera speciosa); 72. Grindelia (Grindelia squarrosa); 73. Grindelia (Grindelia squarrosa); 74. Hawthorn (Crataegus

rivularis); 75. Hawthorn (Crataegus rivularis); 76. Hedeoma (Hedeoma hyssopifolia); 77. Henbane (Hyoscyamus niger); 78. Hollyhock (Althea rosea); 79. Hops (Humulus neomexicanus); 80. Hoptree (Ptelea trifoliata); 81. Horsetail (Equisetum arvense); 82. Hound's tongue (Cynoglossum officinale); 83. Juniper (Juniperus communis); 84. Juniper (Juniperus communis); 85. Larkspur (Delphinium geraniifolium); 86. Ligusticum (Ligusticum porteri); 87. Ligusticum (Ligusticum porteri); 88. Lomatium (Lomatium dissectum); 89. Lomatium (Lomatium dissectum); 90. Madrone (Arbutus arizonica); 91. Madrone (Arbutus arizonica); 92. Marsh marigold (Caltha leptosepala); 93. Monarda (Monarda citriodora); 94. Monarda (Monarda fistulosa); 95. Monarda (Monarda pectinata); 96. Monardella (Monardella odoratissima); 97. Mullein (Verbascum thapsus); 98. Mullein (Verbascum thapsus); 99. Nettle (Urtica dioica subsp. gracilis); 100. Nettle (Urtica dioica subsp. gracilis); 101. Oak (Quercus gambelii); 102. Oregongrape (Berberis repens); 103. Ox–eye daisy (Leucanthemum vulgare); 104. Ox–eye daisy (Leucanthemum vulgare); 105. Pedicularis (Pedicularis procera); 106. Pedicularis (Pedicularis racemosa); 107. Pine (Pinus ponderosa); 108. Pine (Pinus ponderosa); 109. Pipsissewa (Chimaphila umbellata); 110. Pipsissewa (Chimaphila umbellata); 111. Plantain (Plantago major); 112. Pulsatilla (Pulsatilla occidentalis); 113. Pussytoes (Antennaria parvifolia); 114. Pyrola (Pyrola elliptica); 115. Rattlesnake plantain (Goodyera oblongifolia); 116. Rattlesnake plantain (Goodyera oblongifolia); 117. Red osier dogwood (Cornus sericea); 118. Red raspberry (Rubus idaeus var. strigosus); 119. Red raspberry (Rubus idaeus var. strigosus); 120. Red root (Ceanothus fendleri); 121. Red root (Ceanothus leucodermis); 122. Red root (Ceanothus greggii var. perplexans); 123. Ribes (Ribes cereum); 124. Sagebrush (Artemisia tridentata); 125. Scarlet pimpernel (Anagallis arvensis); 126. Self heal (Prunella vulgaris var. lanceolata); 127. Shepard's purse (Capsella bursa–pastoris); 128. Silk tassel (Garrya wrightii); 129. Silk tassel (Garrya wrightii); 130. Skullcap (Scutellaria galericulata); 131. Sneezeweed (Hymenoxys hoopesii); 132. Spearmint (Mentha spicata); 133. Spruce (Picea pungens); 134. Spruce (Picea pungens); 135. Squawroot (Conopholis americana); 136. St. John's wort (Hypericum perforatum); 137. St. John's wort (Hypericum scouleri); 138. Stachys (Stachys pilosa); 139. Sweet cicely (Osmorhiza depauperata); 140 Sweet cicely (Osmorhiza depauperata); 141. Sweet clover (Melilotus officinalis); 142. Sweet clover (Melilotus albus); 143. Toadflax (Linaria vulgaris); 144. Usnea (Usnea spp.); 145. Usnea (Usnea spp.); 146. Uva–ursi (Arctostaphylos uva–ursi); 147. Valerian (Valeriana arizonica); 148. Valerian (Valeriana edulis); 149. Valerian (Valeriana edulis); 150.

Verbena (Verbena macdougalii); 151. Verbena (Verbena bracteata); 152. Western mugwort (Artemisia ludoviciana); 153. Wild cherry (Prunus virginiana var. demissa); 154. Wild cherry (Prunus virginiana var. demissa); 155. Wild cherry (Prunus serotina var. rufula); 156. Wild iris (Iris missouriensis); 157. Wild iris (Iris missouriensis); 158. Wild rose (Rosa woodsii); 159. Wild rose (Rosa woodsii); 160. Wild strawberry (Fragaria vesca); 161. Wild strawberry (Fragaria virginiana); 162. Wild violet (Viola canadensis); 163. Willow (Salix exigua); 164. Yarrow (Achillea millefolium); 165. Yellow pond lily (Nuphar polysepala); 166. Yellow pond lily (Nuphar polysepala).

ACKNOWLEDGMENTS

In some ways writing a book is like building a castle. Only instead of a fortification made from rock through the channeling of physical labor, it's an effort of the mind conveyed through pen and paper. For both it's often a glacial process that can take years (8 years for this one) to complete. A builder has his favorite tools and design resources. Writers on medicinal plants have their favorites too.

I'm continually thankful to have access to the University of Arizona's Health and Science Library's database/journal collection. The research I've been able to conduct has significantly influenced this book (and my others); the bibliography section lists only a small sampling of the full–length articles derived from the UA system.

For online classification and distribution information the SEINet, USDA plants, BONAP, and eFlora websites were especially helpful. Instead to manually flipping through King's American Dispensary or Felter's Materia Medica, I often found myself at Henriette Kress's website where she has the same texts well represented. Very handy. Thank you.

Michael Moore was the first to expound on many of these plants using the western scientific perspective, and for this my gratitude to him is constant. Additionally, I have a tremendous degree of appreciation for my fellow critical–thinking botanical practitioners whom strive to keep the flame of reason burning from the lamp of herbal knowledge. The darkening winds of pseudoscience and psychobabble continue to pose a threat to its light.

The majority of photos within are my own; however, for a number of them credit goes to the following. #115. Rattlesnake plantain (Goodyera oblongifolia), #117. Red osier dogwood (Cornus sericea), and #45. Usnea (Usnea spp.) were photographed by Alexander Yelich. Creative Commons/Public Domain photos include: 'Lomatium dissectum' by Walter Siegmund, CC BY–SA 3.0 [#88. Lomatium (Lomatium dissectum)] and 'Pulsatilla occidentalis – white pasqueflower' by brewbooks, CC BY–SA 2.0 [#112. Pulsatilla (Pulsatilla occidentalis)].

The cover illustration of Wild cherry (Prunus virginiana var. demissa) comes from Forest Trees of the Pacific Slope by George B. Sudworth (1908); illustrator unknown.

INTRODUCTION

By and large the advancement of conventional medicine has left medicinal plant application in the dust. That doesn't mean the latter is without value. After all, the cost of any gain in territory is ultimately a loss of territory. It just means we are left with the scraps.

The scraps: medicinal plants are optimally used when geared towards self–limiting and functional problems, as opposed to the main course of advanced illness. If a problem can be benefited by changes in diet, exercise, or other lifestyle alterations, then chances are the reader will find herbal application of value. Broadly, sensible medicinal plant use is best thought of as a strong and directed lifestyle change. This is the nature of most herbs, not just the ones profiled here.

The best description for this book: a modern treatment of an archaic subject. If this is the reader's first foray into herbal medicine my suggestion is to begin with reading a single profile of a familiar plant. Expand to related plants within the same family (there will be medicinal similarities) or unrelated plants that may address the same problem, but likely in a different way. Let the corollaries begin to take shape and with continued application and study the bigger picture will begin to emerge.

Sometimes the straight–forward approach is best, e.g. an antimicrobial expectorant for wintertime bronchitis or a healing vulnerary for an abrasion. However, for more complicated issues there is often a secondary layer of treatment that addresses not only the symptom, but the cause: female reproductive issues benefited by hepatic–oriented herbs, inflammatory conditions treated with gentle laxatives, or hypertension addressed with nervous system sedatives. This indirect approach to treatment is essentially constitutional herbal medicine. For example, primary herbal medicine may suggest: take a laxative when constipated. However, for the same problem constitutional herbal medicine suggests: reduce stress via a nervous system sedative, which will in turn increase intestinal activity.

With the exception of a handful of species, this book does not discuss the use of kitchen herbs. Beyond the obvious (the majority are not found growing wild) most of these are pedestrian and best thought of as beverage teas with slight medicinal overtones. Not that there is anything wrong with this, it's just that the following plants should be approached with a bit more prudence. Their unknowns and potencies tend to be greater than a kindly cup of Ginger or Chamomile.

The Rocky Mountains, middle New Mexico to Canada, is the book's main coverage area; however, since plants are mainly discerning to two principle factors, temperature and hydration, and not necessarily geography, the majority of species will be found additionally south to the high mountains of southern Arizona and southern New Mexico (and southern California) and then west to California's Sierra Nevada and Oregon and Washington's Cascade Range. To the east coverage essentially ends at the start of the Great Plains, but even here the occasional outlier mountain chain often reliably hosts many of these plants. The expansive basins between the western mountain chains (Basin and Range) are not especially plant-diverse; however, I believe the reader will be satisfied with representative medicinal species such as range plants, Bitterbush and Sagebrush. Even Balsamroot and Lomatium, two significant plant medicines, are more likely to be found in exposed environments.

Overall the plant life of the western mountains does seem to exhibit a number of interesting population patterns. From Ligusticum and Populus species to Pine family trees, there are more balsamic plant medicines in the mountains than in surrounding areas. The Heath family urinary tract medicines are small and some even herbaceous (Pipsissewa, Pyrola, Uva-ursi, and Bilberry) as opposed to Madrone and Manzanita, larger plants that grow to the south and west and lower in elevation. The mountains also have higher densities of bitter tonic Gentian family plants and Rose family astringents than other areas. Beyond these interesting trends, overall the western mountains have a deep bench of botanical medicines, covering nearly all organ systems and their atonic/tonic states, certainly more so than the Deserts or Plains.

I've written this book, not necessarily with the herbal true believer (or the naysayer) in mind, but for the person who is reasonable and understands how to employ critical thinking skills. Being open-minded to this beautiful bastard of a subject is important; however, some healthy skepticism is too. If it is understood that herbal medicine is like an underdog: normally he comes in last, but occasionally he surprises with an upset victory, then I believe Medicinal Plants of the Western Mountain States will serve the reader well.

FORMAT EXPLANATION

Plant Names

Each profile is headed by the main common name, followed by a current scientific name in italics, the accepted author in regular text, and synonyms. Secondary common names follow. The main common name assigned to each plant is generally accepted as the most common and longest in current usage.

It is important to note that most common names as well as many scientific names for any given plant change from generation to generation. No name is set in stone. Botanical classifiers can be fickle in applying and reapplying nomenclature depending on the classifying systems/politics of the day. When you know the plant, you know the plant, names be damned.

Description and Distribution

Look to these sections for the plant's botanical description, growth tendencies, and geographical range. When pertinent, state–to–state location, elevation ranges, topographies, and micro–climates are also covered.

Chemistry

In this section, each plant's known chemical composition is listed. Readers will note that some profiles have a shorter chemistry listing than others. This is not due to a lack of compounds, but rather of available research.

Medicinal Uses

The plant's effect on organ systems, tissue groups, and symptoms are described in this section. Application to organic disease syndromes has been keep to a minimum but occasionally it is pertinent – how the plant affects stress patterns and its mechanism of action are preferred.

Plants are multi–directional. Rarely do they affect just one area of the body. They influence physicality by how an organ or tissue group eliminates or detoxifies the compounds they contain. In other words, it is not the plant that is the remedy for the ailment or discomfort, but rather it is what the plant does to the body, organ system, or group of tissues that then affects the problem. For example, an aromatic–bitter herb stimulates secretion and dilates stomach lining vasculature thereby quieting indigestion. Technically speaking, there is no such thing as an herb for a 'stomachache' or for 'arthritis'...but there are numerous herbs that influence these symptoms by their effects on related physiological process.

Indications

Under this listing readers can find the truncated medicinal use (or what symptoms indicate each plant's use) for each plant. If '(external)' is not by the indication, then that application is designed for internal use.

Collection

Depending on the plant, virtually any part can be medicinally potent. Mostly though, roots, bark, leaves, flowers, seeds, and sap or exudate provide the strongest medicines. Stems, branches, and core wood are less likely to give benefit. The former parts are functional, having an array of chemical processes taking place within them. The latter parts are structural, serving mainly as a skeletal support for the functional parts – much like our bodies.

When preparing to collect medicinal plants, beyond having the obvious implements (shovel, knife, pruners, etc.), it is sensible to first have an understanding of the process and to at least intellectually grasp what the activity entails. The reason why there exists today such a booming herbal market is because collecting plants is hard (roots and bark) and tedious (flowers, leaves, and seeds) work. The average consumer just does not have the time for the activity...and you may not either. If this is the case, then purchase the herb instead. With today's abundance of home–grown 'microbrew' herbal product lines, I guarantee some herbalist has even the most obscure medicinal plant in this book for sale.

Of course, plant collecting is not like ditch–digging (well...it occasionally can be), but still, there needs to be a degree of 'stick–with–it–ness' in order to successfully complete the process. A basic understanding of natural environments and a degree of ecological sensitivity are also of equal importance (most herbal medicine enthusiasts are low on 'stick–with–it–ness' but off the chart on ecological sensitivity). The following list of guidelines/questions will help in determining when, where, and how to properly collect plant medicines.

» First and foremost, be sure that the plant of interest has been accurately identified.
» Is the plant threatened, endangered, on 'at–watch' lists, or just locally scarce? If so it may be better to find an alternative herbal medicine or make a trip to more abundant picking grounds.
» What are the local/state/federal policies in your area regarding plant collection? Will a ticket be issued if discovered by authorities or do

» 'personal collection' laws exist?
» If harvesting on private land have arrangements with the owner been made? You'll likely find a majority of land owners interested in the subject and if they are respectfully approached you may have a reliable gathering area for years to come.
» Are seasonal conditions proper?
» Are the plants healthy and without insect and/or microbial damage?
» Are sources of contamination close by? It is best to collect away from roadsides, city and town areas, industrial sites, agricultural areas, and heavily traveled foot trails.
» Is the plant being collected properly? Take your time and enjoy the experience. The goal should not be quantity, but quality and thoroughness.
» Clean up before leaving – fill in holes, and if preparing medicines in the field, spread around core wood and other unusable plant materials in order to lessen the visual impact of collection.
» Not collecting the plant due to other–than–optimal circumstances is always an option.

Drying Plants

» Dry plant materials out of direct sunlight. Herbage can be placed loosely in paper bags or laid well–spaced on cardboard flats. Small bundles of leafing tops, with the topmost portions of the plant hanging down are secured from ceiling rafters until dry.
» Once dry, garble the leaves and flowers from the stems; discard the stems (unless otherwise directed).
» Chop roots into ¼"–½" pieces or longer longitudinal strips. Both these and bark strips dry adequately if well–spaced.
» For quicker drying or to ensure no mold growth occurs if in a humid environment, a dehydrator can be used.

Preparations

Readers will find this section either joined with the dosage heading or listed independently if there are important details that need to be relayed separately from the plant's dosage. See the main Preparations section for complete instructions on how to prepare a DPT (dry plant tincture), FPT (fresh plant tincture), infusion, decoction, etc.

Dosage

The dosage listings in this section are meant as starting points for an average–weighted adult. Depending on weight and sensitivity, in order to achieve the desired result, dosage may need to be decreased or increased.

For children and infants reduce the dose according to weight. For example, if a dose for a 150lb. adult is 30–60 drops 3 times daily, then for a 50lb. child, 10–20 drops 3 times daily is the correct reduction. All percentages for DPT and fluidextract listings apply to alcohol and glycerin contents.

It is important to note that like herbal medicine in general, dosing crude herbal medicines is not a precise science. The variables that come into play when attempting to achieve an effective dose for most herbs are myriad. Most herbs have a wide safe range (unless otherwise noted) and can be increased (within reason) until their therapeutic effects become apparent.

Cautions

If the following precepts are adhered to when using medicinal plants there will be little to fear from potential adverse reactions.

» Quantity: a little will help, a lot may harm. Any plant properly dosed can be medicinal. The same plant may be toxic in larger amounts.
» As a society, we are over medicated. If taking pharmaceuticals or OTC medicines for a particular problem, throwing an herb or two into the mix to affect the same organ or tissue group may be OK…or not. Do some interaction research before playing herbal doctor, or consult with a professional versed in such matters.
» Herbal medicines during pre– and post–operation times may conflict with existing medical programs/physician recommendations. Be extremely cautious when considering herbs that influence clotting time or that are strongly sedating or stimulating.
» Children, the elderly, and those with sensitive constitutions tend to be more prone to adverse effects with larger herbal doses.
» If any herb causes sickness, headaches, diarrhea, nausea, dizziness, or other unwanted sensations, then lessen the dose or discontinue the herb. In my experience, most 'cleansing reactions' are actually toxic reactions from taking too much of or the wrong herbal medicine. Most herbal 'mega–doses' are only going to sicken the recipient. So much more can be achieved with moderation and consistency.
» If an herb affects the mother to be, then it is affecting the fetus. The

herb's activity is usually delivered to the baby through breast milk as well. While pregnant or nursing limit herbs that have strong physiologic activities. In these times think of food as medicine.

» Aside from the fundamental social and moral wrong of abortion, and the medical procedure's link to breast cancer, a number of herbs discussed in this book have abortifacient potential. As a rule, they are unreliable and if used in sufficient quantity are apt to cause harm to the 'mother' as well.

A Note on Formulas

This book is lacking formulas for a reason: one size does not fit all. If you think the situation calls for a formula, then keep it simple. A formula comprised of over five or six herbs is likely to cause more physiologic chatter than therapeutic direction. A well–formulated mixture should be direct, elegant, and unfettered. Keep in consideration the multi–systemic nature of herbs. They usually affect more than one organ system. When it comes to designing formulas: don't elaborate. Edit.

Excessive polypharmacy is rampant in the natural supplement industry. Read the label of most herbal supplement combinations; if the ingredient list is filled with numerous herbs then that formula has absolutely no direction, and only can help someone through placebo or by creating a little physiological 'noise' in the body by its elimination through various pathways.

PREPARATIONS

Introduction

Medicinal plant preparation[1] can be summed up in one simple premise: how an herb is prepared is of equal importance to what herb is dispensed. Superior plant medicines are made that way by a delivery method that suites each particular plant being utilized. When a plant medicine has been potentiated through proper preparation its activity becomes more distinct and less will be needed for an effective dose.

In determining which methods are optimal for delivery, each plant should be taken on a case by case basis. That said, groupings or corollaries that help in preparation specifics become more evident when focus is placed on a particular plant's family or related constituent groups. Chances are Marshmallow, Mallow, and Globemallow, all Mallow family plants, will be best prepared through water–based preparations. Not only are they closely related botanically but their chemistries are similar; therefore, preparations will be similar, if not identical. Torchwood family plants (Myrrh, Frankincense, Guggul, and Elephant tree), due to their resins and non–polar compounds, should be tinctured with a higher percentage of alcohol. In essence: botanically related plants are often chemically related and consequently preparations (and uses) are related.

It is often forgotten that up to the mid–20th century, half of what doctors prescribed (and pharmacists filled), were plants or derivatives thereof. Prior to WWII, the national formulary and US dispensary (both standard references for doctors/pharmacists) had more print related to whole plants, their derivatives, and related preparations, than synthetically created drugs.

It is a misconception that the area of herbal preparation (herbal medicine for that matter) is uncertain and untried. For over a span of two centuries, preparation (and use) was developed, expanded upon, and peaked (then withered due to its replacement with modern medicines). Just as there is no need to reinvent the wheel, there is no need to alter traditional (and often simple) plant preparation technique in the name of the latest exclusive, propriety, or specialized preparation process that usually was developed as a marketing point anyway.

What follows are the main preparations standard in past and present–day herbal medicine. They are simple and time–tested methods designed to achieve the most from each plant.

---

1   I've kept this section (and Format Explanation) largely unchanged from what's found in Medicinal Plants of the American Southwest. If it's not broken, don't fix it.

Bath
1. Draw a hot bath.
2. Add 1 gallon of tea to the bath water.
3. Soak until the water has cooled, or otherwise directed.

Capsule
Capsules come in various sizes with 'o' (250 mg.), 'oo' (500 mg.), and 'ooo' (1000 mg.) being the most common. To fill simply immerse the two halves in an herbal powder, then fit the capsule together. Encapsulation machines speed up the process. They are available in various designs by different makers.

Cough Syrup
Method 1: Honey Steep
1. Take 5½ ounces of finely chopped, fresh plant material; pack into a pint mason jar and fill to the top with honey.
2. Secure the lid and set aside for several weeks. Squeeze or press the honey from the herb and bottle the infused honey.
» *Ratio: 1 part herb (weight) to 2 parts of honey (volume).*

Method 2: Tincture in Honey/Glycerin Base
1. Mix together 8 ounces of the appropriate tincture(s) with 4 ounces of honey and 4 ounces of glycerin.
2. Bottle.
» *Ratio: 2 parts tincture (volume) to 1 part honey (volume) to 1 part glycerin (volume).*

Method 3: Tincture with Simple Syrup
1. Mix together 8 ounces of tincture(s) and 8 ounces of simple syrup.
2. Bottle.
» *Ratio: 1 part tincture (volume) to 1 part simple syrup (volume).*

Considerations
These preparations do not need to be refrigerated. Method 2 and 3 are basically diluted tinctures and are stronger than the honey steep. 1–2 teaspoons is an average adult dose, verses 1 tablespoon for the honey steep.

Douche
1. Make a half–strength tea.
2. Cool until warm.
3. Add ½ teaspoon of table salt per pint of tea in order to increase the solution's salinity.
4. Use as directed.

Considerations
Like any water–based preparation, be sure to make this herbal solution fresh daily. No need to potentially add bacterial or fungal elements to sensitive tissues by using old tea. For a preparation that is less disturbing to vaginal flora, *see Sitz Bath*.

Eyewash
Method 1
1. Make 1 pint of tea with distilled or filtered water through the properly designated method (infusion, decoction, etc.)
2. Strain well through a paper towel or cloth.
3. Add ½ teaspoon of table salt.
4. Stir until dissolved.
5. Apply as needed.

Method 2
1. Add 10 drops of appropriate tincture to 2 ounces of isotonic water (¼ teaspoon of table salt to 1 cup of distilled or filtered water).
2. Apply as needed.

Considerations
It is important to make any non–preserved eyewash solution fresh daily.

Fluidextract
First introduced into the U.S.P. of 1850, the fluidextract is an official pharmaceutical preparation. More concentrated than a tincture it is 1:1 in strength, meaning each milliliter of extract contains a representation of 1 gram of dried herb (i.e. 1 ounce of fluidextract will be derived from and have the potency of 1 ounce of dried herb).

Not all plants lend themselves well to fluidextracts, but the ones that are suited for this preparation are mentioned in each plant profile. To make a fluidextract a basic tincture needs to be made through percolation. It is then concentrated to a 1:1. Essentially fluidextracts enable a lower drop dose, and are convenient if making formulas. See *Herbal Medicine: Trends and Traditions* for step–by–step instructions.

Fomentation
1. Soak a cloth or towel in a warm herb tea.
2. Squeeze the excess tea from the cloth.
3. Apply the cloth to the affected area.
4. Re–soak and apply as needed.

Hydrosol
Also called floral water, a hydrosol is created through essential oil distillation. Actually considered a by–product of the distillation process, it is composed of the condensed steam (water) that was initially in contact with the plant material. Filled with hydroscopic volatile compounds and traces of colloid–formed essential oil, hydrosols share some therapeutic characteristics with essential oils; the main exception being potency. Dilute and mild, hydrosols can even be used as replacements for standard teas. Often they are used as facial sprays or washes. Additionally, they make a fine replacement for the water portion when making ointments.

Liniment
A liniment is essentially an externally applied tincture. Isopropyl alcohol can be used instead of ethyl alcohol for this preparation (do not use isopropyl alcohol internally). Due to alcohol's dermal penetrating ability it is common for liniment combinations to contain one or more analgesic/antiinflammatory oriented herb.

Oil, Essential
Typically prepared through steam distillation, an essential oil represents the volatile or aromatic fraction of a particular plant. Non–polar terpenes make up the bulk of any essential oil constituent list.

It is important to note that essential oils differ greatly from herbal oils. Two very different processes are employed to reach two very different finished products. The two are not interchangeable.

Pure essential oils can be used both externally and internally. Because they represent a potentiated fraction of a plant care should be taken when they are used, especially when ingested. Undiluted they represent some of the strongest topical medicines we employ. As antiinflammatories, analgesics, and antimicrobials/antivirals they excel. Applied undiluted to sensitize tissue/mucus membranes they may cause some irritation; diluting 100–200% with a carrier oil (olive, almond, etc.) usually is sufficient in reducing this tendency. They can be added to an herbal oil in a wide range of ratios – just enough to impart a fragrance, or enough to be the main topical agent.

Ingested, essential oils should be approached with prudence as toxicity due to overdose is a pertinent issue. Unlike tinctures, where 30–60 drops (for many plants) is a normal therapeutic dose, 1–3 drops for an essential oil is roughly equal in potency. For this preparation, several drops are placed in a gelatin capsule and then swallowed. See Spirit for another internal preparation utilizing essential oils.

Most plants with a distinctive smell can be used as essential oils: many plants in the Mint, Sunflower, Cypress, and Pine families are well utilized. Although this preparation excludes many other constituents (vitamins/minerals, glycosides, and most alkaloids) due to their nonvolatile nature, if used properly the right plant can be better directed and potentiated.

Essential oils are easily added to tinctures. They are particularly useful, like fluidextracts, when keeping volume low is important.

When purchasing essential oils the label will typically state 'not for internal use'. This has more to do with the potential of toxicity from a high dose rather than any innate poisonous quality. Check that they are not preserved or diluted with synthetics (some 'natural' perfumes).

For those inclined to personally render essential oils, there are many distillers on the market today. Most fall into two camps – the 'lab equipment' type and the old–school copper type. Both work; if nothing else the decision to purchase one or the other is often based on size and visual appeal. *See Hydrosol for a useful distillation by–product.*

Oil, Herbal

Herbal oils are applied topically for their interaction with the epidemic/keratin (surface) layers. They soften the skin, retain the active medicine, and provide a limited protective coating, enabling skin conditions to better respond to the herbal medicine within the oil. Herbal oils are the base for both ointments and salves. Ointments are better at penetrating; salves at protecting.

Vegetable oils can be broken into several classes depending on viscosity or thickness and to what degree they dry or thicken when exposed to air. Olive, almond, and peanut oils are thicker than most, and create less of a film when exposed to air. Mustard seed, canola, sesame, sunflower, pumpkin, soy, and corn oils thicken to a moderate degree, but are less viscous. Hemp, linseed (flax), safflower, sunflower, and walnut oils are the least viscous, and upon air contract, produce a gummy film.

Rancidity is a factor with all fats. If an herbal oil is being stored for over several months use olive as the base oil. It is greatly resistant to oxidation and rancidity. Even compared to grapeseed, known for its high antioxidant activity, olive oil will be found more stable.

Once made store the oil in an air–tight, darkened glass container. Refrigeration is not necessary, but nonetheless should be kept at cool temperatures.

Method 1: Alcohol Intermediate
Best for herbs that are high in volatiles, resins, and other non–polar constituents, this method stands out as one of the better herbal oil techniques, demonstrated by the vibrant color imparted to the oil.

1. Mix 1 ounce of dried, coarsely powered herb with ½–1 ounce of 190 proof ethyl alcohol.
2. Cover and let stand for an hour.
3. Pour 7 ounces of olive oil into a blender.
4. Add the alcohol–saturated herb.
5. Blend on high for 15 minutes or until blender container is very warm to hot.
6. Strain the oil/herb through a piece of cloth.
7. Discard the herb and bottle the oil.
» *Ratio: 1 part herb (weight) to ½–1 part 190 proof ethyl alcohol (volume) to 7 parts olive oil (volume).*

Method 2: Wilted Herb
This method works best for herbs that become less potent upon fully drying. Here we are taking advantage of the herb's fresh state but need to reduce the water content to lessen possible microbial fermentation.

1. Wilt the plant to half of its original weight; this often takes 8–12 hours.
2. Chop or dice the herb. Be careful not to make a puree, as this will release too much water into the oil, encouraging fermentation.

PREPARATIONS

3. In a jar combine 1 ounce of chopped herb in 7 ounces of olive oil.
4. Mix thoroughly.
5. Seal and let stand in a warm (90–100 degrees) place, out of direct sunlight, for 14 days. Covered, exposed to the sun or next to a stove or heat duct are some good places.
6. Strain, but do not press the oil from the herb.
7. Let stand until any residual water and the oil completely separate. Pour off the oil, or with a basting syringe collect the oil apart from any water layer.
8. Bottle the oil. Discard the water.
» *Ratio: 1 part herb (weight) to 7 parts olive oil (volume).*

Method 3: Old Standard
1. Combine 1 ounce of dried, powdered herb with 7 ounces of olive oil.
2. Using a blender thoroughly mix the combination.
3. Pour into a sealable jar.
4. Seal and let stand in a warm (90–100 degrees) place, out of direct sunlight, for 14 days. Covered while exposed to the sun or next to a stove or heat duct are some good places.
5. Agitate the mixture several times a day.
6. After 14 days, blend (electric blender) until the container is very warm–hot.
7. Strain the oil from the powdered herb through a piece of cloth.
8. Discard the herb and bottle the oil.
» *Ratio: 1 part herb (weight) to 7 parts olive oil (volume).*

Method 4: Heat
This method is particularly useful when the alcohol intermediate technique is not preferred. Use this method with plants high in stable oleoresins, such as Cayenne pepper, Ginger, or Myrrh.

1. Combine 1 ounce of dried, powdered herb with 7 ounces of olive oil.
2. Mix thoroughly and place the mixture in a sealable jar. Secure the lid.
3. Submerged in a heated pot of water, heat to 140–160 degrees for 4–5 hours.
4. Remove from heat and let stand for an additional 4 hours.
5. Strain and bottle.
» *Ratio: 1 part herb (weight) to 7 parts olive oil (volume).*

Ointment

Ointments are best used when there is call for a penetrating topical medicine. They affect a deeper array of tissues (compared to salves) but need to be applied more often.

1. Combine 7 parts base oil (almond/olive/pre–made herbal oil) with 1 part beeswax.
2. Slowly heat until the beeswax is dissolved in the oil.
3. Let the oil–beeswax mixture cool until it starts to faintly harden on the sides of the container. At this point you should be able to put your finger into the oil without it being too hot.
4. In a blender pour 12 parts of distilled water/herb tea/hydrosol (it is bet to have this mixture ready to go in a blender before the oil–beeswax begins to cool).
5. Blend on low.
6. Slowly pour the oil/beeswax mixture into the blender.
7. Blend for only 10–15 seconds (the mixture should have a creamy consistency).
8. Blot any extra liquid from the top of the ointment.
9. Mix in any additional essential oils at this point (1 ml. per 5–7 ounces or so).
10. Scoop into containers and refrigerate.
» *Ratio: 7 parts herbal oil (volume) to 1 part beeswax (weight) to 12 parts water/tea/hydrosol (volume).*

Considerations
Depending on what tea/hydrosol or essential oil is added, the refrigerated ointment will last without spoilage for several months – some longer.

Poultice
Method 1: Basic
1. Moisten with warm water and knead a pre–determined amount of dried and powdered herb with warm water until a porridge–like consistence is reached.
2. Apply directly to the affected area, or cover the area first with muslin cloth, then apply.
3. Secure poultice with a covering and/or bandage.
4. Change 2–3 times daily, or when cool.

Method 2: Field Poultice
1. Bruise and/or puree the fresh plant.
2. Apply to affected area and secure.
3. Change 2–3 times daily.
4. A 'spit poultice' can be quickly made by chewing the intended herb (make sure it is internally non–toxic) and applying it to the affected area.

Powder

Depending on the part of the plant some dried materials are harder than others to powder. Roots, bark, and stems are more difficult than leaves, flowers, and lightweight parts. For lighter materials, an average blender with a metal or glass container is adequate; for tougher materials a vita–mix works well, or an industrial grinder/mill. Once the plant is powdered it can then be used as a dust, or as a starting point for DPTs, poultices, etc.

Salve

1. While slowly heating 7 ounces of an herbal oil add 1 ounce of beeswax.
2. Let the beeswax slowly dissolve.
3. While still hot, pour the mixture into containers.
4. As the salve cools, it will solidify.
» *Ratio: 7 parts herbal oil (volume) to 1 part beeswax (weight).*

Considerations
Salves will be best applied when there is need of a protective skin coating.

Sitz Bath

Best used for skin, trauma (post–delivery for example), and bacterial/fungal conditions of the genital, anal, and related pelvic tissues, a traditional sitz bath uses a small 'sitting tub'. The updated version of the traditional sitz bath is more superficial in design. It is a small tub of sorts that fits over a toilet bowl. Accompanying this is a gravity–fed solution bag and tubing for specific area application. For simple washes this modern version of the sitz bath is fine. But for more effective treatments longer soaking times will necessitate the traditional design.

1. Prepare a half–strength or full strength tea.
2. Apply/soak until tea is cool.

Spirit

A spirit is simply an essential oil diluted with a specific amount of alcohol. This preparation is mainly designed to make essential oils more palatable for internal use. It also makes essential oils more suitable as formula ingredients.

1. Take 1 part essential oil and dilute with 9 parts 190 proof ethyl alcohol.
2. Mix; bottle; store.
» *Ratio: 9 parts alcohol (volume) to 1 part essential oil (volume).*

Suppository

Suppositories are preparations made for either vaginal or rectal insertion (less commonly for the urethra). Two types of suppositories are covered here. The first has a glycerin/gelatin base and works well with tinctures and fluidextracts as the added medicinal agent. The second type is Cocoa butter based and is better suited for added herbal oils and essential oils.

Method 1: Glycerin/Gelatin
1. Mix together 6.5 parts glycerin with 2.1 parts of tincture or fluidextract.
2. Heat for several minutes using low temperatures.
3. Add 1.4 parts of powdered gelatin.
4. Mix thoroughly and remove from heat.
5. Pour into suppository molds and let cool.
» *Ratio: 6.5 parts glycerin to 2.1 parts tincture/fluidextract to 1.4 parts gelatin (all totaling 10 parts).*

Method 2: Cocoa Butter
1. Using low heat melt 1 part Cocoa butter.
2. Add ½ part herbal oil and mix together.
3. Add any essential oil at this time (1 ml. per 5–7 ounces of oil is a good starting point).
4. Pour into suppository molds and let cool.
» *Ratio: 1 part Cocoa butter to ½ part herbal oil.*

Considerations
» The ratios presented here are meant as guides and can be altered if the suppository's consistency needs to be changed.
» Placing the suppositories in a refrigerator or freezer for a short period of

- Suppositories are best used before bed when the body is in a horizontal position.
- If at any time the suppository causes irritation, discontinue or change the recipe.
- Pharmaceutical grade gelatin, suppository molds (both the disposable plastic type and the aluminum/metal block type) are available through pharmacy suppliers. Check on-line or with compounding pharmacies.

Syrup, Simple

Simple syrup is called for in some respiratory formulations and in any other formula where a preparation's sweetness and soothing qualities are called for.

1. In a pot combine 32 ounces of refined white sugar and 16 ounces of water.
2. Slowly heat and stir until the sugar is fully dissolved. Occasionally 1 or 2 additional ounces of water will be needed to fully dissolve the sugar.
3. Let cool and bottle. The syrup does not need to be refrigerated.
- *Ratio: 2 parts sugar (weight) to 1 part (volume) water.*

Considerations
- Any tea can be converted into a syrup by simply adding sugar in the proper ratio. Senna, Marshmallow, Wild cherry, Rhubarb, and Ginger are a number of classics. Tinctures/fluidextracts can also be added to simple syrups, usually in a 1 part to 1 part ratio.
- Other sweeteners will ferment and spoil if used without added alcohol.

Tea

Tea preparations are best applied to plants that have a large array of water-soluble compounds. Plants that are being used for tannins, starches, minerals, and other polar compounds are best taken as teas. All plants are dried first and then infused or decocted.

Making tea with a fresh plant is a waste. Intact, living plant cells are adept at holding on to their vital cellular compounds, not giving them up to water. Through drying this force is disrupted – cell walls are broken making the plant's various constituents permeable to water. Make tea or any water-based preparation fresh daily.

Infusion
1. Bring 1 quart of water to a boil.
2. Turn off heat.
3. Stir in 1 ounce of dry, fragile plant materials – leaves, flowers, thin stems, etc.
4. Cover and steep for at least 15 minutes.
5. Uncover and strain.
» *Ratio: 1 part herb (weight) to 32 parts water (volume).*

Decoction
1. Bring 1 quart of water to a slow simmer.
2. Stir in 1 ounce of thicker, dried plant materials – bark, roots, stems, pods, etc.
3. Cover and simmer for at least 15 minutes.
4. Turn heat off.
5. Steep for 15 minutes.
6. Uncover and strain.
» *Ratio: 1 part herb (weight) to 32 parts water (volume).*

Cold Infusion
1. In a mesh tea bag or colander suspend 1 ounce of dried plant materials in 1 quart of water.
2. Steep over night at room temperature. Strain.
3. Make fresh daily.
» *Ratio: 1 part herb (weight) to 32 parts water (volume).*

Tincture, Overview
» Plants that are high in volatile oils, complex starches, and other non–polar constituents are best prepared through tincturing.
» A 1:2 FPT (fresh plant tincture) means that in each fluid ounce of tincture produced there is contained the therapeutic constituents of ½ ounce of fresh herb. The herb/menstruum ratio generally corresponds to this as well: 1 part of fresh herb to 2 parts of menstruum. A 1:5 DPT (dry plant tincture) means 1 part of dried herb to 5 parts of menstruum or in each fluid ounce of tincture produced there is contained the therapeutic constituents of ⅕ ounce of dried herb.
» A 1:2 FPT is equal in strength to a 1:5 DPT. Since the dried plant lacks water it is being added back into the menstruum to properly extract the

plant's constituents.
- » The alcohol percentage of the FPT is high. What is being relied upon in this tincture preparation is the hydroscopic (hygroscopic) activity of alcohol. The alcohol literally dehydrates the fresh plant. It pulls all of the plant's constituents/cytoplasm out into the surrounding alcohol. The result is a highly potent, intact representation of the fresh plant. FPTs with lower alcohol contents are inferior; water limits the pulling activity of alcohol.
- » 1:2 for a FPT and 1:5 for a DPT are standard ratios originated by chemists in western medicine's past when plants were the main medicines.
- » Depending on the plant, lower tincture and extract ratios (1:1 or 2:1, etc.) are not necessarily better or stronger. One characteristic of a good quality tincture is its lack of particulate matter, or sediment. Often many plants respond poorly to a 1:1 or more concentrated preparations because their constituents are not able to remain in suspension and 'salt out' through being too concentrated. This limits the body's ability to properly absorb the preparation.
- » All tinctures are made with 190 proof ethyl alcohol (with the exception of several herbs that are extracted well with vinegar – see Acetum Tincture), commonly called Everclear. Look to liquor stores or the liquor section of grocery stores. Availability varies from state to state.
- » Glycerin and vinegar (with several exceptions – see Acetum Tincture) are incredibly poor solvents. Even store–bought liquid glycerin 'extracts' begin as alcoholic extracts. The alcohol is then removed and the condensed extract is added to a glycerin medium and sold as a 'glycerite', 'glycerin tincture', etc. The best use for glycerin, associated with tinctures that is, is its addition to an alcoholic menstruum. Its job here is not as a solvent, but to inhibit the formation of unwanted complexes. That is, it keeps a high tannin–content tincture from forming into a curd–like gelatinous mass. Compared to glycerin and vinegar, even water (tea) is a far superior extractive medium.

Tincture, Dry Plant
Method 1: Maceration
1. Place 2 ounces of dried and powered plant material in a glass jar.
2. Add 10 ounces of alcohol/water mixture – see each plant's preparation/dosage for the correct alcohol/water percentage. (If a plant calls for 60% alcohol then add 6 ounces of grain alcohol and 4 ounces (40%) of water).

3. Combine with the powdered herb in a glass jar. Secure lid and then shake well for several minutes.
4. Let stand for 2 weeks – shaking every day for 5 minutes.
5. Press the tincture from the marc. Or squeeze by hand using a large piece of flannel or cheese cloth.
6. Discard the marc.
7. Bottle the tincture.

» *Ratio: 1 part dried herb (weight) to 5 parts menstruum (volume).*

Considerations
» When using this tincture method with high tannin–content plants the menstruum should consist of 10% glycerin. This inhibits the tannins from binding together and with other constituents.

Method 2: Percolation
Percolation is a tincturing technique regarded as superior to maceration. Fresh menstruum with full extractive potential is always in contact with the powdered herb; by the time it drains from the cone to be caught below it is 'full' with compounds. The concept is the same when percolating coffee.

Powdered and moistened herb is packed into a glass cone or funnel. This is suspended over, via a stand, or inserted into, a suitable receiving container. Menstruum is added topside into the large opening of the cone. As it descends, the menstruum's flow rate is controlled by a cap or valve. The menstruum that is caught in the receiving vessel is now the percolate (or tincture). *See Herbal Medicine: Trends and Traditions for step–by–step instructions.*

Method 3: Vinegar (Acetum Tincture)
Using either the maceration or percolation technique, vinegar (apple cider vinegar is fine) is used as a solvent. Only useful for several herbs such as Artemisia and Lobelia, its main drawback is a short storage time.

Tincture, Fresh Plant

It is important that the alcohol percentage of the fresh plant tincture is high: what is being relied upon is the hygroscopic (water attracting) activity of alcohol on fresh material. Diluting the alcohol with water or using a lower proof alcohol (vodka, etc.) will result in a poor–quality tincture. *See Tincture, Dry Plant* for the preparation that utilizes lower alcohol percentages.

Method 1: Old standard
1. Place 2 ounces of fresh, chopped plant material in a glass jar.
2. Add 4 ounces of alcohol.
3. Secure the lid. There is no need to shake the mixture. After 14 days, press or squeeze the tincture from the herb.
4. Discard the marc (spent herb).
5. Bottle the tincture.
» *Ratio: 1 part fresh herb (weight) to 2 parts 190 proof ethyl alcohol (volume).*

A Simplified Method
1. Place 5½ ounces of fresh, chopped plant material in a pint mason jar.
2. Fill to the top with alcohol.
3. Secure the lid and follow the instructions mentioned previously.
» *Ratio: 1 part fresh herb (weight) to 2 parts 190 proof ethyl alcohol (volume).*

Considerations
» Filling the jar to the top with alcohol will not amount to exactly 11 ounces (or 2 parts), but it will be close enough.
» After the jar is sealed and several days have passed often the alcohol fully settles to where the level is below the jar's lip. Remove the jar's lid and top–off with alcohol. Secure the lid. Press after the initial 14 days.

Wash

A wash is simple a topically applied herb tea. Using a spray bottle for this preparation in cases of sunburn or skin inflammation for example is a handy way of applying an herbal wash.

Wash, Nasal

The principal use of this preparation is as wash for the sinuses. It is a somewhat bizarre experience that goes against instinct (inhaling water in through the nose, instead of blowing it out). But the result is worth the strangeness, particularly if there is a sinus infection.
1. Make an isotonic solution by adding ½ teaspoon of table salt to 1 pint of warm water or an appropriate tea.
2. Pour the solution into a bowl. It should be shallow enough so liquid is close to the bowl's lip.
3. While plugging one nostril, submerge the open nostril into the solution.
4. *Slowly* inhale through the submerged nostril.

5. The solution will be drawn in through the nostril and collect in the mouth.
6. Spit out the solution.
7. Change nostrils and repeat.

Considerations
- In acute conditions this wash can be repeated every hour or so.
- A special container called a 'neti pot' is made for this application. It is basically a miniature watering can. It holds no significant advantage over simply using a bowl.
- Be sure to use distilled or at least 'purified' water. Although rare, upper respiratory tract infections due to water-borne microorganisms have been reported with contaminated water sources.

MATERIA MEDICA

Agastache
Lamiaceae/Mint Family

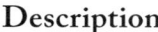

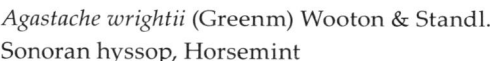

Agastache pallidiflora (A. Heller) Rydb.
Bill William's giant hyssop, Giant hyssop, Purple horsemint, Purple hyssop

Agastache urticifolia (Benth) Kuntze *(Agastache glaucifolia)*
Nettleleaf hyssop, Horsemint, Giant hyssop

Agastache wrightii (Greenm) Wooton & Standl.
Sonoran hyssop, Horsemint

Description

Agastache is a small to medium-sized perennial herb. Square stems, opposite leaves, and vertical growth are several characteristics that unify all species[2]. Additionally, some (not all) species have a minty fragrance.

1½'–3' in height with numerous stems, Agastache urticifolia's leaves tend to be arrow shaped, toothed, finely hairy below, and 2"–3" long. Its white–purple/rose flowers develop in spiked clusters. Similar in height, A. pallidiflora's leaves are also 2"–3" long and triangular. The flowers form in dense spikes and are whitish to rose–purple. A. wrightii's leaves are also triangular, several inches in length, and about half as wide. The rose–purple flowers form in interrupted spikes.

Distribution

A circumpolar, Eurasian–centered genus, in this country the majority of Agastache species are found throughout the southwest mountains. Additionally, outlier populations are found in many parts of the West.

Significant in range, Agastache urticifolia is found from British Columbia, Canada and Montana, south to California, Nevada, Utah, and western Colorado. Adaptable and abundant, it grows in a wide array of habitats: from woodlands to open flats and hillsides.

2   One common name used for various species of Agastache is Hyssop. Although Agastache and Hyssopus (true Hyssop) are both members of the Mint family and share several medicinal traits, for clarity's sake, I believe it is best to keep names for these two groups separate.

Agastache pallidiflora and A. wrightii are mainly Arizona and New Mexico plants. A. pallidiflora's range also extends to southern Colorado and the Trans–Pecos region of Texas.

Chemistry

Agastache (general): volatiles: chavicol, α–limonene, menthone, methyl eugenol, bornyl acetate, spathulenol, cadinol, β–caryophyllene; flavones: luteolin, apigenin, acacetin.

Medicinal Uses

A little–known herbal medicine, Agastache[3] effectively addresses a number of complaints. Like others in the Mint family, the tea is soothing and carminative to an upset stomach, indigestion, or post–vomiting nausea. Its array of stimulating aromatics tends to dilate gastric capillary beds while simultaneously imparting a mild anesthetic effect. This net influence is best suited for individuals whom suffer from chronic or subacute gastritis and/or dyspepsia, whether from long–term alcohol abuse, dietary indiscretions, or even constitutional weakness. Start with 2–4 ounces of the tea as needed. Due to Agastache's (or potentially any Mint) gastric stimulation, occasionally some irritation may be noticed with its use. If this is the case, try Western mugwort or even Chamomile instead.

Agastache is a diaphoretic. It reliably promotes sweating when there is a dry fever. Its strength is similar to a strong cup of hot Spearmint tea. Additionally, some find the plant mildly sedative – a nice combination (sudorific) when sick and in need of rest.

Women usually find Agastache mildly stimulating to menses yet also spasmolytic. For period cramps, it's not as strong as Western peony or Cramp bark, but it will nonetheless provide relief to minor pain and spasm, especially if pelvic circulation is subpar.

Both Agastache mexicana (Mexican agastache) and A. rugosa (Korean mint) are used for a number of mild cardiovascular complaints. These species contain fair amounts of tilianin (and related flavonoids). Interestingly, western (and Mexican) species of Agastache are more closely aligned (botanically and chemically) with Asian species (A. rugosa) than species found

3   One of the more common species that flourishes throughout the northern United States is Agastache foeniculum or Anise hyssop. Along with minty tones, its scent and flavor are distinctly Anise/Fennel–like. Although subtler, a number of other American species also have Anise–Fennel–Licorice (or Lemon) characteristics.

in the eastern United States. This means western species have some potential when applied to mild hypertension and arterial cholesterol/plaque formation. A sensible hypothesis is Agastache's daily use as a cardiovascular antioxidant/protectant.

Most western North American species of Agastache are sedative to nervousness and anxiety. Not as muscularly tranquilizing as Valerian or Pedicularis, use Agastache when in need of a calming agent, possibly in response to emotional surges or hysterical outbursts. Here it combines well with Lemon balm or even Pulsatilla[4].

Indications
» Dyspepsia with gas and bloating
» Gastritis with poor gastrointestinal circulation
» Fever, dry skin with mental agitation
» Amenorrhea/Dysmenorrhea with poor uterine circulation
» Anxiety/Nervousness

Collection
Snip the upper half of the herb when in flower or at least when the leaves are healthy and vibrant. Once dry, garble the leaves and flowers from the stems; discard the stems. Alternately, strip the leaves and flowers from the stems and use these parts fresh.

Preparations/Dosage
» Herbal infusion: 4–8 oz. 2–3 times daily
» FPT/DPT (50% alcohol): 1 teaspoon 2–3 times daily

Cautions
An occasional 4 ounces or so of the tea is fine during pregnancy – more may cause some unwanted spotting (pulegone has been reported for a number of species). When used as a diaphoretic, Agastache may cause a short–term spike in body temperate before triggering surface capillary bed dilation and subsequent perspiration. This makes it best in low to mid dry fevers. Consider Coral root or Aspen for fevers of higher temperatures.

---

4   Add 10–15 drops of Pulsatilla fresh plant tincture to a base of Agastache tea. This combination is both simple and powerful. Use it for depressive histrionics, especially if a perception of bodily coldness is a symptom.

Agrimony
Rosaceae/Rose Family

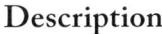
Agrimonia spp.

Agrimonia gryposepala Wallr. *(Agrimonia eupatoria var. parviflora, A. macrocarpa, A. parviflora var. macrocarpa, Eupatorium gryposepalum)*
Common agrimony

Agrimonia striata Michx. *(Agrimonia brittoniana, A. striata var. campanulata, Eupatorium brittonianum)*
Roadside agrimony, Woodland agrimony

Description
A member of the Rose family, Agrimony is a small to mid–sized herb. Blending into the surrounding understory, the plant's leaves are its most distinctive feature. Consisting of varying sized toothed leaflets, they are arranged along the leaf stem in an odd–pinnate pattern where sets of significantly undersized leaflets separate larger leaflets. The small, 5–petaled, yellow flowers form in elongated racemes. They are followed by small prickle–covered seed capsules.

Distribution
Agrimony is most common throughout the eastern and central United States. In the West, it is principally a plant of the upper mountains. Look to streamsides and wet forest margins where some sunlight passes through the surrounding trees and shrubs.

Chemistry
Coumarins; flavonoids: apigenin, isoquercetrin, luteolin, kaempferol, quercitrin, quercetin, rutin; tannins; terpenoids.

Medicinal Uses
European species of Agrimony have a long history of use as mild and well–tolerated urinary tract astringents. Our species are no different in application, and like other Rose family plants, it is Agrimony's array of tannins and related flavonoids that provide its tightening and antiinflammatory effects on tubular–urinary tissues. One of the plant's specific indications is mucus

in the urine. Relatedly, if the urine is cloudy (indicative of mucus) and/or strong smelling (typical symptoms of a urinary tract infection), the plant's soothing and astringent qualities will likely give relief.

As a lithotropic agent, it is an old remedy. Combined with Lobelia and/or Gravel root, obstructions of the urinary tract are more easily passed and corresponding tissue trauma is quieted. Although not completely reliable, Agrimony is often stated to be of use to the aged whom are troubled by incontinence. In these situations (beginning stages), try the tea or tincture if urinary tissues are lax and without tone.

Women will benefit from Agrimony if suffering from heavy menstruation. It is the plant's tannin group that is responsible for its menses–diminishing effect. Minor postpartum bleeding also tends to lessen due to the plant's mild uterine lining astringency. There is probably little Agrimony will do if the situation is caused by diminished levels of estrogen/progesterone (perimenopause).

Mild vaginitis responds well to the warm tea when it is applied as a sitz bath. Although not particularly antimicrobial, it will be found soothing to inflamed tissues.

Indications
» Cystitis/Urethritis/Nephritis, chronic with cloudy–odiferous urine
» Lithiasis
» Incontinence, urinary, age–related
» Menstruation, heavy
» Postpartum bleeding/As a postpartum tonic
» Vaginitis (external)

Collection
Gather Agrimony with or without flower development in the spring or summer when new leaf growth is apparent.

Preparations/Dosage
» Herbal infusion: 4–8 oz. 2–3 times daily
» FPT/DPT (50% alcohol): 1 teaspoon 2–3 times daily
» Sitz bath: as needed

Cautions

Agrimony is a benign herbal medicine. There are no significant cautions for its use. Excessive amounts may lead to mild stomach upset.

Alfalfa
Fabaceae/Pea Family

Medicago sativa

Medicago sativa L *(Medicago tunetana)*
Lucerne

Description

Alfalfa is a 2′–3′ tall, herbaceous, short–lived perennial. Erect to decumbent, the plant's stems are variable in pattern. Its trifoliate leaf arrangement is typical of many plants of the Pea family. Each leaflet is ½″–1½″ in length and lanceolate to obovate. The flower clusters are arranged in racemes at branch ends. Individual flowers are bilaterally symmetrical and a shade of purple. The corolla is ¼″–½″ in length. The tightly–coiled pods each contain 10–20 small, ovoid, yellow–brown seeds.

Distribution

Due to the plant's worldly distribution, its exact Eurasian place of origin remains uncertain. It's a common waif (and crop plant) throughout the western United States. Look to disturbed soils: field edges, grassy areas, dirt roadsides, etc.

Chemistry

Crude protein; lignins; isoflavones; miscellaneous nutrients.

Medicinal Uses

As a mild remedy for nutritional deficiencies, Alfalfa is an excellent source of absorbable minerals. It combines well with Red raspberry leaf or Horsetail as a tea used when there is weight loss due to gastrointestinal–centered illness and/or various forms of anorexia. Whenever malnourishment and tissue–wasting is a factor, Alfalfa will do some good.

The treatment of a number of other conditions has been historically linked to Alfalfa. I don't believe the plant is the best choice for the following, but it may be worth trying if all other avenues have been exhausted. Some find that the herb/seed reduces arthritic inflammation, stimulates lactation, and on occasion, diminishes perimenopausal hot flashes. The last two effects are likely attributed to a hormonal influence produced by the plant's isoflavonoids.

Indications
» Anorexia
» Deficiency, nutritional
» Malnourishment, due to organic or functional issues

Collection
Gather and dry the herb normally. Compared to commercial grades, recently wildcrafted Alfalfa will almost always be of superior quality.

Preparations/Dosage
» Herb infusion: 4–8 oz. 2–3 times daily

Cautions
Just as Alfalfa is a superb tea for nutritional deficiencies, due to its tendency of absorbing trace minerals from the soil, it can also be problematic if collected in contaminated areas. The plant picks up a fair share of copper, lead, cadmium, and nickel; therefore it is best to know the soil's history prior to collection.

Other Uses
Alfalfa is an important feed for stock and is also used in field soil conditioning.

Alumroot
Saxifragaceae/Saxifrage Family

Heuchera L.
Roundleaf alumroot, Littleleaf alumroot, Pink alumroot, Coralbells

Heuchera spp.

Description
Herbaceous and perennial, Alumroot's initial growth is mostly basal. The leaves are ovoid and lobed/toothed with long petioles. Each flower is composed of a 5–lobed calyx and 5 (or less) smaller petals. The arrangement is usually a yellow/whitish–green affair and spike–like. Heuchera sanguinea, commonly known as Coralbells, is a visually–appealing exception – the flowers are deep pink–red. Most species have creeping–rhizomatous rootstocks, sheathed by old leaf base growth.

Distribution
A common plant throughout the West, Alumroot is usually found in gravely soils, scree, or the soil pockets of rock walls. Some appear to need not much more than a finger–hold sized ledge to thrive.

Chemistry
Flavonoids; ellagitannins; gallotannins.

Medicinal Uses
Alumroot's use is alluded to by the root's pinkish (sometimes whitish) inner coloration and astringent taste. When chewed, it is drying and constricting to surface membranes (a common reaction to tannin–oriented plants). This makes the chewed root the most basic (and effective) preparation for mouth sores, bleeding and inflamed gums, and even a sore throat. However effective, most people find this crude method impractical, at least for daily use. The gargled tea or tincture placed in a little water is a more convenient way to proceed.

Internally, the same preparations are astringent to the gastrointestinal tract. From esophageal and stomach irritations related to acid reflux to intestinal inflammation from a bout of food poisoning, Alumroot will be found calming. It particularly excels when imbibed as a strong tea for the nearly resolved, yet the still nauseating, effects of Campylobacter spp. or Salmonella spp. (food poisoning). Though many herbs (Barberry or Simaruba family plants) will have stronger antimicrobial effects, tannin–source plants such as Alumroot are fine as soothing–binding agents used near the conclusion of these diarrhea causing bacterial infections. Additionally, mucus and/or blood tinged urine from a urinary tract infection will diminish with Alumroot. However, herbs like Juniper, Cypress, or Thuja will better address the infection[5].

Similar to the chewed root's application to oral afflictions, use the freshly mashed root, salve, ointment, or wash for scrapes, cuts, burns, and other minor issues with associated bleeding. Not especially pain–relieving, Alumroot used in this fashion is simply an external coagulant, like Oak, Geranium, and other tannin–based plants.

Use a sitz bath of the half–strength tea for minor vaginal inflammations. Not particularly antibacterial, its best indication is regional tissue irritation and itchiness. Used this way it also works well as a postpartum application for passive hemorrhaging and delivery–traumatized tissues.

Indications
» Inflammation, oral
» Gums, bleeding/inflamed
» Pharyngitis
» Inflammation/Irritation, gastrointestinal tract
» Diarrhea, from dietary indiscretions or nearly resolved bacterial infections
» Infection, urinary, minor
» As a topical astringent (external)
» Vaginitis (external)
» As a postpartum sitz bath (external)

Collection
An uncomplicated plant to collect, much of Alumroot's root mass is above ground, or nearly so, making the gathering process easy. Depending on growth habit and environment, many species' roots grow between easily moved rocks. Once exposed simply snip the creeping rhizomes.

5   Be aware of flank pain, associated spasms (kidney stones), and lower back soreness (kidney infection). Depending on the severity of the situation, herbal medicine may be inadequate in treating these potentially serious conditions.

The plant is often precariously located on steep rock–strewn slopes and cliff faces. Indeed, it always seems that the better–quality plants are the most difficult to reach!

Preparations/Dosage
» Decoction: 4–6 oz. 2–3 times daily
» FPT/DPT (50% alcohol 10% glycerin): 30–60 drops 2–3 times daily
» Wash/Fomentation/Sitz bath: as needed

Cautions
If dosing and duration are sensible there is little overall caution for Alumroot. However, as with any tannin–based medicinal plant, standard cautions are as follows. Limit its use with urinary tract issues to about one week; any longer and kidney irritation may result, though large quantities over several days may irritant the kidneys, with or without an infection. An occasional cup or two of the tea is not a problem during pregnancy, but continued daily use should be avoided. Excessive use may cause some minor gastrointestinal and hepatic irritation as well.

Angelica
Apiaceae/Carrot Family

Angelica spp.

Angelica L.
Lyall's angelica, Gray's angelica, Small leaf angelica, Rose angelica, etc.

Description
Most species of Angelica are robust and large growing herbaceous perennials. Adding to the plant's physical stature are its hollow stems, inflated sheathing petioles, and multiple leaf divisions. The compound umbel–type flower clusters are white or yellow (though some species have pink, red, or purple flowers). Individual flower parts are 5–divided. The seeds are oblong or round, ribbed, and aromatic when crushed.

Distribution
Out of the two dozen or so Angelica species listed for America and Canada, nearly half have ranges within California, Oregon, or Washington. The

Rocky Mountain region is the second main area for the genus. Angelica ampla and A. grayi are found throughout the southern Rockies. A. pinnata covers much of the southern and middle Rockies and A. roseana is found in the middle and parts of the northern Rockies.

Most western species grow best in the moist soils of coniferous/montane forests or coastal areas (for a number of Pacific species), and often in proximity to drainages and streams.

Chemistry

I am unaware of an extensive chemical workup for any of the western species. As a reasonable substitute the following is a listing for Angelica archangelica. Prominent essential oils: α–pinene, β–pinene, α–fenchene, myrcene, α–phellandrene, β–phellandrene, limonene, cis–β–ocimene, trans–β–ocimene, terpinyl acetate, α–copaene, α–humulene, germacrene–d, β–bisabolene; furanocoumarins: angelicin, archangelicin, archangelin, bergapten, imperatorin, isoimperatorin, oxypeucedanin, phellopterin, psoralen, xanthotoxin; fatty acids: valeric acid, angelic acid; lactone: muscolide.

Medicinal Uses

Due to a similar chemical makeup, North American Angelica species can be essentially patterned after the medicinal use of the main Old World species: Angelica archangelica[6], also known as Angelica officinalis or Archangelica officinalis. Although some minor variation can be expected, any species that is strongly aromatic will be an effective medicine.

Both the seeds and roots are used as a gastrointestinal carminative. Drink several ounces of the tea, the tincture in a little water, or even chew on a small hand full of seeds for the relief of indigestion, especially if accompanied by fullness, bloating, and nausea. Some find the chewed seeds alone an effective and quick–acting therapy for simple heartburn or gastritis.

Angelica is also well–applied to intestinal issues. Cramps with accompanying flatulence (colic for babies or young children) is a specific for the plant. From transverse colon spasm (borborygmus) to simple lower intestinal cramps from poor quality or spoiled food, Angelica will be found spasmolytic.

6   Angelica sinensis or Dong quai, utilized in TCM and adopted by western herbalists, has some similarity to western Angelicas. Unlike Angelica sinensis though, western Angelicas have a negligible or much reduced influence on reproductive hormones.

Women find Angelica spasm–relieving if suffering from first/second day period cramps especially if topical warmth feels beneficial. Furthermore, it is indicated if pelvic cramping tends to cause parallel intestinal spasm or diarrhea. Try it alone or combined with other reproductive antispasmodics such as Western peony, Cramp bark, or Yellow pond lily.

As a lung herb, Angelica is best used if in need of a stimulating expectorant. The plant's volatile fraction does a fine job of loosening bronchial mucus, particularity in chronic lung complaints. Most species of Angelica also tend to counter bronchial inflammation and airway constriction, meaning asthmatics will find the plant (especially root preparations) opening and antispasmodic.

Angelica is a useful diaphoretic. The hot tea is best for a low to moderate fever that has not yet broken. To trigger diaphoresis, a nearly fool–proof approach is to drink a hot cup of Angelica tea while taking a hot bath or shower just before bed. Have a change of bed clothes/bedding ready as the fever should break later that same night or early morning.

One frontier for Angelica (Angelica archangelica) is its application to Alzheimer's disease and related dementia. Angelica's furanocoumarin fraction has demonstrated (human studies) good cholinesterase inhibitory activity. Essentially, Angelica keeps acetylcholine (and butyrylcholine) in cerebral synapsis longer, therefore potentially slowing the disease's progression.

Indications
- Nausea
- Gastritis
- Spasm/Cramp/Colic, gastrointestinal
- Cramp, uterine
- Bronchitis, thickened phlegm
- Asthma, with constriction and inflammation
- Fever, dry skin
- Alzheimer's disease

Collection
Gather the entire root, either pre– or post– stalk and flower formation, usually in the early spring or fall. Collect the just–beginning–to–ripen, yet still green, seeds in the spring to summer.

Preparations

The fresh root may be found mildly acrid. If this is the case, dry the root first and then prepare it as a dry plant tincture or tea. The steam distillation of Angelica excludes most furanocoumarins and contains many volatiles, so this process will not yield the best preparation if in need of the plant's lung antiinflammatory or cholinesterase influences.

Dosage

» FPT/DPT (60% alcohol): 30–60 drops 2–3 times daily
» Standard/Cold infusion: 2–4 oz. 2–3 times daily
» Essential oil (seed): 1–2 drops taken in a capsule 2–3 times daily
» Spirit: 10–20 drops 2–3 times daily

Cautions

Avoid Angelica during pregnancy due to its stimulating effects on reproductive tissue blood flow. The plant also contains significant amounts of furanocoumarins, many of which have therapeutic uses, but some too are linked to photosensitivity (sun exposure dermatitis). Unlike a number of Cow parsnip species (also high in furanocoumarins), Angelica is traditionally considered non–problematic in this department. However, I believe it wise to approach the plant with some caution if ingesting it with other sun–sensitizing compounds (SSRIs for instance).

Apache Plume
Rosaceae/Rose Family

Fallugia paradoxa

Fallugia paradoxa (D. Don) Endl. ex Torr. *(Fallugia micrantha, F. paradoxa var. acuminata, Sieversia paradoxa)*
Poñil, Feather rose, Feather duster bush

Description

A mid–sized shrub, Apache plume is perennial, deciduous, and many–branched. Older stems exhibit exfoliating bark, whereas the younger branches/stems are covered with gray/white woolly hair. The leaves are pinnately divided into 3–7 oblong lobes. They are green above and lighter–woolly beneath. The flowers are 5–petaled, conspicuous, and white. They range from unisexual to bisexual. After pollination, each seed develops a persistent style, which forms as a long feathery tail 1"–2" in length; this is considered the plant's most distinctive feature and a basis for its common name.

Distribution
A Southwestern plant of mid to high elevations, look for Apache plume between 3500'–7500'. It ranges from southern California and southern Nevada to much of Arizona, New Mexico, southern Colorado, and western Texas. It is not exclusively a desert plant in these regions, but a denizen of grasslands, Oak woodlands, and upper desert transition zones.

Chemistry
Flavonoids; ellagitannins; gallotannins.

Medicinal Uses
Apache plume shares most of its medicinal qualities with other Rose family plants. And like the others, its uses are based upon its flavonoid–tannin complexes. Use the plant as a mild and uncomplicated internal and external astringent.

For the urinary tract, the tea is the best preparation. It reduces irritation, inflammation, and mucus/blood tinged urine. Although most find it symptomatically soothing, stronger disinfectant herbs are likely needed if there is pronounced infection.

For women, the tea reduces excessive menstrual bleeding. Menorrhagia caused from diminishing estrogen/progesterone levels is not reliably influenced, but if the situation is caused from idiosyncratic cycle fluctuations, drink 2–3 cups a day from the first day (or a day before) of menses until the period's end. The tea can also be prepared as a sitz bath for vaginal irritations and vaginitis. It combines well with Tree of heaven if there is parasitic element.

Loose stools and diarrhea caused from disagreeable food or stress are lessened by the tea. Additionally, most will find the tea as a sore throat gargle soothing and antiinflammatory. A crushed leaf poultice (or wash) is reducing to the redness and irritation of minor insect stings, scrapes, and sunburn.

Indications
» As a general astringent

- » Urinary tract, irritation/inflammation
- » Menstruation, heavy
- » Vaginitis (external)
- » Diarrhea
- » Sore throat (gargle)
- » Insect bites/Scrapes/Sunburn (external)

Collection
Apache plume's leaves are the main medicinal portion, but the flowers and wispy–tailed seeds are also fine if gathered all together. Be sure to discard the larger stems, as these parts are essentially inert.

Preparations/Dosage
- » Herbal infusion: 4–8 oz. 2–3 times daily
- » FPT/DPT (50% alcohol): 1 teaspoon 2–3 times daily
- » Sitz bath: as needed
- » Topical preparations: as needed

Cautions
Gastrointestinal upset is possible with excessive amounts. There are no significant cautions for sensible use.

Arnica
Asteraceae/Sunflower Family

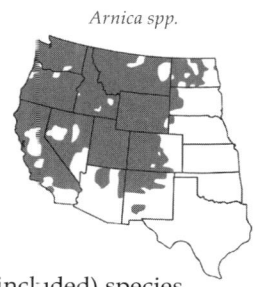

Arnica spp.

Arnica L.
Broadleaf arnica, Chamisso arnica, Foothill arnica, Hairy arnica, Heartleaf arnica, Mountain arnica, Spearleaf arnica, etc.

Description
Nearly a dozen (more if the Pacific Coast states are included) species of Arnica exist throughout the western mountains. Sharing a majority of characteristics, they are small to medium–sized herbaceous perennials with mostly opposite leaves and traveling rhizomes. Glandular, mildly aromatic, with a yellow to yellow–orange flower of varying ray and disc florets,

western Arnicas are usual enough to miss but unique enough to remember once some of the plant's characteristics are committed to memory.

Distribution
Arnica is a circumboreal montane oriented genus. High mountain, subalpine and alpine meadows, clearings, and grassy streamsides are its usual places. Occasionally the plant is found in dappled–shade intermittent forest areas, but rarely in heavily shaded woods.

Chemistry
For Arnica montana (other species similar): sesquiterpene lactones: guaianolides: helenalin; pyrrolizidine alkaloids: tussilagine, isotussilagine; flavonoids; caffeoylquinic acids; polysaccharides: fucogalactoxyloglucans, arabinogalactans; terpenoid: loliolide.

Medicinal Uses
Western species of Arnica, as long as they are glandular and somewhat aromatic, are fine replacements for the official herbal medicine, Arnica montana[7]. Arnica is best applied to painful conditions characterized by subacute/chronic inflammation and pain – issues that were once acute but now have become older and less 'fiery'. Because the plant stimulates tissues and excites immunological mediators, it is less suited for the treatment of new injuries characterized by an array of heightened immunological responses. Essentially, use it for painful injuries when the healing process has stalled or slowed.

Apply Arnica salve, ointment, or liniment to poorly healing sprains, muscle pulls, contusions, and bruises, all with unbroken skin. One exception is the diluted ointment – use it on bedsores, poorly healing wounds, post–operative incisions, and other breaks that would benefit from the plant's tissue stimulation and healing properties. A frequently overlooked application, Arnica is often found calming to arthritis, especially if it is aggravated by the cold.

Although it does not match Arnica's specific subacute/chronic treatment sphere, some people do find it reducing to acute pain, though less reliably. My suggestion is to try Arnica if it is the only herb on–hand. If it

---

[7] To be accurate, Arnica montana will be found slightly more energetic and stimulating than local plants. A. cordifolia is one of the more popular replacement species.

is ineffective, use standard acute pain topical herbs (Tobacco, Datura, Henbane, or Lobelia are good choices).

For chronic pharyngitis, 10–20 drops of Arnica tincture in an ounce of water can be gargled. Hoarseness from stressed vocal cords, a common problem of singers and orators, is addressed by the mixture. The addition of Ligusticum or Yerba mansa will be of benefit as well.

Lastly, Arnica's forgotten use as a cardiovascular stimulant, is an interesting footnote. Small doses of the tincture were once used internally to treat acute heart weakness linked to age, cardiovascular disease, or other episodes that were dependent on diminished heart function. However, due to today's greater understanding of how vascular inflammation is linked to cardiovascular disease, this historical use of Arnica may not be its wisest application. In these situations, Hawthorn or Selenicereus is a more kindly-acting heart tonic.

Indications
» Pain/Inflammation, subacute/chronic (external)
» Muscle pulls/Strains/Contusions/Bruises (external)
» Poorly healing wounds/Bedsores (external)
» Pharyngitis, chronic (gargle)

Collection
The flowers are the most commonly used portion of Arnica, but as long as the species (and part) is glandular, it too can be used.

Preparations
The fresh plant, especially the fresh flower, is the strongest and most potent part, but it is more apt to cause irritation when applied topically as a poultice or liniment. The dried flowers (and other parts) used topically in various forms, are less apt to be problematic.

Dosage
» FPT/DPT: (65% alcohol): 10–20 drops 1–3 times daily (gargle)
» Liniment/Ointment/Oil/Salve: as needed

Cautions
Be aware of tissue irritation with prolonged topical application. For internal use (cardiovascular application...be cautious), dilute the tea or tincture in

a moderate amount of water. This will ward against gastrointestinal upset. Discontinue internal use if restlessness or excitability develops. Arnica should not be taken internally by children or by women who are nursing or pregnant.

Other Uses
Homeopathic preparations of Arnica are altogether different than those of herbal Arnica. Due to composition and potency differences they should not be considered interchangeable. Homeopathic Arnica is used more liberally due to 'stronger' preparations containing no actual Arnica constituents. Moreover, homeopathic Arnica can be ingested without caution internally, as well as applied externally. It is commonly used in sizable amounts for acute trauma but rarely when the situation is chronic.

Asparagus
Liliaceae/Lily Family

Asparagus officinalis

Asparagus officinalis L.
Common asparagus, Garden asparagus, Sparrowgrass

Description
A 3'–6' tall rhizomatous perennial, Asparagus' initial growth is comprised of flexible sprouting stems (edible phase). Becoming more woody and finely branched with age, the plant at maturity appears wispy with its scale–like and inconspicuous leaves. The small, mostly solitary, green–white male and female flowers form on jointed pedicels. The female flower develops into a ½" diameter red berry.

Distribution
Although an Old World native, in America Asparagus is found feral in the lower 48. Look for it as an escapee from garden or crop cultivation. It's common to field sides, grassy flats, and other areas where the soil has been disturbed.

Chemistry
Asparagus root: carotenoid: zeaxanthin; flavonoids: kaempferol, quercetin, rutin; lignans; spirostanol saponins: yamogenin–2, sarsasapogenin; officinalsin–2; inulin; various starches and sugars.

Medicinal Uses
Of significant European (particularly French) repute, Asparagus was once used widely for its diuretic properties. Although not particularly modifying to urinary tract infections, the root tea is a choice herbal remedy for gout, related joint inflammation, uric acid–type kidney stones, and generally overly–acidic urine (imagine a traditional cold season western European diet of beef, wheat, and wine).

Used as a preventative, Asparagus is best taken at the very first sign of a gout related flare–up (sensitive big toe, etc.). Even though the tea will still be of benefit if used alone during an episode, its corrective effect will be greater if there is also an adoption of dietary changes: the reduction of red meat, organ meats, alcohol, legumes, and other urate–forming foods while increasing hydration with pure water.

Other Asparagus species are used in Chinese medicine and Ayurveda. Although there are some application and chemical similarities, these exotic species are not quite comparable with A. officinalis.

Indications
» Gout and related joint inflammation
» Kidney stones, uric acid–based
» Acidic urine, general

Collection
Gather the sub–surface laterally growing rhizomes. Non–compacted soils will make collection less of a chore and in some cases the roots can be simply pulled up by hand.

Preparations
The root tea is the traditional (and most effective) preparation. For convenience, the fresh or dry plant tincture can be used too, but be sure to drink a cup or two of distilled water with the dose as proper hydration also benefits

overly–concentrated urine situations. Unlike Asparagus shoots, the roots are nearly inodorous[8], and should not result in sulphur–smelling urine.

Dosage
» Decoction: 4–6 oz. 2–3 times daily
» FPT/DPT (50% alcohol): 30–60 drops 2–3 times daily

Cautions
There are no cautions with normal usage.

Other Uses
As a vegetable, clip the emerging shoots in the spring. They should be flexible and non–woody. If allowed to grow, the shoots develop into the plant's stems. They are inedible. Purple cultivars of Asparagus are much higher in antioxidant pigments (anthocyanins/anthocyanidins) than standard types.

Aspen
Salicaceae/Willow Family

Populus tremuloides Michx. (*Populus aurea, P. tremula subsp. tremuloides, P. tremuloides var. aurea, P. tremuloides var. magnifica, P. tremuloides var. vancouveriana*) American aspen, Quaking aspen, Tremble, Álamo temblón

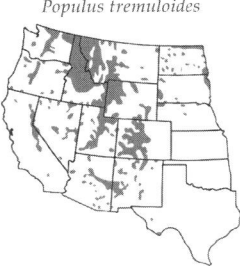

Populus tremuloides

Description
Aspen is a narrow–crowned deciduous tree reaching heights of 50'–100'. One of its more distinctive characteristics is its thin whitish–green, cream–colored bark (though towards the base it is more grayish–brown and furrowed). The leaves are round–ovate and pointed with entire or serrulate margins. They are green, but become golden–yellow in autumn. Male and female flowers form separately in catkins. Extensive colony–stands develop due to rhizome/shoot growth. The tree is called Quaking aspen due to its leaf patter in a breeze.

8   Asparagus shoots contain asparagusic acid. Some people metabolize this compound into methanethiol, dimethyl sulfide, and other sulfur compounds, which are responsible for 'Asparagus–urine'.

ASPEN

Distribution

A very common tree, Aspen is found both intermingled with conifers and in pure stands, especially if the area has been recently logged or marred by fire. In these environments, the root networks easily re–sprout and create new groves in relatively short periods. In fact, along with a number of Oak species, Aspen is an important tree in initiating forest re–growth after fire or logging.

Chemistry

Coumarin: scopoletin; flavonoids: eriodictyol, methylaromadendrin, naringenin, rhamnocitrin; phenolic glycosides: salicin, salicortin, salireposide, salicyloyltremuloidin, tremulacin, tremuloidin; sterol: β–sitosterol.

Medicinal Uses

Aspen belongs to a trinity of Willow family trees that have overlapping (if not identical) medicinal uses. The grouping includes Aspen, Cottonwood (Populus angustifolia and other species), and Balsam poplar (Populus balsamifera/trichocarpa). Bark uses for all three trees (and the majority of Salix species) are the same.

Prosaic in application, Aspen symptomatically addresses painful conditions. The tree's bark has the greatest aspirin–like/antiinflammatory effect (the leaves can be used as a half–strength preparation). Drink the tea for issues ranging from arthritic flare–ups to acute injuries. Even the diffuse tissue and muscular pains of fibromyalgia are often quieted. Essentially, if it hurts, a cup or two of Aspen tea may not cure, but it will ease.

Like other salicin–containing plants, the tea lowers an elevated temperature without potentially causing an initial diaphoresis related spike. Aspen is doubly indicated when temperatures are high and there exists attending tissue/muscular aches and pains (flu).

Although not as strong as Gentian, some find its mild bitter tonic activity of benefit if plagued by indigestion, gastrointestinal stasis, and associated feelings of stomach fullness after meals. Try a strong cup of tea 10–15 minutes before meals; the addition of an aromatic–carminative herb will increase Aspen's effectiveness.

Minor urinary irritation/inflammation is soothed by Aspen leaf buds. Their best application is not necessarily as an antimicrobial, but a soothing diuretic. Try them in transitory kidney and lower urinary inflammations;

even low–level prostatic irritations that cause bladder sensitivity are often calmed.

Like Cottonwood, the leaf buds can be used as a weaker, half–strength substitute for Balsam poplar buds. A liniment, salve, ointment, or oil derived from the semi–resinous leaf buds is well–applied locally to headache pain and most other inflammations and swellings: contusions, sprains, sore joints, etc. These same preparations are also externally applied to burns and scrapes. Part soother and part antimicrobial agent, it moderately reduces sensitivity and inhibits bacterial growth. See Balsam poplar for the main Populus bud medicine.

Indications
bark
» As a general aspirin–like antiinflammatory
» Fevers, moderate to high
» Indigestion, asecretory

leaf buds
» Irritations, urinary and prostatic
» As an antimicrobial/anodyne agent (external)

Collection
Select a group of small trees or saplings. From the larger trunks, saw or prune away several secondary branches (or cut the saplings entirely). After sawing the branches/saplings into manageable 1′–2′ lengths, remove the young–unfissured bark with a knife (or sometimes the bark can be stripped with fingers alone after an initial knife cut). Discard the core wood, smaller branches, and leaves (or keep the leaves for a half–strength preparation).

Preparations/Dosage
» Bark decoction: 4 oz. 2–3 times daily or externally as needed
» FPT/DPT (75% alcohol) of leaf buds: 30–60 drops 3–4 times daily
» Liniment/Oil/Salve/Ointment (leaf buds): as needed

Cautions
The internal use of Aspen bark joins Cottonwood and Balsam poplar with similar potential cautions. Theoretically (and theoretically should be stressed) Aspen's phenolic glycosides may potentiate anti–coagulant pharmaceuticals, though to my knowledge there is no in–vivo evidence to

support this. Another extremely remote caution is Aspen's concurrent use with feverish children (Reye's syndrome).

Avens
Rosaceae/Rose Family

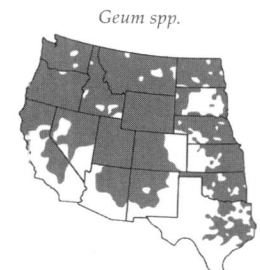

Geum spp.

Geum L.
Large–leaved avens, Old man's whiskers, Prairie smoke, Ross's avens, Water avens, White avens, Yellow avens

Description
A Rose family herbaceous perennial, at first glance Avens appears commonplace and similar to many other leafy green herbs. Upon closer inspection though, Avens' uniqueness becomes apparent. The plant has deeply divided leaves with larger leaflet divisions intermingled with smaller ones. Agrimony and a number of Potentilla species also display this pattern. The flowers rise above the basal leaf growth on extended slender hairy stalks. They are 5–petaled, perfect, and (mostly) yellow. The majority of species form globe–like and faux–spiny seed clusters. They are not prickly; however they easily cling to clothing.

Distribution
A common plant of world–wide disbursement, look for Avens in mid–high elevation mountainous areas. It is usually encountered along small streams, fens, and wet–boggy meadows. Horsetail and Nettle are common companions.

Chemistry
Flavonoids; ellagitannins; gallotannins.

Medicinal Uses
Avens' uses and qualities are shared by any number of related plants: Agrimony, Wild rose, and Cinquefoil are several of note. The plant is therapeutic due to its phenolic glycoside content. That is to say, it contains an array of flavonoids and tannins that tighten and constrict surface tissues.

Use Avens as a soothing astringent for the urinary tract. If the urine is cloudy (denoting mucus) and/or strong smelling, both suggesting a possible infection, the tea is indicated. For extra disinfectant action combine Avens with Juniper, Thuja, or Cypress, otherwise the herb used alone should be fine for simple area irritability and/or mild infection.

Assisting in urinary stone/gravel passage, Avens can be used in conjunction with Lobelia and/or Gravel root as one part of a lithotropic combination. Employed this way, Avens serves as a urinary tissue antiinflammatory and mild hemostatic. The latter two herbs are the urinary tract antispasmodic element of the combination.

Like Agrimony, try Avens for incontinence in older individuals whom suffer from general area laxity. Its effectiveness tends to be erratic. However, for those who are just beginning to show signs of weakness, the tea will encourage area tone.

Women will see benefit in its use for heavy menstruation. Here too it is the plant's astringent attributes that are responsible for its menses abating effects. Although there is little Avens will do if the situation is caused by diminished levels of estrogen/progesterone upon entering perimenopause, the tea works well if used during menses to clarify the end of the period. Minor postpartum bleeding also will abate due to the plant's mild uterine lining astringency.

Mild vaginitis responds well to the tea when it is applied as a sitz bath. It's not particularly antimicrobial, but it will be found soothing to inflamed tissues. A stronger approach for trichomoniasis infections are Simaruba family plants – Crucifixion thorn or Tree of heaven.

Indications
- » Dysuria
- » Hematuria
- » Incontinence, in the aged
- » Menstruation, heavy
- » Vaginitis, mild (external)

Collection
Gather the new herbaceous growth from spring through summer. Leaf, flower, thin stems, and seed are all usable.

Preparations
As with most Rose family plant medicines, the tea is the best preparation.

Dosage
- » Herbal infusion: 4–8 oz. 2–3 times daily
- » FPT/DPT (50% alcohol): 1 teaspoon 2–3 times daily
- » Sitz bath: as needed

Cautions
There are no cautions for Avens with normal usage.

Balsam Poplar
Salicaceae/Willow Family

Populus balsamifera, trichocarpa

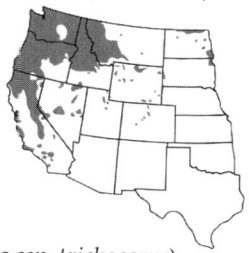

Populus balsamifera L. (*Populus balsamifera* ssp. *balsamifera*, *P. balsamifera* var. *candicans*, *P. balsamifera* var. *subcordata*, *P. candicans*, *P. tacamahacca*)
Balm of gilead buds, Balsam poplar buds, Poplar buds, Tacamahac

Populus trichocarpa Torr. & A. Gray (*Populus balsamifera* ssp. *trichocarpa*)
Black cottonwood, Western balsam poplar

Description
Both species of Balsam poplar are very close in botanical association. In fact, some botanists consider them subspecies rather than separate species. Although both trees share a majority of physical qualities and are easily confused, identification is made easy by them having very little geographical overlap[9]. The other Populus' (Aspen and Cottonwood) have different enough leaf shapes/sizes as to not be easily mistaken for Balsam poplar.

On mature trees the bark is furrowed and grayish–brown. The winter leaf buds are reddish, resinous, and pleasantly balsamic. They can be nearly an inch long, but are usually less. The leaves are narrowly ovate to ovate with rounded to cordate bases. The leaf margins are serrate (lesser so with

---

[9] The main area of overlap for the two species is the northern Rocky Mountain axis: from southern Alaska to northwestern Wyoming. Here they are even known to hybridize with each other resulting in Populus x hastata.

Populus balsamifera). Like other Populus' the leaves change from green to golden in the fall. Male and female flowers develop in catkins and form on separate trees.

Distribution

In the West, Populus balsamifera is principally a tree of the Rocky Mountain region: Colorado, Wyoming, Montana, and Idaho. Encountered in isolated pockets, look to rich woods, forest edges, mountain slopes, and drainage sides. The tree's main area is in the Northeast, north–central parts of the United States, and most of Canada to Alaska.

More likely to be encountered in the western mountains, Populus trichocarpa's density and coverage are much greater than that of P. balsamifera's. From Alaska and British Columbia to Washington, Oregon, Idaho, Montana, and northern–middle California, it's a common tree. Even the mountains of Nevada, Utah, and southern California support occasional groups. In northern latitudes look to lake sides and other bottomlands. The southern growers are found in higher elevation mountainous areas.

Chemistry

Volatiles (buds): α–pinene, β–pinene, myrcene, cineol, γ–terpinene, terpinen-4-ol, α–terpineol, α–bergamotene, β–farnesene, δ–cadinene, trans–nerolidol, α–bisabolol; bark: salicin, salicortin, pyrocatechol, trichocarpin, trichocarpigenin, salireposide, salicyloylsalicin, trichocarposide, populin, dihydromyricetin.

Medicinal Uses

Populus balsamifera (referred to in older texts as P. candicans) is considered the main source tree for Balsam poplar buds. P. trichocarpa is as useful and historically was also gathered, though to a lesser extent. Even P. nigra (European black poplar) was once recognized by the National Formulary as a source. Broadly speaking, Balsam poplar buds, a.k.a. Balm of gilead buds, belongs to any highly resinous Populus species or cultivar, though only several were officially recognized.

The therapeutic effects of Balsam poplar buds are essentially derived from two types of compounds. The first group, found in most other Willow family trees, is a combination of glycosides, mainly salicin and populin. These glycoside compounds (and derivatives) provide most of the buds (and bark) analgesic and antiinflammatory effects. The second group, which is more unique to resinous Populus species, is an array of balsamic and aromatic terpenes, not entirely dissimilar from conifer oleoresin. Here we have Poplar bud's stimulating and antimicrobial influences. Due to these two groups of intermingled compounds and related therapeutic effects, Poplar bud's application is somewhat broad.

Topical use as an anodyne ointment or salve is its principle application. Most specific for chronic or subacute pain, it can also be used for acute afflictions, though if there is excessive tissue redness and swelling, its application (undiluted) is generally contraindicated. External preparations are well used for rheumatic/arthritic conditions (benefited by warmth) and chronic muscular/connective tissue afflictions (tendinitis, bursitis, sports injuries, etc.). Try Balsam poplar buds on chronic neuralgias (unbroken skin) be them from injury or latent viral infection (here it combines well with equal parts of St. John's wort). The liniment (externally applied tincture) is well used in combination with the internal bark tea of Aspen, Willow, or Cottonwood (or even the bark of Balsam poplar) to reduce the dull throb of most headache types. For hemorrhoid relief, use Balsam poplar bud salve, oil, or ointment combined with equal parts of Henbane (see preparations below). As a burn dressing, mixed with equal parts of Aloe vera gel, Balsam poplar bud ointment is pain reducing, antiseptic, and stimulates cellular regeneration of damaged tissue.

The bud's internal effects are best represented by either the fresh or dry plant tincture. As a stimulating antimicrobial agent to the urinary tract, small but frequent doses are of help in resolving dysuria (painful urination) affecting the bladder and urethra. The bronchial region is similarly affected. Take the tincture as a secretion–producing expectorant. It tends to dislodge tenacious phlegm making expectoration more productive and the entire region less sore. The tincture in warm water is gargled for sore throats and laryngitis; additionally, most find its anodyne qualities of value especially if the simple act of swallowing causes throat discomfort.

Lacking the aromatic terpenes of the bud material, Balsam poplar bark is used like any other Willow family tree bark – as a reliable, broadly acting antiinflammatory agent. From acute sport's injuries to rheumatic pain, a strong cup of Balsam poplar bark tea will prove symptomatically relieving. As a useful fever reducer, drink the decoction to lower temperature and quiet muscular and tissue pains commonly associated with the flu and related wintertime viruses. The bark tea taken before meals is a useful gastric stimulant. Its tonic activity is mainly imparted through its bitterness. Lastly, like the buds, the bark is also a urinary tract medicine, only without the tissue stimulant and antimicrobial influences. Mildly diuretic, use it in chronic inflammatory disturbances of the area. Its use in long standing kidney inflammation and prostatitis is worth noting.

Indications
leaf buds
- » As an analgesic (external)
- » As an antiseptic (external)
- » Infection, urinary tract
- » Pain, urinary tract
- » As a stimulating expectorant
- » Pharyngitis/Laryngitis

bark
- » As an analgesic
- » Fever, to lower
- » Indigestion
- » Irritations, urinary and prostatic

Collection
Gather the sticky leaf buds from late winter to early spring when they are at their resinous peak. If the resin is abundant enough, where the buds and twigs are both coated, gather the entire branching end. The occasional flower catkin collected with the mix is fine, though it is best to discard the majority of them. This resin covering quickly fades as the tree's leaves begin to unfurl and form. If possible, gather the buds (or entire branch ends) while temperatures are freezing, or close to it, as this will keep the collected parts from sticking to hands, bags, etc. If harvesting in non–freezing temperatures, the buds/resin covered twigs can be brought home and then placed in a freezer until the resin hardens. This will make processing (bud separation from branches/twigs much easier).

Like other Willow family trees, Balsam poplar bark can be gathered year–round, though the springtime (pre–leafing) or fall (post–leafing) unfissured bark will be best.

Preparations
For topical uses, resin covered material can be prepared both fresh and dried. If the buds/twigs are heavily coated with resin, then the fresh rendering

process can be used. However, if they are not heavily coated then it is best to proceed with the dried bud technique.

In a large pot, cover the fresh buds/twigs (be sure to record the weight of the material before starting) with water. Simmer the material for an hour. Turn off the heat and add to the pot the same volume of olive oil as the material weighed. Stir several times and let the mixture cool. Carefully decant the oil–infused resin from the water segment. The rendered resin–steeped olive oil can now be used topically as is, or converted into a salve or ointment. As long as all of the water was removed from the oil prior to bottling, it will store well without refrigeration.

Preparations for the dried material are just as beneficial for topical use, though procedures do differ. Cover the dried buds (or buds and resin covered twigs) with 7 parts of olive oil and apply a low heat for 8–10 hours. Let cool, strain, and bottle. A stronger oil can be made by powdering the buds and then using the alcohol intermediate oil technique as discussed in the main preparation section.

For a general topical anodyne preparation, the following adaptation of an old European formula will be found of use. Coarsely powder 1 part of dried Henbane leaves (Belladonna, Datura, and/or Black nightshade were once used too, and are fine substitutes if Henbane is unavailable). Mix in 1–½ parts alcohol; cover the combo in a container and let stand for 24 hours. Add 2 parts of dried and powdered Balsam poplar buds. Add 21 parts of olive oil, mix well, and apply a low heat for 8–10 hours. Strain (discard the 'marc') and add 1–2 parts beeswax to the oil if a salve is desired. Pure coconut oil (or lard or clarified butter if being applied to burns) can be used in place of olive oil (and beeswax). The latter mediums will remain solidified at room temperature, making beeswax unnecessary.

The bud oil can also be used as a rancidity/microbial growth inhibitor when making ointments. The base oil segment comprised of 10%–20% of bud oil is usually all that is needed to extend shelf life. For internal uses the buds/resin coated twigs are tinctured fresh or dry.

Dosage

» Bark decoction: 4 oz. 2–3 times daily or externally as needed
» FPT/DPT (75% alcohol) of leaf buds: 20–40 drops 3–4 times daily
» Liniment/Oil/Salve/Ointment (leaf buds): as needed

Cautions

For potential Balsam poplar bark contraindications see Cautions under Aspen or Cottonwood. Used in excess the bud tincture may irritate the kidneys and upset the stomach – normal for any high resin containing herbal medicine. Large internal doses are unwise during pregnancy.

Balsamroot
Asteraceae/Sunflower Family

Balsamorhiza sagittata (Pursh) Nutt. *(Balsamorhiza helianthoides, Espeletia helianthoides, E. sagittata)*
Arrowleaf balsamroot

Balsamorhiza sagittata

Description
Balsamroot is an herbaceous perennial. Forming in wider than tall clumps, nearly all of the plant's leaves develop basally on long petioles. The young leaves are silver-velvety below and green above. Once mature they become more uniformly green. Reaching lengths of about 1', they are generally arrow-shaped. The solitary flowers form on long stems and are quite showy when in full bloom. Distinctly Sunflower-like, they reach sizes of 3" across. Balsamroot's achenes (seeds) are of fair size and also Sunflower-like.

Distribution
Balsamroot, like most other Balsamorhiza species, is a Great Basin grower. Oregon and Washington, east of the Cascades, California, east of the Sierras, Idaho, Montana, Nevada, Utah, and the western half of Colorado hold the greatest concentrations of the plant. Preferring basins, clearings, scrub, and hillsides, the plant is usually found in full sun exposures.

Chemistry
Flavonoids: kaempferol, quercetagetin; sesquiterpene lactones: guaianolides, heliigolides, germacranolides.

Medicinal Uses
Balsamroot's use, like many American herbs, comes to us first from American Indian application. The majority of Great Basin roving tribes considered

it an important medicine, especially for the lungs: the Blackfoot, Cheyenne, and Paiute are just several groups with well-recorded usages for the plant.

A bit of an herbal anomaly, many of its chemical and therapeutic qualities are more closely aligned with a number of Carrot family plants rather than the Sunflower family. In fact, if it helps with remembering what Balsamroot does, think of its activity as being related to (but weaker than) Lomatium or Ligusticum.

The main medicinal part of the plant is the root. Semi-resinous and mildly aromatic, its central area of influence is of the lower respiratory tract. Use the tincture, the most efficacious preparation, in cases of acute to subacute bronchitis with thick and difficult to expectorate phlegm. Like others in Balsamroot's class, the root's non-polar constituents tend to loosen and thin stubborn mucus, making expectoration more efficient. If started at the first sign of sickness, just when a throat tickle/irritation seems to descend into the lungs, the herb often means the difference between a 3-4 day episode versus a 2-week episode. Most people also find it lessening to an irritative cough, particularly if the honey-based syrup is used.

It is well known that either a bacterial or viral element plays its part in most bronchial conditions (barring autoimmune/genetic/structural abnormalities, but even here harmful organisms often colonize in response to a compromised environment). So, it is no wonder that the root does well in these situations: its antibacterial/antiviral influence is broad and effective. From the flu to the common cold, if the problem is lung centered, Balsamroot will likely help.

It has been postulated that Balsamroot is a direct immune stimulant. Even though the plant does have some constituent similarities with Echinacea, a well-documented immune stimulant, take this premise not as gospel, but rather possibility. Since there are no in-vivo studies on the matter, and all we really have to go on is observation and sensible deduction, it is my belief that Balsamroot does not directly increase white blood cell activity (like Echinacea), but instead influences it indirectly through its local effect on bronchial tissue, i.e. dust cell activity is augmented due to increased bronchial fluid transport. Many herbs do this. Lomatium, Ligusticum, Grindelia, and Yerba santa are a few that come to mind. In other words, if there is a lung infection, balsamroot most likely stimulants bronchial immunity, but only because it amplifies nearly all other parameters. To suggest it fights infection due to some direct innate or acquired immune stimulation (regionally or systemically) I believe is inaccurate.

The leaves (half to quarter strength) or roots of Balsamroot are made into any number of topical preparations for their disinfectant qualities. Apply it to cuts, scrapes, bites, or other skin afflictions that have become infected. Antiseptic, antiinflammatory, and mildly anodyne, topical preparations are beneficial to a wide array of self–limiting conditions.

Though not an often–reported application for Balsamroot, it almost certainly affects the urinary tract, not unlike many other resinoid–oriented lung herbs, such as Yerba santa or Grindelia. If the usual suspects (Manzanita, Uva–ursi, Madrone, or Cranberry) have failed in relieving the discomfort of a chronic bladder infection, try Balsamroot.

Indications
» Bronchitis, acute/subacute
» Pharyngitis
» Skin afflictions, as an antiseptic
» Cystitis/Urethritis, as an antiseptic

Collection
Balsamroot's roots can be sizable. Older plants will involve some labor–intensive digging. Less dedicated collectors should choose younger plants with smaller roots.

Preparations
Depending on season, geography, and rainfall, Balsamroot will be more or less hydrated – as evidenced by the root's exudate. If well–hydrated, the fresh plant tincture is the preferred preparation method. If the roots are drier and less resinous, cut and dry them first, then tincture the roots using the dry plant tincture method. Whatever technique is decided upon, be sure to remove the outer corky–dried protective bark layer from the roots before drying/tincturing.

Dosage
» FPT/DPT (65% alcohol): 30–60 drops 2–3 times daily
» Standard/Cold infusion: 4–6 ounces 2–3 times daily
» Syrup: 1 tablespoon 3–4 times daily

Baneberry

Ranunculaceae/Buttercup Family

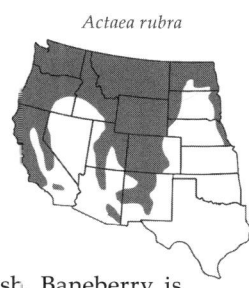

Actaea rubra

Actaea rubra (Aiton) Willd. *(Actaea spicata var. rubra, A. arguta, A. eburnea, A. rubra subsp. arguta, A. neglecta, A. rubra var. dissecta, A. viridiflora)*
Red baneberry, Snakeberry

Description
Like its more popular eastern relative, Black cohosh, Baneberry is an herbaceous perennial. The plant's multiple ternate leaves are sharply toothed to lobed. The white flowers develop in racemes. The red berries usually mature in late summer. White–fruited variants (Actaea rubra forma neglecta) sometimes occur – they are a nice surprise when encountered in the forest.

Distribution
From the Northeast, Baneberry stretches west through the Great Lakes region, skipping most of the Plains, ending with its greatest bulk in the Rocky Mountains and points west and north. It's even found abundantly throughout most of Canada to Alaska. Preferring sloping montane environments, the plant is usually found under the cover of Douglas fir and other conifers, often next to or above intermittent streams.

Indiana, New York, Ohio, and Rhode Island list Baneberry as threatened, endangered, or of a related status. Although some is surely mistakenly picked by unknowing Black cohosh collectors, over harvesting for medicinal use is not a factor in the plant's (middle to east) scarcity. It's simply at the edge of its range in these areas.

Chemistry
For Black cohosh (Baneberry is similar): triterpene glycosides: actein, cimigenol, cimiracemoside a, cimicifugoside h–1; phenolic constituents:

cimicifugic acids a and b, fukinolic acid, cimifugin, cimiracemates a and b, piscidic acid, caffeic acid, ferulic acid, isoferulic acid.

Medicinal Uses

When writing of the medicinal virtues of Baneberry, I write of Black cohosh, and vice versa. Although there are no particular in–vivo studies confirming the two plant's correspondence, empirical observation and constituent similarities suggest both are near duplicates in activity (as are most Actaeas). American herbalists familiar with Baneberry have been using it as a replacement for Black cohosh since the 1990s.

Use Baneberry for the relief of mild to moderate pain, particularly if weak circulation and a sense of bodily chilliness are features. Arthritis–like discomfort throughout the body, often from the onset of a cold or flu, is alleviated as are diffuse muscular pains sometimes described as fibromyalgia. As a mild vascular stimulant, Baneberry's effect on pain syndromes is especially applicable when a local or systemic deficiency underlies any painful episode.

Women are benefited by taking the plant through its ability of reducing perimenopausal complaints. Hot flashes, heart palpitations, sleeplessness, moodiness, and (potentially) bone–loss (all symptoms of estrogen deficiency), have all been shown to lessen under the plant's use. It is also well used as a uterine stimulant when menses is sluggish and warmth to the area feels beneficial.

For migraines, like relatives Clematis, Anemone, and Pulsatilla, Baneberry is beneficial. Although not typically as strong as these other plants, it too is vasodilatory. Dosed properly, as a preemptive, Baneberry will relieve vascular constriction and therefore lessen the rebound over–vasodilation that normally coincides with the intense pain of a migraine episode.

Broadly speaking, Buttercup family plants that are used therapeutically have some medicinal overlap (except the Aconite–Delphinium complex – be very cautious of these). All share sedative and vasodilatory properties. Baneberry is to Black cohosh, what Anemone is to Pulsatilla.

Indications

- » Pain, arthritis–like
- » Pain, muscular, with vascular deficiency
- » Perimenopausal complaints
- » Amenorrhea/Dysmenorrhea, with area congestion

- » Depression, dependent upon hormonal fluctuations and vascular deficiency
- » Headache, migraine type, to preempt

Collection

Baneberry, like Black cohosh, is a rhizome/root medicine[10]. It is composed of a single (usually) main laterally–growing short rhizome surrounded by a tangle of much smaller anchoring roots. Being close to the ground's surface, the entire plant can be successfully uprooted with a well–placed shovel insert and gentle pry. Before moving on be sure to examine the area for any remaining rhizome pieces that may have broken away.

Preparations

Like Black cohosh, Baneberry is remarkable in that its potency is well preserved even after drying. Besides minimal degradation, all major triterpene glycosides within the root remain intact (even after decades). Additionally, the roots take well to both fresh and dry methods of tincturing. The root tincture and tea (both Baneberry and Black cohosh) have a Licorice–like taste, which likely points to a number of chemical (glycosides) and therefore medicinal (reproductive/perimenopause) similarities with Licorice.

Dosage

- » FPT/DPT of root (80% alcohol): 20–30 drops 2–3 times daily
- » Fluidextract of root: 5–10 drops 2–3 times daily
- » Capsule (00) of root: 1–2, 2–3 times daily

Cautions

With overuse, be attentive to a peculiar deep–seated vascular irritation, usually localized to the arms and legs. It is not permanent and dissipates quickly when the dosage is stopped or lessened.

Do not take Baneberry during pregnancy due to its effect on the uterine environment and luteinizing hormone. Moreover, do not use the plant if there is existing liver inflammation or with pharmaceuticals that irritate the liver.

---

10   It has been suggested that the leaf material of Baneberry (and Black Cohosh) has similar yet diminutive medicinal value. Although I initially supported this view, I now believe otherwise: leaf and root uses do not overlap or potency levels are so disparate that they cannot be reasonably compared.

To err on the side of caution I recommend against taking Black cohosh/Baneberry in concordance with any related breast or uterine hyperplasia or cancer. There just is not enough research to recommend these plants as an active cancer therapy.

Barberry
Berberidaceae/Barberry Family

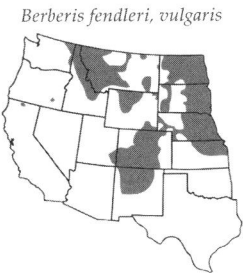

Berberis fendleri, vulgaris

Berberis fendleri
Colorado barberry, Fendler barberry, Western barberry

Berberis vulgaris
European barberry, Common barberry

Description
Colorado barberry is a mid-sized shrub reaching heights of 6' (usually less). The leaves are narrowly elliptic with entire or slightly toothed margins. The plant's stout spines develop at leaf cluster bases. The mature stem bark is distinctly reddish-brown (Common barberry is gray). The yellow flowers form in clusters of 6–10 and give way to a group of slightly elongated red berries.

A large bushy shrub, growing to heights of 12', Common barberry's leaves are ovate with serrated margins. They develop in clusters of 2–5 and originate from alternating nodes, where there is a confluence of items: the 3-parted spines originate from the area, as do the flowers, which are arranged in drooping panicles. Individually they are 6-petaled, yellow, and ¼" in diameter. Like Colorado barberry, the berries ripen from late summer to autumn, and are oblong and red.

Distribution
Colorado barberry's core area is the southern Rocky Mountains. Although outlier populations exist, the plant is abundantly found from Santa Fe, north through the San Juan Mountains, then to southeastern Utah. Mixed conifer canyon bottoms/sides are Colorado barberry's usually places.

Common Barberry's native range is from Europe and western Asia to northwestern Africa. The plant exists in America due to ornamental plantings. It has expanded to current populations (troublesome in some states) due to escapees. Although in the West it is encountered less frequently than in the Northeast and Midwest, look for the plant in disturbed soils: streamsides, trailsides, and secondary roadsides. It is often found growing feral in close proximity to older established plantings (it was once commonly cultivated as a hedge–divider shrub).

Chemistry

Berberis general: isoquinoline alkaloids: oxyacanthine, berberine, columbamine, corydine, isocorydine, glaucine, jatrorrhizine, magnoflorine, obaberine, obamegine, palmatine, thaliporphine, thalrugosine; lignan: syringaresinol.

Medicinal Uses

In western herbal medicine, Barberry (Berberis vulgaris) represents the best–known and likely longest–used berberine–oriented plant of the Barberry family. Consider it the standard bearer of the group (with Oregongrape essentially identical in use, just not quite as popular).

There are not many other botanicals that rival Barberry's broad antimicrobial activity. Dozens of bacterial and fungal strains are inhibited by the plant. Some of the more common strains that are known to present clinical symptoms that call for Barberry's use are: several Bacillus species known to cause food poisoning; Escherichia coli (urinary tract and intestinal infections); both Staphylococcus and Streptococcus strains (responsible for a myriad of systemic and local infections); at least four Salmonella species (also a causative factor in food poisoning and intestinal infections). Candida albicans, Trichophyton mentagrophytes, and Microsporum gypseum are several fungal strains that Barberry inhibits.

For systemic infections Barberry combines well with Echinacea or Myrrh. Even for topical involvements, the same applies, though the plant also can be used alone with good results. Of course, serious infections (systemic infections usually are) will be most efficiently treated with conventional antibiotics, barring allergy or bacterial resistance.

Although bitter, it makes an effective gargle for bacterial–derived pharyngitis. The nasal wash or repeated gargle is a sound treatment for sinusitis as well. Combined with internal use (along with Echinacea or Myrrh), its upper respiratory cold–fighting power should not be underestimated.

Applied to vaginal Candida infections, as a sitz bath/douche, Barberry is effective. Likewise, thrush in babies and children will be remedied with topical application. Fungal infections that affect the skin and nails respond particularly well to long soaks in the root decoction.

Food poisoning from a variety of pathogens will be remedied. Not only is Barberry, like Oregongrape, directly inhibiting to these microbes, it also reduces the harmful effects of related endotoxins. Combine Barberry with Field mint or Monarda if there is nausea or intestinal cramping; with Slippery elm or Checker mallow if irritative diarrhea is present.

Although Simaruba family plants such as Crucifixion thorn and Tree of heaven, due to their array of quassinoids and tannins, will prove better medicines for traveler's diarrhea (amebiasis) and even giardiasis, Barberry is a worthy second choice, as it too is inhibiting to these infections.

The tea or tincture is a simple bitter tonic. Stimulating to gastric secretions, use it in uncomplicated asecretory indigestion. It is best taken 5–10 minutes before meals.

Like many other bitter herbs, Barberry is a hepatic stimulant. As a chologogue/choleretic the plant triggers bile manufacture, ultimately providing more of this digestive substance for lipid breakdown and assimilation. If plagued by general feelings of sluggishness, frontal headache, and nausea, all upon eating a high–fat meal, the tea will particularly be of use. Occasionally the plant will benefit suffers of anorexia by enlivening the gastrointestinal tract and promoting hunger sensations. Of course, psychological issues should be addressed in tandem.

Underlying the plant's bile augmentation is its hepatic antioxidant activity. Reducing to cellular inflammation, Barberry is decidedly useful to hepatitis sufferers. Elevated hepatic enzyme levels tend to lower with the plant's use. Although Barberry's hepatoprotective influence is not as strong as Milk thistle's, the plant can still be used with therapeutic results in many situations where there is liver distress.

Through Barberry's effect on the liver, it has a marked influence on inflammatory skin conditions. Poorly healing skin, reactive dermatitis, eczema, and acne are some of the plant's main indications. Barberry's healing effects are most likely due to its augmentation of hepatic detoxification pathways: the liver's activity of neutralizing hepatic/systemic/local metabolites and toxins is increased. Topical use of the ointment/oil/salve builds on the plant's internal effects. Due to Barberry's reduction of dermis over–proliferation, even psoriasis with its related scaly skin patches responds well to its application.

Another interesting effect of Barberry is its influence of liver suppression in mild cases of hypothyroidism[11]. It can be used with conventional thyroxin therapies.

As an eyewash, the isotonic tea is useful for bacterially–derived conjunctivitis. Another eyewash preparation (described in the main Preparations section under Eyewash) for Barberry is 10 drops of tincture added to 2 ounces of isotonic water.

Lastly, with the addition of Bayberry or Yerba mansa, Barberry can be considered a Goldenseal of sorts. The former plants provide tissue stimulation. Barberry provides the berberine aspect of Goldenseal. Together they serve as a decent replacement for this overused, yet potent plant.

Indications
» Food poisoning
» Infections, systemic/local
» Pharyngitis
» Sinusitis/Common cold
» Candida/Thrush infections (external and internal)
» Fungal infections affecting skin and nails (external and internal)
» Amebiasis/Giardiasis
» Indigestion/Poor protein and fat digestion/assimilation
» Hepatic sluggishness or inflammation
» Poorly healing skin/Dermatitis/Eczema/Psoriasis (external and internal)
» Hypothyroidal induced hepatic deficiency
» Conjunctivitis, bacterial (eyewash)

Collection
Common barberry, being a substantial woody bush, will have similar semi–woody roots. Its subterranean mass is composed of one or several larger tap roots and many secondary spreading lateral or semi–lateral roots. On larger bushes, lateral roots can be gathered alone, ensuring the plant's continuation

---

11 In overt and particularly sub–clinical hypothyroidism, liver functions are often slowed due to insufficient or ineffective T3 (triiodothyronine) and/or T4 (thyroxine) levels. Poorly healing skin and nails, slowed intestinal movement, and increased allergic reaction, are several of the more common presentations.

and future harvest. Colorado barberry is usually a smaller shrub with an abundance of sub-surface roots. It is easier to gather.

Drier locales will produce roots with less water content. They are fine for tea or the dry plant tincture. Hydrated roots, collected in wetter seasons/soils, can be dried and used in the aforementioned ways, or prepared through tincturing fresh.

Preparations/Dosage

- Root decoction/Cold infusion: 4–6 oz. 2–3 times daily
- FPT/DPT (40% alcohol): 30–60 drops 2–3 times daily
- Capsule (00): 1–2, 2–3 times daily
- Fluidextract: 10–20 drops 2–3 times daily
- External preparations: as needed

Cautions

Considering Barberry's significant therapeutic activity, its cautions are few. Normal doses will not create any problem. However, one exception is berberine's possibility of causing hemolysis in babies with G6PD (glucose–6–phosphate–dehydrogenase) deficiency. Also, extremely high doses may erratically affect blood pressure, and common sense tells us – do not use it (or any hepatic stimulant) if there is a biliary blockage.

Both plants are hosts for Puccinia graminis, a stem rust (fungus) troubling to a number of grain crops. It appears as a flaky–warty rust–colored crust on the stem/leaves. An occasional patch does not affect the root, but if the plant is covered, it's probably best to forgo its collection.

Other Uses

Both species have edible fruit. They tend to be mildly sweet–sour, sometimes with a hint of bitter. They're pleasant tasting when fully ripe and also make a fine jam/jelly base.

Bilberry
Ericaceae/Heath Family

Vaccinium myrtillus (Vaccinium myrtillus subsp. *oreophilum, V. myrtillus* var. *oreophilum, V. oreophilum)*
American bilberry, European bilberry, Myrtle blueberry, Whortleberry

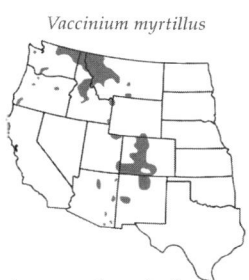

Vaccinium myrtillus

Description
As a small understory sub–shrub, Bilberry stands between 1' and 2' high. Its leaves are distinctly angled, ¾"–1" long, and ovate with serrated margins. Its urn–shaped flowers are solitary and develop from the leaf axil areas. The juicy dark blue fruit are ¼"–½" in diameter.

Distribution
Bilberry is found in montane and subalpine Spruce/Fir/Lodgepole pine forests. It ranges from British Columbia to Arizona and New Mexico. It is additionally found throughout Europe and parts of Asia. It's common to temperate zones of the Northern Hemisphere.

Chemistry
Anthocyanins/anthocyanidins: cyanidin, delphinidin, peonidin, petunidin, malvidin; flavonols: kaempferol, quercetin, myricetin, isorhamnetin; hydroxycinnamic acids: p–coumaric acid, caffeic acid, ferulic acid.

Medicinal Uses
Bilberry's traditional use, which tends to be overshadowed by the fruit's effect on blood vessels and capillary beds, is as an astringent for the gastrointestinal and urinary tracts. For mild diarrhea/loose stools, the leaf tea is astringent enough to act as a binding agent. Although not quite as strong as the leaf, the fruit tea can also be used in a similar manner. It is better tolerated by children and infants due its sour–sweet taste. The plant's tannins and anthrocyanins are also mildly antibacterial, furthering its usefulness in treating microbial oriented diarrhea.

Bilberry leaf is a specific renal astringent. It lacks the harshness and antimicrobial strength of other Heath family plants, such as Uva–ursi, but when there is low–grade renal inflammation of a constitutional nature, causing low specific–gravity urine, the tea has a corrective influence. Use it if abnormally high levels of vital elements are found in the urine, such as protein and glucose, which if persist, have a weakening effect on the body.

Due to the fruit's anthocyanidin/anthocyanin fractions, it has a marked influence over smaller blood vessels, especially capillary beds. Fruit preparations stabilize vascular membrane surfaces in response to injury or oxidative stress. Vascular ulceration, extremity pain, heaviness, edema, and even hemorrhoids will show improvement with its internal use. Raynaud's syndrome and diabetic neuropathy are also good applications for the fruit.

Bilberry fruit is best known today as an eye–centered preventative medicine. As an antioxidant, apply it to any ocular disturbance which involves free radical/oxidative damage (most autoimmune/age–related problems). Macular degeneration and cataract formation may not be corrected by Bilberry, though with internal fruit use, their progressions are certainly slowed. On a more prosaic level, Bilberry supplementation has shown to improve night vision, visual acuity, and light sensitivity.

Like other flavonoid and anthocyanin/anthocyanidin containing fruit, Bilberry speeds the healing of damaged tissue. Taken internally, the fruit reduces inflammation and collagen breakdown – two important factors in wound/injury healing.

Indications
- » Diarrhea
- » Urine, low–specific gravity
- » Vascular disorders, peripheral
- » Raynaud's syndrome
- » Ocular disorders, as an antioxidant
- » Night vision, to improve
- » Wounds

Collection
The leaves should be gathered in the spring or early summer before the fruit develops. Once dry, garble the leaves from the stems. Discard the stems. Dry the fruit with a dehydrator, otherwise mold growth may occur.

Preparations
The infusion method will be best for both the leaf and fruit. The other preparations are secondary, yet still of some use (see Dosage). Even though

standardized extracts are commercially available, whole-plant preparations will prove effective, especially if applied towards gastrointestinal and urinary complaints. If the fresh fruit is available, in place of other supplementation, 1–2 oz. should be eaten daily.

Dosage
» Leaf/Fruit infusion: 4–8 oz. 2–3 times daily
» FPT/DPT (50% alcohol) of leaf: ½–1 teaspoon 2–3 times daily
» Fluidextract of fruit: 20–30 drops 2–3 times daily
» Capsule (00) of powdered fruit: 2–4, 2–3 times daily

Cautions
Loose stools may result from excessive intake of the fresh fruit.

Other Uses
Not only can Bilberry fruit be eaten raw, it is also a fine candidate for jams, jellies, and juices. Its edible (and medicinal) uses are essentially the same as American blueberry (Vaccinium corymbosum), and other blue-fruited Vaccinium species.

Birch
Betulaceae/Birch Family

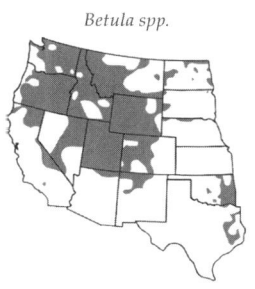

Betula spp.

Betula glandulosa Michx.
Bog birch, Dwarf birch, Resin birch

Betula occidentalis Hook.
Mountain birch, Water birch, River birch

Betula papyrifera Marsh.
Paper birch, Canoe birch, White birch

Description
Betula glandulosa is a large shrub. Its ascending growth is supported by brownish-barked branches and resinous-glandular twigs. The leathery leaves, 1"–2" long by 1" wide, are rounded with serrated margins. They

typically are resinous and gland–dotted (below). The male and female flowers develop in small catkins.

Also a large shrub (occasionally a small tree), Betula occidentalis' brownish–bronze twigs are resin–dotted. The 2"–3" long, coarsely serrated, ovate leaf has a rounded–truncate base and acute tip. The flowers develop in catkins.

Betula papyrifera is a small to medium–sized tree. The bark on younger branches is reddish brown and smooth, but on mature parts, it becomes creamy–chalky white and exfoliates in thin sheets. The leaves are the largest of the three species profiled. They are elliptic–ovate in shape, acute–tipped, 4"–6" long, and have serrated margins. The catkins are 1"–2" long.

Distribution

Betula is common to circumboreal forests of the Northern Hemisphere. From Greenland, Alaska, and much of Canada, Betula glandulosa ranges south through most of the Rockies to central Utah and Colorado. It grows abundantly around water where soil hydration is extremely high. Montane/subalpine bogs, fens, and various wetlands are its usual places.

From western/central Canada, Betula occidentalis is found south to northern Arizona and New Mexico. It too has a substantial presence in the Rocky Mountains. It's the most southerly grower of the group. Also a riparian shrub, look to mountain streamsides. Red osier dogwood is a regular companion plant.

Betula papyrifera ranges through most of Alaska and Canada. Aside from a number of north–central and northeastern states, the tree's southern limit reaches Washington, northern Idaho, and Montana (its reported to occur naturally only where the average July temperature is no higher than 70 degrees). Not nearly as water–oriented as the other two species, Paper birch is associated with a wide array of habitats: from bottomlands to open forests and rocky hillsides.

Chemistry

Betula papyrifera: triterpenes: betulin, lupeol, acetyl oleanolic acid, betulinic acid, oleanolic acid, β–sitosterol; flavonoids; hydrolyzable and condensed tannins.

Medicinal Uses

Western growing Birches differ slightly in medicinal activity from the better-known aromatic Birches of the Northeast (Betula lenta and B. alleghaniensis). Western species lack the methyl salicylate (Wintergreen–like smell) found in these others, which makes them poor aspirin–type, pain-relieving antiinflammatories.

Rich in tannins and triterpenes (betulin, lupeol et al.), use Birch as a tissue healing intestinal astringent. Diarrhea and lower bowel disarray, with or without spasm, especially with chronic/subacute inflammation, will be curbed. It has potential too if used in ulcerative colitis and related autoimmune intestinal complaints.

Birch has equal merit as a urinary tract astringent. Mildly antiseptic, diuretic, and tissue healing, use it on mild to moderate infections with associated mucus–tinged urine.

For Birch's topical application, make a base oil from the bark (and/or leaf) using the alcohol intermediate technique. Through this process the oil will contain fair amounts of betulin (and other triterpenes). It can then be used as is or converted into a salve or ointment for the betterment of eczema, psoriasis, and poorly healing wounds and ulcerations.

Indications

» Diarrhea/Inflammation, intestinal, chronic/subacute
» Infection, urinary, mild–moderate
» Eczema/Psoriasis/Poorly healing wounds and ulcerations (external)

Collection

Birch bark, twigs, and leaves are all useful. Its tannin/flavonoid content is highest in the bark, lesser so in the leaves. The resinous qualities (betulin) are highest in the bark and twigs (if glandular), but ultimately, it's best to judge when on–site: the more resinous any part is, the better medicine it will be.

Preparations

Water preparations (infusion for leaves, decoction for bark) will isolate more of the tannin/flavonoid compounds, making these preparations closer to Oak tea (astringent) in application. The tincture (and alcohol–intermediate oil method), of whatever part, will produce a triterpene–rich preparation (better for tissue healing).

Dosage
» FPT/DPT of bark (70% alcohol): 20–40 drops 2–3 times daily
» Infusion/Decoction (bark): 2–4 oz. 2–3 times daily
» External preparations: as needed

Cautions
Unfortunately, Birch's high tannin content limits its consistent–everyday use...it's just too tedious on the gastrointestinal and urinary tracts. For internal usage, it's a short–term remedy. External preparations are caution–free.

Other Uses
Due to its high percentage of non–polar compounds, Birch wood/bark is water–resistant (e.g. Birch bark canoe).

Bistort
Polygonaceae/Buckwheat Family

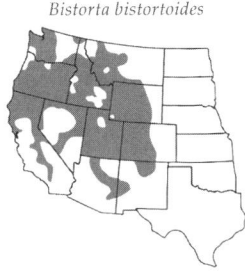

Bistorta bistortoides

Bistorta bistortoides (Pursh) Small (*Bistorta bistortoides var. oblongifolia, Persicaria bistortoides, Polygonum bistortoides, P. bistortoides var. linearifolium, P. bistortoides var. oblongifolium*)
American bistort, Smokeweed, Western bistort

Description
Bistort is a long–stemmed herbaceous perennial. Standing 2'–3' when in flower, its base is mainly composed of long basal lance–shaped leaves. A few smaller sessile leaves develop along the central flower stem/stalk. Both basal and stem leaves have semi–inflated sheaths. Bistort's cylindrical flower clusters are composed of small white–pink inflorescences. When in flower (summer) the plant is distinctive due to its white spikes rising above the surrounding grassy vegetation.

Distribution
From western Canada and California, east to Montana and New Mexico, Bistort is a plant of wet mountain meadows and moist grassy areas.

BISTORT

Chemistry
Flavonoids; ellagitannins; gallotannins.

Medicinal Uses
Bistort belongs to a family well known for its tannins and associated astringency; however, unlike other plants that are recognized for their herbal portions, it is Bistort's root that is the main medicinal part[12].

Use a decoction of Bistort as a tightening mouth and gum rinse. Symptomatically, it addresses spongy and bleeding gums and mouth sores/ulceration (canker sores[13]). Pharyngitis suffers will also derive relief from the gargled warm tea. Likewise, individuals suffering from sinusitis, especially if the situation is chronic with mucus discharge, will benefit from the isotonic nasal wash made with the root tea.

As a reliable intestinal astringent, use 4–8 oz. of the tea if suffering from diarrhea or dysentery. It will slow evacuations, especially if the offending food/organism has at least been partly voided (as evidenced by watery and mostly clear evacuations).

Try the tea (or tincture mixed with a little water) for other gastric distresses such as nausea, gastritis, and even stomach ulcerations, but sensitive people may find Bistort's tannin fraction unpredictable in its stomach settling effect.

Like Geranium, the warm tea is used as a soothing sitz bath for vaginal irritations. As a postpartum toner, it will be found astringing to any residual passive hemorrhaging and inflamed–abraded tissues.

Lastly, the shaved or pureed root is well used as a simple field poultice for stings, insect bites, and rashes. The dried and powdered root as a dust (or a fomentation made with the tea) is used for similar red and weepy inflammations.

Indications
» Mouth/Gum sores/ulcerations (gargle)
» Pharyngitis (gargle)

12 Consider Bistort root about twice as strong as Buckwheat (Eriogonum spp.). Additionally, Bistort is related to Fallopia multiflora (Polygonum multiflorum) also known as Fo–ti or Ho shu wu, a medicinal plant commonly used in TCM. Unfortunately, Bistort's and Fo–ti's uses are unrelated.

13 Canker sores are commonly induced by stress, immune suppression, or even dietary imbalances, and may for some have a viral underpinning.

- » Sinusitis, chronic (nasal wash)
- » Diarrhea/Dysentery
- » Nausea/Gastritis
- » Irritation, vaginal (external)
- » As a postpartum toner (external)
- » Insect stings/bites/Rashes (external)

Collection

The root of Bistort is not far beneath the ground's surface. Fairly easy to dig, especially in boggy soils, the plant's root has the fascinating appearance of a small gnarled fist. Once gathered, discard the stem and foliage.

Preparations/Dosage

- » Decoction: 2–4 oz. 2–3 times daily
- » FPT/DPT (30% alcohol, 10% glycerin): 30–60 drops 2–3 times daily

Cautions

There is little concern of toxicity with normal short–term use (several days to one week). Longer term use may lead to gastrointestinal and/or renal irritation, which is normal for the extended use of any tannin–containing plant. During pregnancy, several days of Bistort is not a concern; however, several weeks of use may be. There are no cautions for its external use.

Bitterbrush

Rosaceae/Rose Family

Purshia tridentata (Pursh) DC. *(Tigarea tridentata)*
Antelope bitterbrush

Description

As a perennial shrub, Bitterbrush's stem bark is gray to brown and exfoliating on older branches. The leaves develop in fascicled groups. Individually they are wedge–shaped and 3–cleft. The upper leaf sides are green. The lower sides are white–tomentose with prominent veins. The flowers are somewhat showy for an otherwise drab bush: both the yellow petals and sepals are 5–numbered. The seed capsules are cone–shaped.

Distribution
With several minor exceptions, Bitterbrush is found from around the Continental Divide to all points west. It is absent from the lower elevation Southwest and Pacific coastal areas. In all other western regions where it is cold and dry, Bitterbrush is likely not far away. It often grows with Sagebrush and is very common in the Great Basin Desert.

Chemistry
Cucurbitacins, flavonoids, volatiles.

Medicinal Uses
Rarely used today, Bitterbrush (and other Purshia species) has a significant ethnobotanical accounting. Klamath, Navajo, Paiute, and Shoshoni basic medicinal uses for Bitterbrush were strikingly similar. Traditionally a strong leaf (or entire young branch) tea was used as a laxative or an emetic.

Smaller therapeutic doses tend to be stimulating to gastrointestinal function and can be used like any other bitter (see Gentian or Green gentian). Also, small to moderate amounts of the leaf (or root) are surprisingly useful as an antibacterial expectorant and mild cough suppressant. It can be used in a wide range of bronchial complaints when there is need of an agent that loosens phlegm, reduces coughing, and inhibits microbes. If the bitterness of the tincture is overwhelming (even mixed in a little water) try combining it with equal portions of Yerba santa – an herb that fits many bronchial complaints as well, but also is superb at masking bitter flavors.

Use the ointment, salve, or oil as antibacterial dressing for scrapes, cuts, and abrasions. These non–emergency external injuries will heal more quickly with the plant's external application.

Indications
- » Indigestion, asecretory
- » Bronchitis with a dry cough
- » Scrapes/Cuts/Abrasions (external)

Collection
Snip the last couple of feet from a new branch end. The flower and leaf collected together is best, but if not in season, leaf growth alone is fine. If using Bitterbrush for tea, garble the flowers and/or leaves from the branches once dried. Discard the branches.

Preparations/Dosage
» FPT/DPT (75% alcohol): 20–40 drops 2–3 times daily
» Standard/Cold infusion: 2–4 oz. 2–3 times daily
» External preparations: as needed

Cautions
It is not wise to use Bitterbrush in conjunction with most gastrointestinal inflammatory problems (gastritis/active ulcer). A chemically complex plant, it also should not be used (internally) while pregnant or nursing. Small amounts with children for seasonal bronchitis is not a problem (though getting them to ingest it will be) – just keep dosages reasonable.

Bogbean
Menyanthaceae/Bogbean Family

Menyanthes trifoliata

Menyanthes trifoliata L.
Buckbean, Marsh trefoil, Trefoil

Description
An aquatic/semi–aquatic, rhizomatous, creeping, perennial, Bogbean produces glabrous, 3–leaflet, succulent, oblong leaves. They are 2"–4" in length and tend to rise just above the water's surface. Also situated above the water are its stalked flower clusters. They are narrow and composed of small, 5–lobed, white, funnel–shaped flowers. The fruit forms as an ovoid capsule.

Distribution
Mountain fens and bogs, and lake, pond, and slow moving stream margins are common places to look for Bogbean. It is locally abundant, yet sporadic throughout the western mountains.

Chemistry
Iridoids: loganin; secoiridoids: foliamenthin, dihydrofoliamenthin, menthiafolin; triterpenoids: menyanthoside; flavonoids: catechins; phenolic acids; pectins; phytosterols.

Medicinal Uses

Even though Bogbean is not a Gentian family plant (it is botanically affiliated though), it shares a majority of medicinal characteristics with members of that family. Accordingly, Bogbean's use as a classic bitter tonic is its smartest application. Use it in simple indigestion due to insufficient gastric secretion. Try several ounces of the tea or a teaspoon or two of the tincture before meals if troubled by food (especially protein) lingering in the stomach. Bloating, related gastrointestinal unease, and even post–feeding mental fog are other symptoms that point to Bogbean.[14]. The plant can also be mixed with an aromatic herb such as Field mint or Monarda for extra vascular stimulation, and therefore increased activity.

Nicely suited as a restoring agent of normal gastric response, use Bogbean daily before meals if recovering from gastrointestinal surgery, feeding tube removal, or even anorexia nervosa/orthorexia. The main premise here is to use the herb in order to reestablish the gut's natural reaction to food.

Like most other bitter tonics, Bogbean is often found mildly lowering to above normal blood sugar levels. Its best application is to individuals whom suffer from postprandial hyperglycemia and/or borderline type–2 diabetes. Combined with some simple dietary modifications (and weight–loss if needed) Bogbean's use before (and/or after) meals may make blood sugar lowering pharmaceuticals unnecessary.

Indications
» Indigestion/Dyspepsia, asecretory
» Gastrointestinal surgery/Anorexia nervosa, recovery
» Hyperglycemia, mild

Collection
Although the above–water leaves are easiest to utilize, all parts of Bogbean are bitter and subsequently useful. Find a patch growing around a body of water and simply gather what is easiest to prune.

Preparations/Dosage
» FPT/DPT (50% alcohol): 20–40 drops 2–3 times daily
» Standard/Cold infusion: 2–4 oz. 2–3 times daily

---

14 Bogbean augments the area by stimulating pepsin, hydrochloric acid, and mucus – all necessary secretions intrinsic to digestion and assimilation.

Cautions
With over use any bitter tonic herb can potentially cause gastrointestinal irritation, nausea, heartburn, and/or diarrhea.

Buckthorn
Rhamnaceae/Buckthorn Family

Rhamnus betulifolia, californica

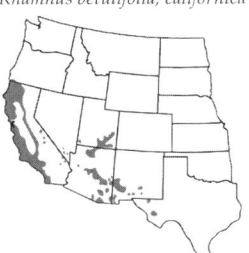

Rhamnus betulifolia Greene *(Frangula betulifolia)*
Beechleaf buckthorn, Birchleaf buckthorn

Rhamnus californica Eschsch. *(Frangula californica)*
California buckthorn, Coffeeberry

Description
Like other species of Rhamnus, these two plants grow to be large shrubs. They are non–spiny and generally have elliptic leaves. The flowers are small, greenish, perfect, and 5–parted. They develop solely or in small axillary clusters on branch ends. The fruit are berry–like and dark–purple to black at maturity. Differences between the two species are as follows: Birchleaf buckthorn tends to be deciduous and only semi–pubescent on leaf undersides. Coffeeberry is a larger plant and has a slightly smaller leaf that is evergreen, thickened, and densely tomentose abaxially.

Distribution
Birchleaf buckthorn is found throughout most of the southwestern states. It ranges from West Texas to southern Nevada. As a mid–elevation/transition zone grower, it's typically found next to creeks and intermittent mountain streams.

Located in similar habitats, Coffeeberry has a significant California distribution. It is also found in southwestern Oregon, southern Nevada, throughout much of Arizona, and finally to southwestern New Mexico.

Chemistry
Anthraquinones; flavonoids; tannins.

Medicinal Uses

Like its better-known relatives Cascara sagrada (Rhamnus purshiana) and Eurasian buckthorn (R. cathartica), Buckthorn is an intestinal stimulant, but unlike other anthraquinone-containing laxatives such as Aloe and Senna, it is less apt to cause irritation and dependency. The tea is best used in chronic constipation when stools are dry and difficult to pass. Taken before bed the plant works with the body's natural hepatic rhythm by making a bowel movement for the morning more likely. Used this way (small-medium amounts) rarely does it cause griping, or a watery stool. Although Buckthorn can be used long-term, intestinal health is best regulated through proper diet, fluid intake, and stress reduction.

The plant's secondary influences also work to remedy constipation: Buckthorn is a bitter tonic, stimulating upper gastrointestinal response. It is also a biliary stimulant. These attributes, in concert with its influence of the large intestine, make the plant a key therapy for upper, mid, and lower gastrointestinal deficiencies.

One lesser known activity of Buckthorn is its arthritis lessening effect. It is not as strong in relieving pain as Creosote bush or Turmeric; however, when applied properly, some find the plant remarkably effective. Suffers of rheumatoid or osteo arthritis whose pain seems to be partly linked to constipation, often find Buckthorn quite relieving. It is no secret how the plant works in these situations: through stimulation of the large intestine and liver, tissue wastes are eliminated more efficiently. This creates a reduction in systemic inflammation and therefore joint pain. Additionally, with the exception of acute pain from injury, most inflammatory conditions, including allergies, fibromyalgia, and autoimmune problems (if chronic constipation is part of the picture), respond well to the plant.

Besides Cascara sagrada, other Rhamnus/Frangula species are likely as useful as the two species profiled here. As long as the inner bark is yellow-orange and tastes somewhat bitter, additional species should prove effective.

Indications
- » Constipation, chronic
- » Liver deficiency
- » Arthritis with constipation
- » Inflammatory conditions, with constipation

Collection
Select a secondary branch with thin and unfissured bark. Using a knife (or sometimes hands are adequate), scrape/strip the inner and outer bark from the core wood.

Preparations
The separated bark should first be aged. Two methods can be employed. One: air dry the bark normally and set it aside for 6 months. Two: place the bark in an oven or a dehydrator and dry it at 120 degrees for 24 hours. The first method is more reliable. The second method should be used mainly if the bark is needed immediately. Either method reduces the gastrointestinal griping potential of the green/freshly dried bark.

Dosage
- » DPT (30% alcohol): 30–60 drops 1–2 times daily
- » Fluidextract: 10–20 drops 1–2 times daily
- » Bark decoction/Cold infusion: 2–4 oz. 1–2 times daily

Cautions
Due to potential uterine stimulation by the plant's anthraquinones, do not use Buckthorn during pregnancy. A laxative effect will be seen in nursing babies if used by the mother. Buckthorn is fine for children – reduce the dosage accordingly by weight. Like other herbs in Buckthorn's class do not use it if there is an active intestinal, hepatic, biliary, or pancreatic obstruction/inflammation. Long–term use may cause dependency.

Other Uses
A common name for Rhamnus californica is Coffeeberry, which likely points to a pioneer use for the fruit as a coffee substitute. Having personally eaten a half–a–dozen or so of the bitter–sweet ripe berries (and suffered the consequences), I suggest enthusiasts dry and thoroughly roast the fruit before consuming any amount as a coffee replacement. Like the bark, for what the fresh fruit lack in central nervous influence (caffeine) they make up in gastrointestinal stimulation (cramping). The dried fruit too can be added to the dried bark for its similar gastrointestinal properties.

Bugleweed
Lamiaceae/Mint Family

Lycopus americanus Muhl.
American bugleweed, Water horehound

Lycopus asper Greene
Rough bugleweed

Lycopus uniflorus Michx. (*Lycopus parviflorus, L. virginicus var. parviflorus*)
Northern bugleweed, Northern water horehound

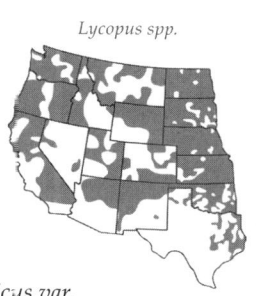

Lycopus spp.

Description
Bugleweed is a non or faintly aromatic perennial herb. Colony forming, most species have sub–surface rhizomes (or stolons). They enable the plant to achieve sizable interconnected stands when conditions are favorable. The leaves are oppositely arranged, and depending on species, are linear to ovate–lanceolate, entire, toothed, lobed, or pinnatifid. Densely forming, the small whitish flowers develop in upper leaf axil clusters. They are cup–shaped, faintly two–lipped, and 4–5 lobed (both corolla and calyx). The small seeds (nutlets) are 3–angled.

Distribution
Except for Nevada, Alaska, and Hawaii, Lycopus americanus is found country-wide. Look to the moist and wet soils of streamsides, pond and lake sides, and ditches. From spotty outposts in Massachusetts and New York, L. asper continues its occasional presence to the northern and western Great Plains where it is found in greater abundance. West of the Continental Divide look for it in isolated but well developed stands. Marsh banks, wet meadows, and around springs are common places for the plant.

Like the others, Lycopus uniflorus is found in and around wet thickets, boggy meadows, and in moistened soils next to springs and pond/lake sides. Its main area is the Northwest: from western Washington and Oregon to Idaho and western Montana.

Chemistry

Lycopus general: polyphenols: rosmarinic acid, protocatechuic aldehyde, protocatechuic acid, lithospermic acid, caffeic acid, cinnamic acid, ferulic acid, apigenin, luteolin, quercetin, isorhamnetin, chlorogenic acid, rutin. Volatiles for Lycopus americanus (totaling less than 0.01%): limonene, linalool, 3–octanol, β–caryophyllene, 1–octen–3–ol, germacrene d.

Medicinal Uses

The medicinal use of western North American Bugleweed is essentially patterned after Lycopus virginicus (eastern North American) and L. europaeus (western European). Some pharmacological and therapeutic variance can be expected between species. In essence though, they can be used interchangeably. One tell–tale sign that any species of Lycopus will likely be medicinally active is an intensely bitter taste[15].

Bugleweed is not definable by any typical Mint family medicinal characteristic set. Not particularly aromatic, nor vasodilatory, like its relatives, Bugleweed's main areas of influence are the nervous system, glandular tissue (mainly the thyroid[16] and tissue groups influenced by this gland), and the cardiovascular system. Additionally, individuals best suited for Bugleweed may not have any diagnosable problem. Physiological tendency or borderline issue best describes the amplitude of what the plant addresses. In overt pathology Bugleweed's efficacy is usually found either ineffective or lacking.

Use Bugleweed if stress responses tend to mirror a thyroid surge (or vice versa). Minor basal temperature elevations, weight loss, rapid yet weak heart action, restless sleep, and night sweats are a solid symptom set indicating the plant. It likely will not do much for true hyperthyroidism, but for borderline stages, or when adrenergic/adrenaline responses either appear like or trigger thyroidal spikes, it often does some good.

---

15 Bugleweed's taste rivals Horehound's (Marrubium vulgare), another very bitter Mint family plant. In fact, this taste similarity gave rise to another common name for Bugleweed – Water horehound.

16 Ongoing since the 1950s, research suggests that Bugleweed has a broad (but weak) thyroid–oriented influence. Due at least in part to its retarding influence of thyroid hormones T3 and T4, pituitary hormone TSH, potentially other pituitary hormones, and thyroid antibodies common to Graves' disease, Bugleweed should be considered a mild thyroid sedative.

More broadly, for individuals with nervous temperaments, it is well used as a unique sedative for sleep disturbances, insomnia, and general anxiousness. The people it best fits will be excitable, have easily flushing skin, and heart action quickly triggered by external stressors – essentially the opposite of a 'slow and steady' temperament.

Used alone for non–organic heart dysfunctions, Bugleweed is often effective. Here too, hypertension, tachycardia, palpitations, and an environmentally–caused unsteadiness are the plant's cardiac indications[17]. For more serious cardiovascular problems (yet still treatable with herbs), where symptoms continue to match its application, it combines well with Cactus (Selenicereus grandiflorus). Furthermore, a Hawthorn–Bugleweed combination will have a broader reach than either used alone, and usually has a more profound blood–pressure lowering effect.

Bugleweed's most unique use (there are no other Mints used in western herbal medicine that have similar effects) is its application as a subastringent. How the plant astringes passive hemorrhaging is unknown, nevertheless sufferers of chronic nose bleeds will see benefit from taking Bugleweed daily. Likewise, if blood–tinged sputum is produced due to bronchitis (especially if there is fever and rapid heart activity), Bugleweed will be of help. It can also be used in league with other lung–affecting herbs that specifically addresses the infection.

Bugleweed should be considered in passive hematuria (blood in the urine) and metrorrhagia (break through bleeding/menstrual bleeding at non–regular intervals). For this last application, women who are entering perimenopause may see a reduction of excessive bleeding with its use, especially if hot flashes are also present (in fact Bugleweed used alone for uncomplicated hot flashes is often very successful[18]). For these excessive menstruation applications, it combines well with overt tannin plants like Krameria or Geranium and even alkaloid dependent vasoconstrictors like Vinca major (Greater periwinkle).

Indications

» Stress (sympathetic nervous system) with hyperthyroidal qualities

17   Bugleweed's recorded antagonism (or down regulation) of heart β–receptor sites presumably is the mechanism of action here. Furthermore, it is sensible to consider the plant's broader adrenergic system sedation is also β–receptor related.

18   This effect is likely due to Bugleweed's dampening of heightened pituitary secretion – see Cautions.

- » Hyperthyroidism, sub–clinical
- » Insomnia/Anxiety with cardiovascular stress
- » Tachycardia/Palpitations with stress
- » Nose bleeds, chronic
- » Hemorrhaging, passive (lungs, urinary, intestinal, reproductive)
- » Bleeding, perimenopause with hot flashes

Collection

Preferably when in flower, gather Bugleweed's new growth. This usually consists of the top several inches of the plant – flower, leaf, and stem. If not in flower, the collection of only leaf material is adequate.

Preparations/Dosage

In at least one clinical study with human subjects[19] Bugleweed (Lycopus europaeus) was observed to have a dose dependent effect. Small to moderate doses reduced thyroid related cardiovascular symptoms (tachycardia, hypertension, etc.) but had little to no effect on circulating T3, T4, and TSH levels. Greater amounts reduced both cardiovascular symptoms and also thyroid–pituitary factors.

Use less than the following recommendations for a subtle approach to sub–clinical/latent hyperthyroidism. Use greater amounts for a more robust approach.

- » FPT: 30–60 drops 2–3 times daily
- » Herb infusion: 4–6 oz. 2–3 times daily

Cautions

Bugleweed has a safe usage history, with very little report of toxicity. However, it is theoretically possible that larger doses may potentiate hypothyroidal conditions. Even though this remains to be proven, I believe a sensible approach is to forgo Bugleweed's use in cases of hypothyroidism or any thyroid condition that is well managed with conventional therapies.

Due to Bugleweed's lithospermic acid content the plant probably has a mild suppressing effect on hormonal secretions of the anterior pituitary (LH, FSH, TSH, etc.), and this may even be partly responsible for its influence of the thyroid, and other regions. Therefore, using Bugleweed in pituitary conditions is also an unknown – some situations it may help, in others, it

---

[19] Scheck, R. and A. Biller. Wolfstrapp herb – an alternative to synthetic antithyroid agents. *Naturamed* 15, 5 (2000): 31–36.

may exacerbate. During pregnancy[20] and when nursing, Bugleweed should also be avoided. With children as a general sedative, there are better suited herbs that lack glandular effects: Chamomile, Passionflower, etc.

Checker Mallow
Malvaceae/Mallow Family

Sidalcea neomexicana

Sidalcea neomexicana A. Gray
Mountain sidalcea, Salt spring checkerbloom

Description
Checker mallow is an herbaceous perennial. Standing 2'–3' high at maturity, its leaves are highly variable in shape. A combination of entire, cleft, or lobed (5–9 segments) leaves (often on the same stem) are not uncommon. The showy 5–petaled rose to purple flowers are raceme forming. 5–9 carpels compose the fruit. The whole plant is more or less pubescent and mucilaginous when crushed.

Distribution
A mid to high mountain grower, Checker mallow is found from Idaho and Wyoming, south to California, Arizona, and New Mexico. It is common to pristine moist meadows and mountain streamsides.

Chemistry
Malvaceae general: various polysaccharides (pectin, mucilage, and starch), namely arabinogalactans; tannins; anthocyanins/anthocyanidins.

Medicinal Uses
In many ways, Checker mallow is the high mountain equivalent to non–native Mallow (Malva neglecta and related species). Like Mallow, it contains very little tannin (unlike desert growing Globemallow and Abutilon species) making its therapeutic influence as a mucilaginous soother more direct.

---

20 It has long been known that thyroid insufficiency during pregnancy is linked to both gestational complications and abnormal fetal/neonate cerebral development. New research suggests that there may also be a correlation between low thyroid levels during pregnancy and autism.

Drink Checker mallow tea as a gentle urinary soother: painful urination and regional tissue irritation is often quieted with its use. The plant should also be tried for random low–level renal inflammations, especially if the usual suspects have been eliminated: dietary irritants (caffeine, artificial sweeteners, food dyes, miscellaneous plant compounds, tannins, etc.), active urinary stone involvement, and/or congenial–genetic nephritis.

Aside from these semi–nebulous indications, the plant is well used in combination with Jumping cholla (Cylindropuntia) root or Gravel root (Eupatorium purpureum) as a kidney stone preventative or as a long–term stone dissolver. To approach kidney stone dissolution this way, first, be sure that there is no active blockage. For one month drink 2–3 cups of diluted tea daily. The elimination of sodas, coffee, and most other caffeine sources is also important, as is the addition of distilled water, which is needed to keep urinary output elevated. Don't be surprised of the stone's breakup and passage with this simple type of therapy.

Checker mallow combines well with Heath family plants (Uva–ursi, Manzanita, or Madrone) and Cypress family plants (Juniper, Cypress, or Thuja). It reduces the potential of renal irritation, particularly if higher or extended duration doses of these plants are used.

Like many other Mallow family plants, Checker mallow is demulcent and soothing to the lungs. Use it when there is bronchial irritation/inflammation in association with bronchitis. Relatedly, the tea, gargled and swallowed is an effective application for sore throats and general oral passageway irritation.

The long–chain starches that give most Mallow family plants their characteristic thickened viscosity are known in the herbal world as mild immune stimulants. I stress *mild* here. Use it as an accent when addressing immune challenges, and only when its demulcent–soothing qualities fit the overall situation.

Indications
» Urination, painful
» Urinary gravel, as a preventative
» Irritation, bronchial
» Pharyngitis

Collection
All herbaceous parts of Checker mallow are utilized: flower, leaf, and flexible stems.

Preparations/Dosage
» Infusion: 4–8 oz. 2–3 times daily

Cautions
There are no cautions for Checker mallow.

Chicory
Asteraceae/Sunflower Family

Cichorium intybus

Cichorium intybus L.
Coffee weed, Chicoria

Description
A weedy short lived perennial herb, Chicory grows to several feet in height and is usually profusely branched. The leaves mature to 2′–3′ in length and are short–petioled to sessile. Though nearly entire when young, they become pinnatifid (much like a Dandelion leaf) with age. The flower heads are numerous and borne singly or in clusters among the upper leaves. The individual florets are fertile and form in radial discs. They are light blue to occasionally white. Like Dandelion, when cut Chicory weeps a white bitter tasting latex.

Distribution
A Eurasian native, Chicory is now naturalized extensively throughout North America. Although it is absent in the lower elevation Southwest, it is common to most other regions/elevations. Preferring disturbed soils, look to field margins, ditches, and secondary roadsides.

Chemistry
Hydroxycinnamic acid derivatives: caffeic acid, chicoric acid, chlorogenic acid; coumarins: aesculetin, cichorin, aesulin; flavonoids: apigenin, luteolin, quercetin, kaempferol, isorhamnetin; sesquiterpenoids: costunolide, lactopicrin, lactucin, lettucenin a, 8–deoxylactucin.

Medicinal Uses

Chicory shares a majority of medicinal attributes with Dandelion. Even in regards to herbal commerce, the two plants are historically intertwined (Dandelion's adulteration with Chicory was once common; however, this was never a major issue due to overlapping uses).

Roasted Chicory root is best known as a coffee substitute (and where quality controls are lacking, as an unbeknownst additive to real coffee). Containing no caffeine, it is a mild gastrointestinal stimulant – two attributes habitual coffee drinkers will find of benefit when attempting to stop its regular use.

As an herbal medicine, non–roasted Chicory root (or seeds) is a mild gastrointestinal/biliary stimulant best used in atonic–deficient conditions. Take the tincture (or better yet, the fluidextract), or tea before meals as a simple bitter tonic. It will increase digestive activity via the stimulation of an array of gastric secretions. Sufferers of asecretory indigestion and digestive stasis will benefit most from its daily use.

As a liver/biliary stimulant, Chicory rivals Dandelion in usefulness. Augmenting to bile production by the liver and its release by the gallbladder, those plagued by poor lipid breakdown and assimilation will notice fewer digestive complaints if it's taken before a rich meal. Even those plagued by chronic gallstone formation should see a noticeable reduction in unwanted symptoms with its daily use.

Suffers of liver inflammation will surely benefit from Chicory's regular application. In many ways rivaling Milk thistle, its use will reliably reduce inflammatory markers associated with hepatocyte oxidation and related hepatitis/cirrhosis, especially in chronic manifestations.

Chicory is surprisingly effective as a wound/incision healer when applied externally. Traditionally used this way in Unani and Ayurvedic systems, the plant's success as a topical medication is most likely related to its modest antibacterial and antifungal properties (and flavonoid content).

Indications

- » Indigestion, asecretory
- » Congestion, Liver/Biliary
- » Poor lipid digestion/assimilation
- » Inflammation, hepatic
- » As a vulnerary (external)

CINQUEFOIL

Collection
Chicory arises from a simple or moderately branched small taproot. Easy to gather, sink a shovel spade-deep into the soil next to the plant, then carefully lever upward. Most if not all of the taproot should come up intact this way. At the root's crown, clip and then discard the stem and foliage (or the foliage can be dried and used like Dandelion leaf tea, i.e. as a mild diuretic).

Preparations/Dosage
» Root/Seed decoction: 2–6 oz. 2–3 times daily
» FPT/DPT of root/seed (40% alcohol): 60–90 drops 2–3 times daily
» Fluidextract of root/seed: 20–30 drops 2–3 times daily
» External preparations: as needed

Cautions
Excessive use may result in mild gastritis. Additionally, the plant is not recommended if there is an active biliary blockage, otherwise Chicory is an extremely safe herbal medicine.

Other Uses
Although slightly bitter, like Dandelion the young leaves are used as a potherb. Fresh or lightly sautéed, add them to salads or other cooked greens. Endive also belongs to the Cichorium genus.

Cinquefoil
Rosaceae/Rose Family

Potentilla spp.

Potentilla L.
Fingergrass, Fivefingers, Goosegrass

Description
Cinquefoil can be loosely divided into three groups: herbaceous palmate–leaved types (Potentilla diversifolia), herbaceous pinnate–leaved types (Potentilla arguta), and at least one larger bush type[21].

---

21 Though it is often assigned to the Dasiphora genus, Potentilla fruticosa is the most commonly used scientific name for this species.

Most Cinquefoils are perennial and have 5-petaled yellow flowers. The majority are also very to somewhat hairy, with some being two-toned in appearance due to a dense underside layering of leaf hair. Many species are adept at both asexual reproduction (runners) and regular seed reproduction. Crossbreeding is common, so species identification can be tedious.

Distribution

With well over fifty species found throughout the western United States the majority of plants are found at higher elevation or in northern latitudes. Forest meadows, pastures, and next to streams are common places for Cinquefoil. Bush cinquefoil (Potentilla fruticosa) is very common throughout the West and is typically found around Pine forest openings.

Chemistry

Flavonoids; ellagitannins; gallotannins.

Medicinal Uses

Like Agrimony, Wild rose, Avens, and most other Rose family plants, Cinquefoil is an uncomplicated mild astringent. One area Cinquefoil reliably influences is the urinary tract. The plant's tannin-derived astringency is found soothing to urethra, bladder, and renal tissues. Painful urination with corresponding mucus in the urine (cloudy) are the main indicators for Cinquefoil's use. If there is a lower urinary tract infection, the plant combines well with aromatic disinfectants like Cypress or Juniper. Its use for incontinence (in early stages when muscle tone is a factor) will be found beneficial. Later in more progressed states, Cinquefoil will do little good.

As a curb for excessive menstruation and mid-cycle spotting, Cinquefoil has a long history of use. It will be found most effective if the situation is due to constitutional tendency or idiosyncratic biorhythm discombobulation. Minor postpartum bleeding also will abate due to the plant's mild uterine lining astringency: use it as a sitz bath and internal tea. Applied this way, mild vaginitis responds well to the plant, and even though it is not strongly antimicrobial, it will nevertheless be found soothing to inflamed tissues.

Indications

- » Cystitis/Urethritis/Nephritis, chronic, with cloudy-odiferous urine
- » Incontinence, in the aged
- » Menorrhagia, idiosyncratic

- » Postpartum bleeding, passive (external and internal)
- » Vaginitis (external and internal)

Collection
Easy to gather, snip the above half (leaf, flower, and stem) with pruners. If collecting Potentilla fruticosa (Bush cinquefoil) simply prune the new leafing branch tips.

Preparations/Dosage
- » Herbal infusion: 4–8 oz. 2–3 times daily
- » FPT/DPT (50% alcohol): 30–60 teaspoon 2–3 times daily
- » Sitz bath: as needed

Cautions
Like other Rose family plants, there is little to no caution for Cinquefoil. Some stomach upset is possible with excessive amounts.

Cleavers
Rubiaceae/Madder Family

Galium aparine

Galium aparine L.
Goosegrass, Catch weed

Description
Cleavers is a creeping or bunch–forming herbaceous annual, preferring shady to semi–shady locations. Its thin angular stems support opposite or whorled leaves. They are lance shaped and sessile. The flowers are small, inconspicuous, and cream in color. The mature seeds are about ⅛" in length. Unlike most other species of Galium (Bedstraw) the whole plant is covered by recurved hairs – weak prickles in fact. They cause no pain, but when brushed against the plant clings to skin and clothing...'Cleavers'.

Distribution
Cleavers is a circumpolar species. Common throughout North America, it is particularly abundant in temperate zones throughout the West. It is almost

always found in moist soils next to rocks, boulders, and larger perennials where it gains some protection from the sun.

Chemistry
Anthraquinones, iridoids, alkanes, flavonoids, tannins, polyphenolic acids, ascorbic acid.

Medicinal Uses
A simple herbal remedy for the urinary tract, use the fresh juice or recently dried plant prepared as an infusion for the relief of painful/burning urination and related irritation of the urogenital area. The traditional indication is a fever along with urinary irritability[22]. For reasons that are somewhat esoteric (the plant is not particularly antibacterial), if these two symptoms occur together, Cleavers is considered specific.

An older use that gets little attention today is the plant's application to poorly healing and inflammatory skin conditions, such as psoriasis and eczema. As an 'alterative', use it if plagued by allergic–type skin conditions.

Cleavers is an age–old European and North American folk cancer remedy, particularly of cancers that have a topical expression (surface tumors, skin cancer, etc.). Over the last couple of decades there have been multiple in–vitro[23] studies showing Cleavers' success in retarding cancerous growth: breast, laryngeal, head, and neck cancer cell lines have all been diminished with its application. As a co–therapy with standard chemotherapy/surgical treatments, Cleaver's use makes sense.

Indications
» Cystitis/Urethritis with fever
» Psoriasis/Eczema

Collection
The plant grows in small upright or vining clumps, making simple hand collection nearly effortless. Grab and prune.

---

22 These two combined symptoms likely denote a moderate to advanced urinary tract infection. Try Cleavers for a day or so – if symptoms do not improve it is wise to resort to conventional antibiotics.

23 Meaning petri–dish, not human, studies.

Preparations
Preparing the infusion is simple enough. To juice the plant, use a 'wheatgrass' juicer (standard juicers are ineffective). For storage, the juice can be frozen in ice cube trays and melted/used as needed.

Dosage
» Fresh juice: 60–90 drops 2–3 times daily
» Herb infusion: 4–6 oz. 2–3 times daily

Cautions
There are no cautions with normal usage.

Coral Root
Orchidaceae/Orchid Family

Corallorhiza spp.

Corallorhiza Gagnebin
Chicken toe, Crawley, Dragon's claw

Description
Easily missed, Coral root's singular (or occasionally multiple) yellow to reddish–purple stem arises inconspicuously from the forest's floor. The leaves are tiny and scale–forming. The flowers develop in spike–like formations and are often purple spotted (Corallorhiza maculata) or purple striped (C. striata). The oblong seed capsules are pendant.

Certainly, Coral root's most interesting characteristic is its coral–like rhizome formation. Developing in small budding ovoid clumps, they are fascinating, both visually (the root tips may also be imagined as appearing like 'chicken toes') and in functionality. They utilize a soil fungus for energy and nutrition. All parts of the plant lack chlorophyll.

Distribution
Occurring throughout most of the western coniferous/mixed forests, look for Coral root in decaying leaf litter. Shaded by overhead trees, it prefers dark and deep woodlands.

Chemistry

Apparently Coral root is not a well–researched plant – my attempts at a listing came up empty handed. At the very least it contains a broad range of flavonoids.

Medicinal Uses

Rarely used today, Coral root was once a preferred sudorific employed by the Eclectic physicians of old. Corallorhiza odontorhiza, native to the eastern part of the country, was their choice plant. As replacements, regional species are locally available and will be found as effective.

The older indications for Coral root still apply today. It best fits individuals whom are immunologically weakened in the bronchial region and exhibit a generally lowered vitality, be it from age, environment, or genetics. Within this constitutional context, it is a specific remedy for sufferers of residual fever arising from a long–standing bronchial infection. Subacute inflammation manifesting as a dry–hacky cough, seasonal bronchitis that has lasted a little too long, or lung–centered influenza that seems to be lingering due to a weakened immune system are indications for the plant. More broadly, use it at the end stage of a lung infection where there still is a nagging–painful cough, bronchial soreness, exhaustion, lack of appetite, and fever.

I believe western species are more sedative than Corallorhiza odontorhiza. They are well used as simples in this department and are related in some ways to other Orchid family nervous system agents such as Stream orchid and Lady slipper.

Insomnia, anxiety, and mental agitation, especially if connected to overwork and exhaustion indicate Coral root. Its central nervous system sedation is somewhat broad: it affects cerebral states of unrest as well as muscular tension.

Not only is the hot tea the stronger diaphoretic preparation, it also is moderately stimulating to menses. If a stress component and lack of pelvic circulation dovetail into suppressed menstruation, Coral root should help.

Indications

- » Debility, respiratory
- » Cough, chronic/irritative
- » Fever, dry skin with bronchial involvement
- » Insomnia/Anxiety with exhaustion

» Menstruation, suppressed

Collection

The roots of Coral root are fairly close to the ground's surface. With a full-sized shovel start digging 8"–10" out from the central stem. Dig down about 1' then towards the stem. The root cluster is usually shaped like a baseball-sized knot that breaks apart very easily. Proceed slowly and with care so the whole root is not mauled while digging. It is not uncommon for unaware collectors to crush the roots if digging begins too close to the stem or in a hurried manner.

Remove all adhering dirt, pebbles, and forest matter with running water. Dry the root pieces with a dehydrator, or tincture the pieces fresh. The above ground parts can also be included in whatever preparation is decided upon.

Coral root is an Orchid, though not a particularly showy one. Most Orchids are not prolific propagators, even in optimal settings (numerous states list varying species of Coral root on threatened/protected lists). Given the plant's inherent environmental fragility and all the other modern day factors (habitat loss, etc.) do be sure that there is a sizable quantity in your area before collecting. Some forest sections will have well established large stands, others will have only a sparse population. Take a couple of plants from a healthy stand. If only several are encountered in a local area, it probably is best to visually admire them only.

Preparations/Dosage

» FPT/DPT (60% alcohol): 45–90 drops 2–3 times daily
» Standard/Cold infusion: 4–8 oz. 2–3 times daily

Cautions

Not much is known about Coral root's chemistry, but factoring its uses with non-toxic related plants, there should be little worry with sensible dosing. Due to its stimulating influences over menses, I caution against its use during pregnancy.

Cottonwood

Salicaceae/Willow Family

Populus angustifolia E. Jame
Narrowleaf cottonwood

Populus angustifolia

Description

One of the smaller Cottonwood's of the West, Narrowleaf cottonwood reaches heights of 50'. Fast growing, this species has a generally narrowed top and ascending branches. The tree's bark is smooth on younger sections, but deeply furrowed around the trunk. The leaf buds, like all Populus', are more or less resinous[24] and mildly balsamic–smelling when crushed. The leaves are finely serrated, pointed, slender, and rounded. Male and female flowers are catkin–forming and develop on separate trees.

Distribution

Cottonwood boasts a significant range throughout the Interior West. In the southwestern states, it is typically a middle elevation grower, but further north, its habitat decreases in elevation. Like other species of Cottonwood, look to stream and creek margins or surrounding flats where the water table is high.

Chemistry

Populus (Cottonwood–type) general: phenolic glycosides: isoferulic acid, ferulic acid, caffeic acid, prenylferulate, prenylcaffeate, pinocembrin, pinostrobin, pinobanksin, chrysin, benzyl–(e)–caffeate, galangin, isosakuranetin, phenylethyl–(e)–caffeate, kaempferol, salicin, salicortin, salireposide, populin, temuloidin, tremulacin.

Medicinal Uses

Although Cottonwood's phenolic glycoside content differs slightly from Aspen (Populus tremuloides) and Balsam poplar (Populus balsamifera), the tree's uses are very similar. The bark tea is a reliable and broadly acting antiinflammatory agent. Whether the pain is from an acute sport's injury or

---

24 This species of Cottonwood has more resinous buds than Populus fremontii (Fremont's cottonwood).

long-standing arthritis, Cottonwood's cyclooxygenase inhibition will prove relieving. If feverish, it lowers body temperature without potentially elevating it first, unlike Elder or many Mint family plants. The bark tea taken before meals is a useful gastric stimulant. Its tonic activity is mainly imparted through its bitterness.

Like many Willow family plants, Cottonwood's leaf buds are a urinary tract medicine. Mildly diuretic, they are indicated in chronic disturbances of the area. Use the bud tincture in long standing kidney inflammation and prostatitis.

Externally the poultice, liniment, salve, or oil made with the leaf buds[25] is curbing to headache pain and the inflammation and swelling of contusions, sprains, arthritic joints, and the like. The salve or oil from the same part is soothing to burns and scrapes. Due to its antimicrobial activity, it will also retard infection.

Indications

bark
- Rheumatic conditions/Injuries
- Fever, mid to high
- Indigestion, asecretory

leaf buds
- Nephritis, chronic
- Prostatitis, chronic
- Pain/Inflammation (external)

Collection

In the spring, when the new leaf buds are starting to develop, find a secondary branch with light, non-fissured, and smooth bark. Cut the branch from its attaching point, then clip and discard all the small branchlets less than a finger-width in diameter. Once the bark is removed dry it in an open paper bag out of direct sunlight. Collect the buds in the spring before the leaves begin to unfurl. They should be semi-sticky and resinous.

Preparations/Dosage

- Bark decoction: 4 oz. 2–3 times daily or externally as needed
- FPT/DPT (75% alcohol) of leaf buds: 30–60 drops 3–4 times daily
- Liniment/Oil/Salve/Ointment (leaf buds): as needed

25 Balsam poplar buds are the main medicine. Use Cottonwood if it is not available.

Cautions
Forgo large doses of Cottonwood if taking anti–coagulant pharmaceuticals. The chance of Cottonwood triggering Reye's syndrome is remote, but it is best to err on the side of caution and not use Cottonwood internally with feverish children.

Cow Parsnip
Apiaceae/Carrot Family

Heracleum maximum W. Bartram *(Heracleum lanatum)*
Masterwort, Wild parsnip, Hogweed

Description
An herbaceous perennial (sometimes biannual), Cow parsnip's basal leaves are divided into three maple leaf–like leaflets. Coarsely lobed and serrated, the mature leaf is between 1'–2' in diameter. Rough to the touch, the large flowering stalk (one per plant) is stout, hollow, coarse, and can reach heights of 6'–8' feet. The compound umbels are composed of white, ½"–sized, radial flowers. The seeds are ½"–¾" in length, flattened, and marked with longitudinal lines. Heracleum (from Hercules) describes the plant's large stature.

Distribution
Although there are dozens of Old World Heracleum species, this is the only native species found in North America. Common throughout the West, look to Aspen and conifers next to streams and drainages. The plant prefers moist and even boggy soils. In the Southwest, it is solely a plant of the high mountains.

Chemistry
Furanocoumarins: psoralen, bergapten, xanthotoxin, isopimpinellin, angelicin, isobergapten, sphondin, pimpinellin; polyacetylenes: falcarindiol; volatiles (general): octyl acetate, octanol, α–pinene.

Medicinal Uses
Heracleum species have been important traditional medicines throughout the ages. Pediacus Dioscorides, the renowned Greek surgeon and doctor to

the Roman Legion wrote of Heracleum sphondylium during first century AD as a cure for epilepsy. Traditional Iranian herbalists still use the seeds of Heracleum persicum as a carminative and pain reducing sedative. The Mi'kmaq and Malecite Indians of eastern Canada once used H. maximum as a lung medicine in cases of bronchitis and the flu.

American herbal doctors of the ninetieth century were keenly aware of Cow parsnip's value as an antispasmodic sedative. It was considered to have both smooth muscle and nerve pathway affinity. Tics, tremors, and associated spasm due to nerve pathway over–stimulation and trauma are the plant's best indications. Mild seizure and convulsant activity, particularly if muscular tension and paralysis–like symptoms exist, also suggests Cow parsnip will be of use. More prosaically, the plant can be used as a simple nervous system sedative taken before bed. Here it will be found specifically calming if muscular tension due to stress is a factor in sleeplessness.

A number of older references state that the plant has some restorative influence when applied to individuals afflicted by paralysis of various kinds. I believe the suggestion that Cow parsnip has a mending effect on completely severed nerves and related paralysis is faulty; however, applied to areas where minor nerve damage has occurred, it will do good. It is possible that herbal doctors of the past observed a relaxing (and movement restoring) effect on tissue affected by hypertonic seizure[26] activity. Excessive neurotransmitter discharge is reduced with internal and external (bath soak) application, therefore normal somatic movement is more quickly reinstated with its usage.

Herpatic neuralgias – the pain and sensation of shingles, herpes simplex virus (trigeminal or sacral) are less reliably influenced. My suggestion is to try it – for some it helps. Even though the topically applied root (usually made into an herbal oil), is the traditional preparation, seed formulations can be used as well. Relatedly, apply the herbal oil (seed or root) to muscular pains and joint aches.

Cow parsnip's in–vitro stimulation of certain immune parameters, interleukin 6 (IL–6) for instance, a well–known cytokine related to macrophage activation, helps to explain its Canadian Indian use as a cold and flu herb and for bronchial–related infectious conditions[27]. Before conventional

26   Most species of Heracleum contain the furanocoumarin bergapten (and related compounds) which demonstrates strong anticonvulsant activity.

27   Another interesting finding concerns sphondin, the main furanocoumarin of Cow parsnip. It has been observed to have a significant reducing effect on bronchial

antibiotics, Cow parsnip was even a popular regional therapy for tuberculosis (the plant's roots have demonstrated strong anti–Mycobacterium activity).

Use root preparations in any viral cold or flu infection, especially if the respiratory tract is affected. Additionally, a wide–array of bacterial (and even fungal strains) are inhibited[28] by Cow parsnip, making its use as potentially worthwhile as Lomatium or Ligusticum, two related Carrot family herbal medicines.

Root preparations (ointment, salve, oil, soak, etc.) should also be considered for their topical influences. From poorly healing wounds prone to infection, to dermal fungal infections (ringworm for instance), its application has merit.

Any plant that has a sizable photosensitizing furanocoumarin content has the *potential* of treating psoriasis, eczema, and vitiligo. Several furanocoumarins (psoralen, bergapten, and xanthotoxin) found in all parts of Cow parsnip are standard treatments for these conditions (internally and/or externally used, then followed by UVA exposure). I mention it here only to offer a more complete view of the plant – even if it is only theoretical. It is possible that the amounts of these particular furanocoumarins in Cow parsnip are just too small or inconsistent to have an appreciable effect.

Additionally, the hot tea will be found diaphoretic if afflicted by an elevated body temperature (dry fever). Many will find it generally carminative if troubled by gas pains and food related stomach cramps. Also, some women find a hot compress along with the internal tea or tincture relieving to menstrual cramps (it is also slightly stimulating to menses).

Indications
» Tics/Tremors/Spasm (internal and external)
» Insomnia/Restlessness with muscular tension from stress
» As an analgesic (external)
» Infection, bronchial, viral/bacterial
» Infection, skin, bacterial/fungal (external)

---

inflammation.

28   Although Cow parsnip's volatile oils add to its antimicrobial nature, it appears that its polyacetylene and furanocoumarin contents are at the heart of it strength.

Collection

Once the seeds develop (late spring/early summer), there is a window of only about one week or so when they are prime for collection. They should be green, yet with visible inner dark stripes. These stripes signal the beginning of the seed's maturation and are a good indicator of this part's potency. When crushed, they should be very aromatic and still hydrated. If collected too early or late they will be inferior.

Although the roots from flowering Cow parsnip can be collected, I recommend gathering this part pre– or post– above ground stalk development – essentially in the early spring or later fall (before the ground is snow covered or frozen). Depending on the plant's age, the roots will be a simple forked tap root (young plant) or a radial ring of finger–width roots stretching horizontally just beneath the ground's surface, anchored by a number of deeper reaching tap roots (mature plant). Both are good medicines. However, older plants will have more material.

Preparations

The fresh plant tincture of either the seed or root[29] is easy enough to prepare: separate and discard the seed stems before tincturing or chop the roots into ¼ inch pieces before submerging them in alcohol. If drying the roots for later use, employ a dehydrator, as mold growth sometimes occurs even if well–spaced on a flat or screen.

The taste of Cow parsnip is at first interesting, then cloying, and finally revolting. The tea especially becomes tiresome quickly. Any long–term, consistent internal dosing will likely entail use of the tincture. It's best to add it to a swallow of water and imbibe it quickly.

Dosage

Although they are not exact duplicates, the roots and seeds are loosely interchangeable; however, consider the roots the main medicinal part. They'll address the majority of issues and should be thought of as the stronger of the two. The seeds, having a greater volatile oil content, better addresses topical pain issues.

» FPT/DPT (60% alcohol) of root: 20–40 drops 2–3 times daily
» Root decoction: 4–6 oz. 2–3 times daily

29 The fresh root tincture can be irritating to gastrointestinal membranes. If symptoms develop from its internal use either take less, dilute it with water, or use the dried plant tincture instead.

- » Topical root preparations: use as needed
- » FPT/DPT (60% alcohol) of seed: 30–60 drops 2–3 times daily
- » Seed infusion: 4–6 oz. 2–3 times daily
- » Topical seed preparations: use as needed

Cautions

Cow parsnip should not be used during pregnancy (or while nursing) due to its complex and active chemical make-up. Plus, most medicinal plants of the Apiaceae group stimulate reproductive blood flow. It is plausible that the plant influences a variety of CNS/PNS neurotransmitter receptor sites, therefore, due to general unknowns, its co-use with pharmaceuticals in nervous system disorders may not be wise. In general, consider Cow parsnip a short to intermediate term use herb.

The furanocoumarin/phytotoxicity issue: all Heracleum species produce furanocoumarins (as do Angelica, Celery, Parsnip, and other Carrot family plants). This group of compounds (some individual furanocoumarins more than others) are notorious for causing dermatitis when sunlight exposure follows plant contact. A number of variables, some unpredictable, factor into potential rash development, but generally, longer topical contact followed by sun exposure increases the chance of an issue. Even though I have never observed a problem with this species of Cow parsnip, and there is little historical record suggesting a problem, my advice is cover up when collecting the plant if concerned[30].

Relatedly, it is possible (but not probable) that sensitive individuals may develop a phototoxic rash or simply dermal sensitivity after external (the steam distilled essential oil contains no or few furanocoumarins) application or with liberal internal use followed by sun exposure. Again, this is an extremely remote caution. If a rash does develop, cleanse the area with a warm soap solution and proceed with other topical treatments. Furanocoumarin rashes are self-limiting.

Other Uses

Occasionally Cow parsnip is listed as a condiment and/or edible plant. Due to the unique aromatics of the seed, it is possible that this part may have been used (in very small quantities – bitter!) as a spice of sorts. The first emerging leaf buds are sometimes too mentioned as a cooked green (boiled

---

30 Heracleum sphondylium and H. mantegazzianum, the two introduced species, are considered much more problematic than native H. maximum.

once or twice and rinsed). Fair enough. I laugh though when I read about the roots, eaten as a roasted 'vegetable'. Being very familiar with the plant, I would consider the roots (and seeds) a food only after all the inner tree bark and old leather had first been consumed. In other words, close to death with nothing else to eat, and only then boiled, rinsed, and roasted repeatedly, would I give it consideration. The seeds and roots of Cow parsnip are not a food. They are a medicine. And the mature leaves? Boil 90% of any fresh plant material long enough, and I suppose the result will be, in the broadest sense, 'edible'.

Dandelion
Asteraceae/Sunflower Family

Taraxacum officinale

Taraxacum officinale F.H. Wigg. (*Leontodon taraxacum, Taraxacum dens–leonis, T. retroflexum, T. sylvanicum*)
Blowball, Chicoria, Lion's teeth

Description
Dandelion is a small perennial arising from a single or branched taproot. Both the leaves and flowers originate from the plant's root crown. Lacking branches, the dark green leaves are between 2"–12" long and deeply lobed. The yellow flower heads arise on hollow stems, which can be several inches in length. The seed clusters are puff–like. Each achene is attached to a parachute–like grouping of silky hair making wind dispersal easy. If damaged, the entire plant exudes a milky sap.

Distribution
This European native is extremely robust and versatile, making the best of what it is given. Found throughout most of the country, lawns, gardens, grassy parks, and roadsides are common places for the plant.

Chemistry
Sesquiterpene lactones: eudesmanolides, germacranolides, guaianolides; phenyl–propanoids; phenolic acids; flavonoids: apigenin, luteolin, chrysoeriol; coumarins: scopoletin, aesculetin, cinnamic acid esters (mono-caffeyltartaric acid, chlorogenic acid, chicoric acid), hydroxycinnamic acid;

triterpenes; β–amyrin, taraxol, taraxerol; carotenoids: lutein; phytosterols: sitosterol, stigmasterol, taraxasterol; polysaccharide: inulin.

Medicinal Uses

Dandelion's use as a gastric and hepatic/biliary stimulant is straight forward. The tea or tincture taken before meals is a reliable bitter tonic. It increases digestive prowess by stimulating an array of gastric secretions. Use the plant if prone to indigestion and combine it with Field mint or Monarda if there is a tendency for bloating.

Augmenting to small intestinal fat digestion, Dandelion is stimulating to bile production by the liver and release by the gallbladder. It tends to be more cooling to the liver than other hepatic stimulants such as Barberry, so its use in liver inflammation, like hepatitis C, is safe and even called for. In fact, alone or combined with Milk thistle, Dandelion reduces liver sensitivity, upper body tightness, and itchy eyes and skin associated with liver inflammation. A cup of roasted or plain Dandelion root tea before breakfast is an effective way of thinning bile so gall stones tend not to develop. 1–2 cups a day over several months will diminish established gall stones from overly concentrated bile.

The root has a substantial inulin content. Due to the body's inability to digest this complex carbohydrate, it enters the colon intact. Here inulin promotes beneficial microflora growth, particularly Bifidobacteria. This in turn stabilizes the large intestinal environment, limiting pathogenic bacteria and their destructive by–products. Use Dandelion in the nefarious 'leaky gut syndrome' – a title meant to describe a symptom picture of skin allergies, joint inflammation, fatigue, and colon instability dependent upon the proliferation of harmful colon bacteria, their by–products, and heightened leukocyte activity. For this purpose, Dandelion can be combined with Yucca. The duo tends to stabilize beneficial flora levels, while binding harmful endotoxins.

The leaf is particularly diuretic. It is indicated in resolving uric acid kidney stones and acts systemically to reduce elevated uric acid levels responsible for gout.

Writing of Dandelion and its virtues, Doctor Geo F. Collier stated in an 1843 issue of The Lancet: "The great objection to its use will be that it costs nothing, and may be made by everyone, without pharmaceutical mystery or expense." Some things just never change.

Indications
- » Indigestion, asecretory
- » Congestion/Inflammation, liver/gallbladder
- » Poor fat digestion
- » Uric acid kidney stones/Gout
- » Poor intestinal health

Collection
Gather Dandelion leaf when verdant and hydrated during the spring and summer. The roots of the plant can be dug all year. However, they are strongest[31] during colder seasons, particularly in the fall when they contain up to 40% inulin. Dry the leaves normally. Split the taproots length–wise prior to drying.

Preparations
The root powder in capsules is the best way to receive the plant's inulin content.

Dosage
- » Root decoction/infusion: 2–6 oz. 2–3 times daily
- » Leaf infusion: 4–8 oz. 2–3 times daily
- » FPT/DPT of root (40% alcohol): 60–90 drops 2–3 times daily
- » Fluidextract of root: 20–40 drops 2–3 times daily
- » Capsule of root (00): 2–3, 2–3 times daily

Cautions
Do not use Dandelion if there is a biliary blockage.

Other Uses
Although slightly bitter, the young leaves are used as a potherb. Fresh or lightly sautéed add them to salads or other cooked greens.

---

31 In low elevations and arid locales Dandelion tends to be diminutive in size and weaker in strength. The high mountain/cold country growers tend to be better medicines.

Dock
Polygonaceae/Buckwheat Family

Rumex L.
Bitter dock, Broadleaf dock, Western dock, Willow dock, Violet dock, Yellowdock, etc.

Rumex spp.

Description
Although herbaceous, Docks are perennial plants with alternating lance–shaped leaves (or at least longer than wide). With entire margins, they are wavy, or in a few cases, almost dentate. Early in the season they are arranged basally; later in the season the stalk leaves tend to be diminutive in size. The small cream to green flowers form in clustered spike–like racemes. The mature seeds are small and brown and are surrounded by a winged encasement.

Usable Docks will have a stout (forked or singular) taproot (not a tuber). If the roots are small and rhizomatous it is likely a Sorrel species of Rumex – good as an occasional leaf edible, but not as a medicine.

Distribution
Dock species are common throughout the West, and indeed throughout many parts of the world. Most species in our area are non–native temperate zone growers, fond of moist and disturbed soils and drainage edges.

Chemistry
For Yellowdock (other species are similar): condensed and hydrolyzable tannins; anthraquinone pigments: nepodin, chrysophanol, physcion, emodin; flavonoids: kaempherol, quercetin.

Medicinal Uses
There are about a dozen Rumex species that fall into the Dock category (excluding Sorrel–types[32]) commonly found throughout the West that can be used like Yellowdock – the official plant medicine. They all share a majority of medicinal characteristics. However, some variation should be expected from species to species. Consider the following description a starting place

---

32   Rumex hymenosepalus (Desert or Wild rhubarb) is also a Dock biotype, but due to its significant tannin content the roots are for external use only.

only to be clarified by each species' consistent use. The main physical attribute to be aware of when evaluating the potency of a Dock species is the root color. The inner root should be yellowish to yellowish–orange. The lighter it is, the less potent it will be.

Dock's primary use is as an intestinal wall tonic. Stimulating and tightening, it has the unique property of reducing subacute/chronic inflammation while structurally tonifying intestinal tissue. Through this influence, it has a beneficial effect on small intestinal fat absorption. Dietary lipid uptake tends to improve as does corresponding skin and lymph irregularities dependent upon faulty assimilation. Use Dock if there is a tendency towards eruptive and scaly skin conditions that appear to be linked to intestinal discomfort and stasis. In addition, lymph enlargements are typically reduced due to Dock's lipid–lymph organizational ability. Dock improves the absorption of fat–soluble vitamins. Consequently, it is often found nutritional to individuals whom are struggling with functional anemia or sub–anemic tendencies.

Externally the fresh poultice of the whole plant (or other topical preparations) is used for many of the same conditions Dock treats internally. Poorly healing ulcers and migrating itchy rashes dependent upon 'bad blood', stress, Poison ivy exposure, or chemical sensitivity are Dock specifics.

Indications
» Skin rashes (external and internal)
» Skin eruptions/Acne with poor fat digestion (external and internal)
» Malabsorption, fat/nutritional

Collection
A general rule of thumb when harvesting Dock: if the root is internally yellow–orange then it will make for a good medicine. Stronger plants are usually found in drier, clay–laden, and dense soils. Dock found partially submerged on streamsides will be inferior.

Preparations
After cleaning the roots, either split them into strips or chop them into ¼" pieces. Dry them normally or use a dehydrator.

Dosage
Like Rhubarb, in small amounts Dock is tonic to intestinal walls. Larger amounts may be found irritating and laxative (with rebound constipation).
- » FPT/DPT (50% alcohol): 30–60 drops 2–3 times daily
- » Fluidextract: 10–20 drops 2–3 times daily
- » Root decoction: 4–6 oz. 2–3 times daily

Cautions
Due to Dock's anthraquinone–laxative principles, large doses should not be used during pregnancy.

Other Uses
The young leaves can be added to salads or cooked as a green.

Dogbane
Apocynaceae/Dogbane Family

Apocynum cannabinum

Apocynum cannabinum L.
Common dogbane, Indian hemp, Prairie dogbane

Description
Dogbane is a small to medium–sized, rhizomatous, colony–forming perennial. Mostly erect in growth, it has opposite and lanceolate leaves. The stems are often reddish, very fibrous, and difficult to break. The small flowers are white and develop in cymes. They are tubular with a 5–lobed corolla and a 5–parted calyx. The seed pods are long, narrow, and often form in pairs. When broken all parts of the plant weep a milky latex.

Distribution
A fairly common and wide–ranging North American plant, Dogbane is found in open meadows, fields, roadsides, dry streambeds, and exposed hillsides.

Chemistry

Steroidal compounds: (20S)–, (20R)–18, 20–epoxycymarin and –epoxyapocannoside, cannogenin, strophanthidin, d–cymaroside, d–oleandroside, d–digitoxoside, d–digitaloside; pregnanes: neridienone a, 6, 7–didehydrocortexone; apocynin.

Medicinal Uses

Dogbane was used up until the early 20th century by alternative doctors as a digitalis–like substitute: it was placed in the same strata as Digitalis[33], yet was thought to better–influence fluid retention and edema from poor heart function more reliably and with less potential for accumulation toxicity.

Although in the past Dogbane was applied to a number of symptoms of overt heart failure (ascites and cyanosis for instance), I believe the present–day use of Dogbane should stay in the realm of addressing functional tendency or early disease. Its primary indication should be fluid retention/edema, especially of the lower extremities, due to imperfect cardiovascular activity. Its use is additionally indicated if the following symptoms accompany any long–term heart condition: chronic indigestion and constipation, fatigue, edematous tissues, and easily labored breathing and cough.

I've observed individuals whom thought they were suffering from sub–thyroid conditions, when in fact they were affected by constitutionally weak hearts, benefited by Dogbane. Often just after one dose, increased visual acuity, a deepness of breath, and better tissue oxygenation are sensed. If the pulse is weak and rapid (and some of the other indications are present) Dogbane will likely improve the overall cardiovascular picture.

It is important to consider though, Dogbane has little –if any– present–day medicinal following. The reason being, for moderate to serious heart disease there exist pharmaceuticals that are far superior in effectiveness, reliability, and safety. However, for sub–heart disease, when pharmaceuticals are not yet necessary (or the negatives outweigh the positives), Dogbane used sensibly, still has a place.

Indications

» Cardiovascular weakness with fluid retention

---

33   Foxglove (Digitalis purpurea and a number of unofficial species), is the source of digoxin, an isolated/purified compound (and older generation heart pharmaceutical).

Collection

If possible, gather Dogbane roots in less compacted soils such as sandy creek sides or field edges. Lacking that luxury, a proper shovel along with some moderate effort will likely be needed. Regardless of soil conditions, multiple above ground stems will signify a greater rhizome mass beneath.

Preparations

Dry the roots and tincture them with equal proportions of alcohol and water. Start with 5–10 drops 2–3 times daily for minor issues. Slowly increase to larger amounts (maximum, 20 drops per dose) for more significant edematous problems.

Dosage

» DPT (50% alcohol): 5–20 drops 2–3 times daily

Cautions

When using Dogbane, it is wise to keep blood pressure monitored as higher doses may cause temporarily elevations with nausea and sweating. If this is the case either reduce the dosage or discontinue Dogbane. The herb should not be combined with standard cardiovascular pharmaceutics. Dogbane is an 'herbal drug' (its activity is dependent upon cardiac–affecting glycosides) and should be used with attention and caution. Do not use it while pregnant or nursing.

Other Uses

Dogbane's fibrous stems are considered one of the vegetable world's best source material for hand woven cordage, rope, etc. This use refers to the common name, Indian hemp.

Elder
Caprifoliaceae/Honeysuckle Family

Sambucus cerulea, melanocarpa, microbotrys

Sambucus cerulea Raf. (*Sambucus caerulea, S. caerulea var. neomexicana, S. caerulea var. velutina, S. cerulea var. cerulea, S. cerulea var. neomexicana, S. cerulea var. velutina, S. glauca, S. mexicana* subsp. *caerulea, S. mexicana* subsp. *cerulea, S. mexicana var. caerulea, S. mexicana var. cerulea, S. neomexicana, S. neomexicana var. vestita, S. nigra* subsp. *caerulea, S. nigra* subsp. *cerulea, S. velutina*)
Blue elderberry, Western elder

Sambucus melanocarpa A. Gray (*Sambucus racemosa var. melanocarpa*)
Black elderberry, Rocky mountain elder

Sambucus microbotrys Rydb. (*Sambucus callicarpa, S. pubens, S. pubens var. arborescens, S. racemosa* subsp. *pubens, S. racemosa var. arborescens, S. racemosa var. laciniata, S. racemosa var. leucocarpa, S. racemosa var. microbotrys, S. racemosa var. pubens, S. racemosa var. racemosa*)
American red elderberry, Pacific red elderberry, Red elderberry

Description
Species/subspecies/variety names, for whatever reason, have always been in a state of flux for American Sambucus. I believe the main binomials listed for the three above species are currently the best descriptors; however, tomorrow they may not be!

A large shrub to small tree (Sambucus cerulea tends to be the largest of the three), Elder has pithy, fast-growing, sucker-type stems. The large, pinnately compound leaves are comprised of 5–9 serrated leaflets. When crushed, they are unpleasant smelling. The flowers form in cymes and are slightly rounded (Sambucus cerulea) or cone-shaped (S. melanocarpa and S. microbotrys). Individually they are small, white-cream in color, and 5-parted. The juicy, small-seeded fruits develop in sizable clusters and are blue (S. cerulea), black (S. melanocarpa), or red (S. microbotrys).

Distribution

Sambucus cerulea is common throughout the coastal and intermountain West. Its greatest density occurs in the western–most portions of California, Oregon, and Washington to Idaho and Montana. Higher mountain areas of Nevada, Utah, western Colorado, Arizona, and New Mexico are additional areas. It is typically found in association with Douglas fir, Pine, and Oak, in forest openings and other sun–exposed places.

Sambucus melanocarpa is primarily a middle and southern Rocky Mountain grower. Also found in the more easterly mountains of Washington, Oregon, and California, it's common to creek sides and moist–soiled flats and hillsides.

Sambucus microbotrys' range overlaps S. melanocarpa's. It too is found throughout the Rocky Mountains. High mountain Arizona, New Mexico (Sangre de Cristos), Colorado, Wyoming, and Utah are its usual places. Additionally, there are isolated stands found further west until the Pacific Coast where it is very common west of the Cascades through to Alaska.

Chemistry

Sambucus canadensis (others similar): triterpenes: α–amyrin palmitate, balanophorin, oleanolic acid; flavonoids: cyanidin, cyanin, quercetin, rutin; monoterpene: morroniside; sterols: campesterol, β–sitosterol, stigmasterol; sambucine.

Medicinal Uses

Elder's use as a stimulating diaphoretic is as old as it is effective. Its application to low to moderate fevers[34] is its most specific indication. Simply put – Elder promotes sweating in febrile states. Users will find the hot tea drunk during the latter part of the day/evening[35] is its most effective preparation and schedule.

For best results, Elder should be combined with commonsense measures such as keeping the body warm with a hot bath before bed and adequate bedding throughout the night. Once a fever breaks, usually in the

---

34 In essence, a fever serves to stimulate immune system activity. It's not an illness, but rather a manifestation of the body's natural defense process. Contrary to herbal diaphoretics, modern conventional approaches (Tylenol, etc.) strive to suppress a temperature and therefore the body's innate infection–fighting mechanism.

35 Body temperature tends to naturally rise throughout the day and into the evening, so using Elder in accordance with the body's natural rhythm only makes sense.

middle of the night, it is best to change perspiration soaked clothes and bedding. Depending on the infection's severity, this routine may repeat for several days before finally resolving. In these cases, Elder combines well with Echinacea, Wild indigo, or other immune stimulants.

There are times when diaphoretic approaches for an infection are inadequate: when a fever is dangerously high, does not resolve after 3–4 days, or when other symptoms delineate a threatening infection. In these situations, the effectiveness of pharmaceutical antibiotics outweighs their drawbacks.

Elder has been found to inhibit varieties of Salmonella and Shigella dysenteriae making its application to gastroenteritis and food poisoning sensible. Although there exist stronger topical herbs, Elder is well applied to external infections (bacterial and fungal), particularly if the affected tissues are edematous, slow to heal, and tend to ulcerate.

The popular use of Elderberry syrup as a cold and flu treatment, which incidentally has only been on the herbal scene since the 1990s, is a textbook example of how product marketing can effectively seed the herbal buyer's mind. Elderberry syrup is a tasty addition to pancakes, but for the serious herbal medicine, only the flower/leaf should be considered.

Indications
» Fever, dry, low to moderate temperature, with lung centered viruses
» As a mild diuretic
» Wounds, edematous, ulcerated, slow to heal, with or without bacterial or fungal involvement (external)

Collection
Prune the last foot or so from the flowering branch ends or collect the flowers and leaves separately. The fruit clusters are collected in bunches and then separated from their small stems.

Preparations
The flowers are simple enough to dry. The leaves though can be problematic. If they are not dried quickly they often mildew, turn black, and become unusable. Be sure to dry them quickly in a warm and arid environment or use a dehydrator.

Dosage
» Leaf/Flower infusion: 2–4 oz. 2–3 times daily, though often less of the

leaf tea is needed as it can be more stimulating

Cautions

Although individual species (and even populations within species) can differ markedly in sambucine and cyanogenic glycoside concentrations, it is best to use flower and leaf preparations (verses the bark which tends to contain higher amounts of these compounds). The berries of Red elderberry (Sambucus microbotrys) should generally be avoided, though they were once rendered safe to eat by various American Indian tribes by applying heat, which degrades their glycoside content (I do not necessarily recommend this, but I've eaten small amounts [1–2 ounces] of the fresh fruit with no problem...more would most likely cause digestive upset).

Some sensitive individuals may find the flower and especially leaf preparations mildly laxative. Like any vasodilating herb, Elder can potentially increase body temperature very briefly before promoting diaphoresis. Be mindful of this when using it in higher febrile states and/or with children.

Other Uses

The berries of blue–black Elder types are sweet and edible. Eat them fresh (limited) or dry them for future use. The dried berries can be stored or rehydrated/used as needed. In fact, the drying process concentrates the berries' natural sugars, making them sweeter than fresh. Combine the dried berries with trail mix or eat them as is. Elder berries are a classic jam/jelly base and can also be fermented instead of grapes to make a wine.

Evening Primrose
Onagraceae/Evening Primrose Family

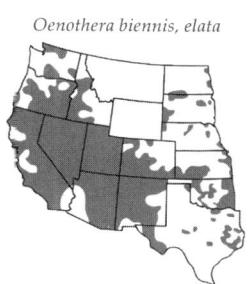

Oenothera biennis, elata

Oenothera biennis L. *(Ongra biennis)*
Field primrose, Tree primrose

Oenothera elata Kunth *(Oenothera hookeri, O. biennis var. hookeri, Ongra hookeri)*
Hooker's evening primrose

Description
Most species of Evening primrose are either annuals or short–lived perennials, though the ones profiled here belong to a select group of biennials. Physical characteristics are very close for both species, so they will be described as a single biotype.

Evening primrose's first year of growth is as a rosette of oblanceolate shaped leaves. They reach lengths of 6"–8" (longer and often red–spotted for Oenothera biennis) and are entire or sinuate–dentate. The plant's second year stalk can reach heights of 5'–6', but usually they are less. The stalk leaves are alternate and shorter than the plant's rosette leaves. The simple to branched stalks are composed of spikes of large 4–petaled yellow flowers that begin to open at dusk and close with the morning sun. In many areas, they are pollinated by nocturnal sphinx moths. The seed capsules are erect, elongated, and contain numerous small reddish–brown seeds.

Distribution
Oenothera biennis is really a plant of northeastern, eastern, and midwestern portions of the United States. Aside from a handful of pockets, it is absent from most of the intermountain western states, though Oregon, Washington, and Montana do have several sizable populations. O. elata has a much wider geographic disbursement. From the Rocky Mountains, to most points west, it's found abundantly.

Both species are commonly found in disturbed mountain/upper elevation soils. Roadsides, trailsides, and areas that have been previously graded are good places to look for either plant.

Chemistry
Phenolics for Oenothera elata: ellagic acid, gallic acid, digallic acid, neo-chlorogenic acid, caffeic acid, p–coumaric acid, o–coumaric acid, myricetin, quercetin, kaempferol, delphinidin, cyanidin.

Medicinal Uses
Evening primrose is a plant of limited medicinal use. It has a disconnected patchwork of therapeutic application with no clear or consistent usage history. It is not a chemically interesting plant (flavonoids/tannins), but nonetheless it is listed in older books (and newer books that copy the old) quite often for a hodgepodge of unrelated issues, as if even then, herbal authors were writing mainly to fill space. The plant's topical use as a freshly crushed/pureed poultice has some merit. If nothing else is available, use it on rashes, insect bites, and sunburn.

Indications
» Rashes/Insect bites/Sunburn (external)

Collection
Gather the basal rosette/lower stalk leaves.

Preparations/Dosage
» Topical preparations: as needed

Cautions
There are no cautions for normal usage.

Other Uses
The late first year and early second year roots of Oenothera biennis were once used in war–torn parts of Europe[36] as a survival 'vegetable'. Chop the roots into ½" or so pieces and then boil, rinse, and re–simmer before adding other soup ingredients (or cook, season, and eat as a simple cooked root). O. elata is used in an identical fashion.

Evening primrose seeds (mainly Oenothera biennis) have become one of the main commercial sources for gamma linolenic acid (GLA). Deficiency

---

36 In Europe Oenothera biennis grows as a non–native import from America. The plant has been recorded as a successful weed for the past several centuries.

of this essential fatty acid has been linked to multiple glandular and inflammatory problems.

Relatedly, the whole seed, garbled from the dried pods, can be ground and eaten as a meal, or sprinkled whole on salads and the like for their nutritional aspects.

False Solomon's Seal
Liliaceae/Lily Family

Maianthemum racemosum

Maianthemum racemosum (L.) Link *(Smilacina racemosa)*
Branched Solomon's seal, Solomon's plume, False lily of the valley

Description
False Solomon's seal[37] is a 1′–2′ tall herbaceous perennial. Forming in colonies from creeping rhizomes, its above ground leaf growth is centered around a single stem (actually multiple stems originate from any one rhizome, but appear singular due to above ground spacing). The leaves are narrow, tapering, sessile, and marked by length–tracing veins. The small, white, 6–parted flowers form in pyramidical clusters. Individually they appear star–like. The mature fruit is the size of a large pea and is red or occasionally purple–spotted.

Distribution
Common to mountain forests throughout the West (and temperate North America), look for False Solomon's seal on moist slopes (often with springs)

[37] A number of popular online databases list Maianthemum's common name as 'False lily of the valley'. Unfortunately, this new common name assignment just muddies the waters. Poisonings become more likely if true 'Lily of the valley' (Convallaria) is thought of as being pharmacologically related to False Solomon's seal (Maianthemum). Convallaria is a drug–like cardiac stimulant and heart toxicities would certainly manifest if taken at dosages recommended for non–toxic Maianthemum. Or inversely, it sends an inaccurate message that Maianthemum is much stronger than it really is. The fact of the matter is, Solomon's seal or Polygonatum (also Lily family) is nearly identical in chemistry and use to Maianthemum, therefore False Solomon's seal for Maianthemum, its traditional common name, makes naming sense.

under open Ponderosa pine and allied conifers. Star Solomon's seal (Maianthemum stellatum) and Fairy bells (Disporum trachycarpum) are two similar-appearing plants that are often nearby, if not intermingled.

Chemistry
General: flavonoids, tannins, steroidal glycosides, starch.

Medicinal Uses
False Solomon's seal's closest medicinal relative is Solomon's seal (Polygonatum multiflorum). The two plants are basically interchangeable.

As a soothing field poultice, crush the leaf or root and apply it to scrapes, rashes, minor cuts, and insect bites. Most will find it mildly antiinflammatory and reducing to tissue irritation. The strong root tea is gargled for sore throats and other oral irritations – it is bland tasting, slightly starchy, and mildly astringent.

The tea also has application as an internal soother. Use it for bronchial, gastrointestinal, and urinary irritations. The lungs are its most consistent area of influence. Apply the root tea (or root syrup) as a simple inflammatory-lessening demulcent.

Indications
» Skin injuries, minor (external)
» Pharyngitis, as a non-antibacterial soother (gargle)
» Bronchitis, as a demulcent

Collection
Search for plants growing in non-compacted soils, usually thriving in leaf-Pine needle chuff. If the chuff is deep enough, simple hand collection is all that is needed. Don't pull on the plant from above, but rather work your fingers under the lateral rhizomes. Compacted soils will necessitate the use of a trowel or shovel. Once gathered, use both the larger rhizome and fine tendrils.

Preparations/Dosage
» Root infusion/decoction: 4–8 oz. 2–3 times daily
» Field poultice: as needed

Cautions
There are no cautions with normal usage.

Field Mint
Lamiaceae/Mint Family

Mentha arvensis

Mentha arvensis L.
Wild mint, Brook mint, Corn mint, Marsh mint, Poléo

Description
Field mint is a 1′–2′ high clump/colony–forming herbaceous perennial. The leaves are opposite and lance–shaped with toothed margins. The flowers are lavender–purple to whitish, two–sectioned, and form in axil clusters. When crushed, Field mint has distinctive minty aroma.

Distribution
As our only native Mentha species, Field mint is found throughout most of temperate North America. Except for much of the Southeast, the plant is common to streamsides, wet meadows, and other moist grassy areas.

Chemistry
Volatiles for Mentha arvensis var. piperascens: α–thujene, α–pinene, camphene, β–pinene, myrcene, 3–octanol, p–cymene, limonene, (z)–β–ocimene, (e)–β–ocimene, γ–terpinene, trans–sabinene hydrate, terpinolene, linalool, menthone, isomenthone, neomenthol, menthol, pulegone, piperitone, geraniol, menthyl acetate, geranyl acetate, β–elemene, β–caryophyllene, germacrene d, γ–cadinene, (e)–nerolidol.

Medicinal Uses
Field mint is a useful stomachic–carminative, ranking somewhere between Spearmint and Peppermint in strength. All forms: the tea, tincture, spirit, or essential oil are used to reduce the gastrointestinal discomfort of gas pains and bloating. Soothing and anesthetic for irritable bowel suffers, Field mint provides relief, especially during the spastic stages of an episode. Reducing to area sensitivity, it is one of our better treatments for pre– or post–vomiting nausea. It won't necessarily inhibit the body from regurgitating

(contaminated food, usually), but with Field mint the episode will be tolerated with less lingering queasiness. Try 1–2 drops of the essential oil swallowed in a capsule (or 10 drops of the spirit in a swallow of water) for these situations, as a smaller volume of liquid (compared to the tea) will be found more agreeable.

Like others of the Mint family, a hot cup of Field mint tea is a reliable diaphoretic. It is useful in breaking a mild to moderate fever where the skin is hot and dry.

Used topically the volatile oils found in the plant, particularly menthol, are pain relieving to headaches. Using a circular motion, rub the oil into the forehead, temples, and nape until a tingling sensation is sensed. If applied in tandem with the proper internal herb for that particular headache, the likelihood of relief increases. The essential oil (with a carrier oil) also makes a decent muscle rub. Its anesthetic effect is useful for sprains, muscle pulls, and other subcutaneous traumas where the skin is unbroken.

In at least one in–vitro study Field mint was observed to produce moderate cholinesterase inhibition. Like Angelica, this effect may be of use to Alzheimer's disease sufferers, as a number of pharmaceuticals are designed to provide symptomatic relief from the disease by preserving synaptic acetylcholine.

Indications
- » Gas pains/Bloating
- » Nausea/Vomiting
- » Fever, with dry skin, mid–low temperature
- » Headache (external)
- » Sports injuries (external)
- » Alzheimer's disease

Collection
Gather the upper herb. The newer growth will typically provide higher amounts and better quality volatile oils, but ultimately let the plant's taste and smell be the guide to its potency. If using the herb for tea or the dried plant tincture, garble the leaf/flower from the stems once dried. Discard the stems due to their lack of oil glands. If the dried herb is strong scented it will be an active medication.

Preparations/Dosage

» Infusion: 4–8 oz. 2–3 times daily
» FPT/DPT (60% alcohol): 30–60 drops 2–3 times daily
» Essential oil: 1–2 drops taken in a capsule 2–3 times daily or applied topically as needed
» Spirit: 10–20 drops 2–3 times daily

Cautions

Due to Field mint's small pulegone quantity, it's not recommended during pregnancy. In susceptible individuals, excessive amounts may cause heartburn and/or gastrointestinal upset.

When used for fevers, Field mint (or any strong diaphoretic) may initially cause a small spike in body temperature before promoting diaphoresis. Be aware of this when using the herb with children.

Figwort

Scrophulariaceae/Figwort Family

Scrophularia L.
Carpenter's square, California figwort, Lanceleaf figwort, Mountain figwort, New Mexican figwort, Pineland figwort

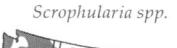

Scrophularia spp.

Description

Most Figworts are large herbs, capable of reaching heights of 5'–6'. The stems are 4–angled, ridged, and stout. The leaves are opposite, petiolate, and generally serrated to divided. Additionally, they are lanceolate, triangular, cordate, or ovate in shape.

The flowers develop in large panicles. Individually they are oval, two–lipped, and generally pea sized (Scrophularia macrantha or New Mexican figwort/Red–birds–in–a–tree is an exception with its larger bright red flowers). The corolla is greenish–purple to reddish–brown. The ovoid seed capsules are filled with numerous small seeds.

Distribution

Mostly a woodland plant preferring rich soils, look to forest margins, next to streambeds, roadsides, or around fire breaks and ski slopes. Although there are an abundance of North American Scrophularia species found country-wide, Asia has the greatest numbers.

Chemistry
Iridoid and phenylpropanoid glycosides.

Medicinal Uses
Figwort's topical influences are soothing and antiinflammatory. Best applied as a crushed fresh plant poultice, the powdered plant (herb and/or root), first moistened, is also fine. Use it as a vulnerary for stings, bites, rashes, burns, and other inflammations. Combined with Penstemon's (nearly identical in use) flowering tops, which are high in structure-enhancing anthocyanins/anthocyanidins, it makes a decent preparation for skin repair and wound healing.

Indications
- Rashes/Bites/Stings (external)
- Wounds/Cuts (external)

Collection
When in flower clip the upper herbage. Use it fresh or dry. The semi-fleshy roots are easily gathered in most soils.

Preparations/Dosage
- External applications: as needed

Cautions
There are no cautions for Figwort.

Fir
Pinaceae/Pine Family

Abies Miller.
Grand fir, White fir, Subalpine fir, etc.

Abies spp.

Description
Fir is a spire to conical shaped evergreen conifer. When young the tree's bark is thin and smooth. With age, it becomes thick and fissured. The leaves (needles) are its best identifying feature: they are singular, flat, linear, and sessile. Curving upward, they create a spiky flat–top. After a needle drops from its branch the remaining scar is smooth and circular (Spruce is raised and rough). The male cones hang from the mid to upper parts of the tree. The female cones are erect and form on the upper branches. Neither cone remains intact longer than a season.

Distribution
Throughout the West, Fir is common to mountain regions. Often mixed with Spruce, Pine, and Douglas fir[38], it is a prolific (and circumpolar) genus.

Chemistry
Abies lasiocarpa (oleoresin): sesquiterpenoids: farnesene, γ–humulene, β–bisabolene, α–selinene, selinadiene, γ–cadinene, δ–cadinene, α–muurolene, sativene, cyclosativene, α–longipinene, longifolene; monoterpenoids: myrcene, geraniol, geranyl acetate, citronellyl acetate, limonene, β–phellandrene, α–terpineol, methyl thymol, borneol, bornyl acetate, α–pinene, β–pinene, δ–3–carene; piperidine alkaloids; resin acids (general): abietic acid, neoabietic acid, palustric acid, pimaric acid, isopimaric acid.

Medicinal Uses
Like Pine and Spruce, Fir is an oleoresin secreting conifer. Fir oleoresin (the resinous sap produced from bark cracks, insect holes, or other injuries) is

---

38 An altogether different genus, Pseudotsuga or Douglas fir, is distinguishable from Fir and Spruce by its female cones. They are a couple of inches in length, do not disintegrate, and have conspicuous 3–lobed bracts (the 'mouse tail').

on par in terms of therapeutic activity with Pine and Spruce oleoresin[39]. Although variations in specific aromatics and other constituents are to be expected, concerning their broad medicinal influences, they are all essentially interchangeable.

A tincture made with the dried (or still soft and gummy) oleoresin is the most reasonable preparation. It lends itself well to dilution and formula–making, which is the best way to internally use any oleoresin medicine. Be warned though, used alone in sufficient concentration, Fir oleoresin is often irritating to tissues. One common result of orally using the tincture alone is the collection of oleoresin around the teeth and gums, resulting in tissue redness and eventual blistering.

Shortly after the oleoresin's ingestion the aromatic lipid–based terpenes are secreted/excreted into the bronchial environment. Their influence dislodges and thins thickened bronchial mucus. The surrounding airspace/lung tissue becomes inoculated with antimicrobial volatiles. Consequently, coughing becomes more productive and bacterial/viral growth is inhibited. Formulated as a cough syrup ingredient, it's best to maintain the oleoresin tincture fraction to 10%–25% of the total volume.

As an antimicrobial, combined with other herbal tinctures, it is well applied to slow–to–resolve lower urinary tract infections. Hollyhock or Checker mallow tea is a good addition to any oleoresin–containing formula: Mallow family herbs are useful at countering any renal irritation that may result from excessive amounts.

Having influence over the gastrointestinal region, the oleoresin tincture (or Fir essential oil) demonstrates success in treating bacterial infections of the small and large intestine (dysentery and/or enteric fever). As part of a formula (or if used solo then mixed with a mucilage), Fir oleoresin (and the essential oil) was even used to resolve cholera infections[40].

Fir oleoresin's internal application is important. However, its external usage is what mainly held the attention of doctors of the past. Again, almost never used alone due to its irritant potential, topically applied oleoresin imparts a stimulating and antimicrobial effect. As a 10% ingredient, the melted oleoresin added to oils or salves makes a superb accent when formulating a

[39] Due to the similarly of uses between Fir, Spruce, and Pine, I have written the most complete monograph under Pine, which should be referred to for a more comprehensive understanding of oleoresin and other conifer applications.

[40] Due to modern antibiotics, this is an extreme usage for any herb today, but sensible application does include its use for intestinal Candida proliferations.

chronic muscle/sport's injury rub. Additionally, it is well used in combinations designed to address old rheumatic complaints aggravated by cold and damp weather.

Small amounts of ascorbate complexes (vitamin C) are found in the needles, seeds, and inner bark of Fir (and most other conifers). Slightly tart, aromatic, and overall pleasant–tasting, a Fir–needle infusion is an efficient way of utilizing its vitamin content. Although this simple preparation only contains micrograms of vitamin C, it's still enough to counter scurvy (which is rare in the First World due to the year–round availability of vitamin C containing foods). Early pioneers and American Indians knew this (though not by present–day definitions), hence the reason for eating conifer needles (or inner bark) throughout the winter months after dried berry stores had become exhausted.

A more practical use for the Fir needle infusion is its application as a wintertime cold and flu tea. Its small ascorbate content, plus the needle's high antimicrobial volatile oil concentration, makes for a useful sore throat gargle or sipping tea if troubled by seasonal infections of the upper or lower respiratory tract. The tea can also be used as a nasal wash in cases of viral/bacterial sinusitis.

Indications
» Bronchitis, non–productive cough
» Infection, urinary tract, chronic
» Infection, intestinal
» As a stimulating/anesthetizing/antimicrobial application (external)
» As a cold and flu tea

Collection
Springtime oleoresin will contain the greatest concentrations of essential oils and hence medicinal activity. The semi–hardened to crystallized nodules are less medicinally active; however, a fair medicine is obtained if both soft and hard oleoresin nodules are mixed together.

The collection of the semi–hardened nodules is easy enough – just pick the pieces from the tree. The fresh oleoresin is a different matter: the use of a putty knife or similar implement and a mason jar will make collection less difficult. After removing the oleoresin from the tree, scrape the lump off on the lip of the jar. If tincturing directly, know the weight of the jar before adding alcohol. By weighing the oleoresin and the jar together, the weight of just the oleoresin can be easily determined and tincturing can proceed with one less step (weigh both, then subtract the jar's weight). Afterward, use a high–proof alcohol to wash hands and tools.

Gather the spring to summertime green needles when still on the tree. When drying them for tea be sure to keep the needles away from direct sunlight and heat – their essential oil content diminishes quickly when exposed to the elements.

Preparations

To prepare an oleoresin tincture (technically a solution) combine 1 part of fresh oleoresin (weight) with 5 parts of alcohol (volume). If hardened nodules are being used, crush or powder them before adding the alcohol. Shake the mixture for several minutes daily for 7–10 days. At the end of this period strain and discard from the solution whatever undissolved oleoresin or sediment remains. Often an additional round of decanting/straining for finer sediment is needed after bottling a week or two later.

When using oleoresin topically keep concentrations to 10% (larger percentages applied to unbroken skin may be fine, but it is wise to make incremental increases if experimenting with formulation). Add 1 part of oleoresin to 9 parts of a base herbal oil. Apply low heat and stir until the oleoresin is totally dissolved. Beeswax can be added at this point if a salve is desired.

Fir needle tea, like Pine and Spruce, is prepared as an infusion. Be sure to cover the steeping tea so the aromatics do not dissipate.

Although Pine needle essential oil is commonly found in health food stores, Fir needle essential oil may take more searching. Like the oleoresin from different conifers, the needle essential oil of Pine and Fir (and Spruce) are basically interchangeable. Whatever tree is decided on, make sure to purchase a pure aromatherapy grade essential oil for both external and internal use.

Added to a base oil or salve at a 1%–2% concentration, Fir essential oil can nearly mimic an oleoresin addition. For internal use, the essential oil should be prepared as a spirit, which can be used alone or added to other tinctures as part of a formula. 1–2 drops (average internal dose) of the essential oil can also be placed in a capsule and swallowed or if using the essential oil for its intestinal effects, a dose can be added to a mucilage base (bran, psyllium, Aloe gel, etc.) and then consumed.

Dosage
- » DPT of oleoresin (95% alcohol): 10–20 drops 2–3 times daily
- » Essential oil (needles, cones, inner bark, or oleoresin): 1–2 drops 2–3 times daily
- » Spirit: 10–20 drops 2–3 times daily
- » Oil/Salve: as needed
- » Needle infusion: 4–6 oz. 2–3 times daily

Cautions
Some will find the internal use of oleoresin causes stomach upset. Although tincture preparations tend to lessen this effect, if plagued by this issue then try ingesting the tincture with food or reduce the dose.

Internal use of the oleoresin or Fir essential oil should be considered a short-term therapy. Dosed properly there is little to fear concerning side effects, but when consumed in excess, liver and kidney inflammations and central nervous system symptoms have been reported. Keep the essential oil out of the reach of children and babies, though as an occasional chest or muscle rub, there will be no problem. Do not use Fir essential oil, the spirit, or any oleoresin preparation internally while pregnant or nursing, though an occasional cup of the needle tea is fine. Lastly, the oleoresin (and the essential oil) is flammable.

Other Uses
All conifer oleoresins were once used extensively as maritime patching and waterproofing agents. Whether sealing canoe bottoms or Spanish galley hulls their application was universal. Though usually mixed with other ingredients, for a primitive patch, simply gather a quantity of hardened oleoresin nodules. Heat until soft, then spread the oleoresin while warm on the item that needs patching. Once cool the congealed oleoresin should take on the consistency of a tacky varnish.

Small nuggets of oleoresin can be burned on a hot plate as an incense, or even 5–10 drops of the oleoresin tincture can be burned similarly. The smoke is aromatic and piney.

Fireweed
Onagraceae/Evening Primrose Family

Chamerion angustifolium (L.) Holub *(Chamaenerion angustifolium, Epilobium angustifolium)*
Great willow herb, Indian wickopy, Narrowleaf fireweed, Rosebay, Wickup

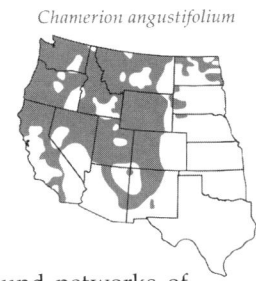

Chamerion angustifolium

Description
A colony–forming plant sprouting from underground networks of connected rhizomes, Fireweed usually grows in dense stands, reaching heights of 3′–4′ (occasionally 6′–7′). The leaves are linear and lanceolate, loosely arranged in spirals, and span from 2″–8″ in length. The somewhat showy lilac–purple flowers form in terminal racemes. They are comprised of four petals and four sepals. The slender capsules are 2″–3″ in length and contain numerous downy–fiber (floss) connected small seeds.

Distribution
Widely distributed throughout the Northern Hemisphere, in western North America Fireweed is best known for its adaptable and initiatory seeding behavior. It is one the first plants to flourish in recently burned, logged, or otherwise damaged forested areas. Intermittent stream edges, forest road margins, and other edge areas where sun exposure is full to partial likely hosts the plant.

Chemistry
Flavonoids: kaempferol, quercetin, myricetin, phenolic acids: ellagic acid, valoneic acid, caffeoylquinic acid, gallic acid, protocatechuic acid, gentisic acid, syringic acid, vanillic acid, isovaloneic acid, cinnamic acid, caffeic acid, ferulic acid, oenothein a and b.

Medicinal Uses
Fireweed's traditional use is as a mild intestinal astringent. Given to young children and babies it is considered an effective and safe counter for loose stools and diarrhea, especially in those with sensitive systems.

Not significantly antispasmodic, Fireweed combines well with most Mints if a degree of smooth muscle sedation is needed (spastic diarrhea for instance). Alone or combined with equal portions of Canadian fleabane, use it as a daily tea to diminish tissue inflammation associated with ulcerative colitis (crones disease). With regular use, area sensitivity and disarray will reduce, as will ulcerative factors.

The late Austrian herbalist Maria Treben popularized a small flowering Epilobium species for the treatment of prostatitis. Today, the exact species she referenced remains a mystery, but herbal gestalt (anecdote + marketing) recommends several species for prostate issues (occasionally Chamerion angustifolium is cited in sales literature too). Given Fireweed's tannin and flavonoid composition, it's possible that this herb is a soothing diuretic; however, its effect on the prostate remains to be seen.

Indications
» Diarrhea, especially children
» Inflammation, intestinal

Collection
Gather the upper portions of Fireweed, preferably in flower, but if only leaf material is available, that is fine too. If Fireweed is gathered further along in the season when the seed capsules are apparent, it can make for a cumbersome–fluff mixture once dried: picture Milkweed or Cottonwood floss intermingled with herbage.

Preparations/Dosage
» Infusion: 4–8 oz. 2–3 times daily

Cautions
There are no cautions with normal usage.

Other Uses
Until the late 1800s, Kaporie tea/chai was a popular beverage in Russia and eastern Europe. Made from the young fermented leaves of Fireweed, its use has all but ceased due to the rise of green and black teas (Camellia sinensis).

Fragrant Sumac
Anacardiaceae/Cashew Family

Rhus aromatica Ait. (*Rhus trilobata*)
Lemonade berry, Skunk bush, Squaw bush, Stinking sumac, Three leaf sumac

Rhus aromatica

Description
Fragrant sumac is an ungainly medium to large sized shrub. Each leaf is comprised of three lobed leaflets. Typically, before the leaves develop the flowers form in dense spike–like clusters. Individual flowers are yellowish and 5–sectioned. When in season, the plant develops red, sticky, and edible–tart fruit.

It is important to recognize the differences between Poison ivy/oak (Toxicodendron) and non–toxic Rhuses (Fragrant sumac and others). Toxicodendron's fruit are whitish as opposed to the red–sticky fruit of non–toxic Rhuses. When a stem or leaf is broken of Toxicodendron, a white, milky, urushiol–containing sap exudes from the break. This does not occur in Fragrant sumac or any other non–toxic Rhus.

Distribution
An extremely variable species, it is found at numerous elevations and grows as high as 7,000'. It is a common shrub throughout the West.

Chemistry
All parts of the plant contain phenolic acids (tannins) and flavonoids. The fruit are high in anthocyanins/anthocyanidins, organic acids (citric/malic acid, etc.), ascorbic acid (vitamin C) and various B vitamins.

Medicinal Uses
Fragrant sumac leaves are astringent due to their tannin content. Soothing to skin irritations and superficial inflammations, use a fresh leaf poultice or the externally applied tea for stings, bites, rashes, and sunburn. The leaf powder applied topically will quickly astringe minor bleeding from cuts and scrapes. As a gargle for sore throats, mouth sores, and receding and bleeding gums, it is efficacious. A strong cup of tea will also prove lessening to episodic diarrhea. The plant's effect on the urinary tract is similar to

FRAGRANT SUMAC

any number of Rose family astringents. Use the tea to limit irritation and mucus-tinged urine. Its mild antibacterial influence likely plays a part in its soothing effect. Due to its negligible water volume and concentrated form, 5–15 drops of the fluidextract before bed was once a treatment for bed-wetting children in the 1800s. According to the literature the therapy often took several months to make a difference.

Other species of Rhus not discussed here can also be used medicinally. In fact, any red-fruited Rhus will have nearly identical uses to Fragrant sumac.

Indications
» Burns/Cuts/Scrapes (external)
» Sore throats/Bleeding gums (gargle)
» Diarrhea

Collection
Clip the leaves from the upper portion of the plant.

Preparations/Dosage
» Leaf infusion: 2–4 oz. 2–3 times daily
» External preparations: as needed

Cautions
Except for daily low-doses, keep consecutive, internal use of the leaf to 1–2 weeks. Longer-term use, as with most tannin-containing plants, may irritate the gastrointestinal and urinary tracts. Its use is not recommended in large amounts (an occasional cup or two is fine) or for any significant duration during pregnancy.

Other Uses
The fruit of Fragrant sumac makes a refreshing tart lemon-like beverage. Prepared as a sun-tea add 4 oz. of fresh fruit to 1 gallon of water. Let the mixture stand for several hours, strain, and sweeten to taste. A tea can also be made by the fruit's infusion in hot water (not boiling). As an edible berry eaten whole, they are dry, mealy, and unrewarding. However, the dried fruit can be powdered and used alone or mixed with Wild rose fruit (hips) powder as a teaspoon-a-day vitamin C rich antioxidant (due to the fruit's tannins, some people may find Sumac powder constipating).

Gentian

Gentianaceae/Gentian Family

Gentiana affinis Griseb.
Prairie gentian, Pleated gentian

Gentiana calycosa Griseb.
Explorer's gentian, Mountain bog gentian

Gentiana parryi Engelm.
Parry's gentian

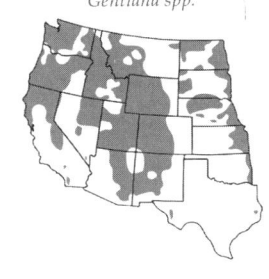

Gentiana spp.

Description
The three species described here are opposite–leaved herbaceous perennials, growing to heights of 1'–1½'. Clump–forming to few–stemmed, Gentian's deep–blue to violet tubular flowers are it most striking feature.

Several–stemmed, Gentiana affinis sprouts from a well–developed root crown. The leaves are lance shaped to ovate and ½"–1" in length. The funnel–form flowers are ½"–1" long, bluish–purple, and develop in the upper leaf axils. The linear seed capsules are about ½" long.

A clump–cluster forming plant, Gentiana calycosa has ovate, ½"–1" long leaves. The flowers are deep–blue and mostly solitary. Like the others, the seed capsules are elongated. G. parryi is multi–stemmed, thick–rooted, and herbaceous in growth. The leaves are lanceolate to ovate. The flowers develop in groups of 1–6 and in terminal or subterminal whorls. They are violet with accenting green bands. The capsules contain smooth brown seeds.

Distribution
From Texas, Minnesota, and Canada, to the Pacific Coast states, Gentiana affinis has a significant range. Look to the moist soils of mountain meadows, grasslands, and foothills. G. calycosa is a mountain–growing plant common to alpine and subalpine areas. Meadows, grassy slopes, and stream banks are its common places. It is found from Canada, Washington, Oregon, and California, east to Montana, Wyoming, and Utah. Limited in distribution, G. parryi is found in southern Wyoming, Utah, and throughout most of the Rocky Mountain region of Colorado. It is a common plant of moist mountain meadows.

Chemistry
Gentiana (general): anthocyanins/anthocyanidins (flowers); flavones; iridoid and secoiridoid glycosides; sterols; triterpenoids.

Medicinal Uses
Considered by many to be the bitter tonic champion of western herbal medicine, Gentian's place is well-deserved, not because it is the strongest bitter, but because it is the purist. It has few secondary attributes that might dilute its focus. For dyspepsia/indigestion related to insufficient gastric secretion, the plant should be considered before others. A dose of tea or tincture before meals will increase proper food breakdown and assimilation via gastric secretory augmentation: essentially Gentian stimulates pepsin, hydrochloric acid, and mucus secretion by the stomach lining. For lowered saliva production that results in a chronically dry mouth, a symptom often related to gastric deficiency, Gentian will be helpful.

For these influences, Gentian is often mixed with an aromatic herb such as Monarda or Field mint for extra vascular stimulation. An aromatic bitter combination is almost always superior to a bitter used alone, though some exceptions include acid reflux or gastritis. In these situations, the combination may prove too stimulating and increase discomfort (try Western mugwort instead).

An often underutilized application of Gentian is as a restorative to digestive response when suppressed (or disrupted) due to anorexia nervosa, orthorexia, temporary feeding tube intervention, and other chronic gastrointestinal traumas. Taken 5–10 minutes before meals (or when a meal should be eaten) Gentian's bitter tonic activity will help to reestablish the body's normal digestive reaction to food.

Another Gentian family plant, Green gentian, will have a more pronounced stimulatory effect on the liver and intestines. Yet Gentian too augments these areas, though indirectly: stimulate upper gastric response enough and lower functions usually follow. Although the plant is only a mild stimulant to hepatic secretions, it is diminishing to liver inflammation. Not quite as profound as Milk thistle or Turmeric, its application as a hepatoprotective in most inflammatory conditions of the area is worthwhile.

Type-2 diabetics and hyperglycemics often find the internal use of Gentian mildly lowering to circulating blood sugar levels. Likely due to the plant's effect on the liver and potentially the pancreas, individuals whom also add diet and exercise changes to their daily routine will see the greatest benefit from Gentian.

Try Gentian topically as an antibacterial/antifungal dressing. The salve or ointment (or the moistened root powder used as a poultice) is a fine preparation, especially for minor injuries that have the potential to become infected.

Indications
- Dyspepsia, asecretory
- As a digestive training aid
- Hyperglycemia
- As an antimicrobial dressing (external)

Collection
Uncomplicated to gather, Gentian's taproot is simple or if belonging to an older plant, forked once or twice. Taste the fresh herbage. If it is bitter it too can be used.

Preparations/Dosage
- FPT/DPT (50% alcohol): 15–30 drops 2–3 times daily
- Root decoction/Cold infusion: 2–4 ounces 2–3 times daily
- Topical preparations: as needed

Cautions
There is little to be concerned about with Gentian. The most likely side effect will be heartburn if used by someone with over-abundant stomach secretions or cardiac sphincter weakness. Individuals suffering from a gastric or duodenal ulcer may also experience some digestive irritation, but in many instances, bitters help here too. If nausea, gastritis, liver tenderness, or diarrhea occurs lessen the dose or try another herb.

Geranium
Geraniaceae/Geranium Family

Geranium caespitosum E. James ex Torr.
Pineywoods geranium, Wild geranium

Geranium richardsonii Fisch. & Trautv.
White geranium, Richardson's geranium

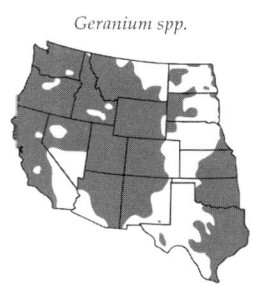

Geranium spp.

Description
Both plants profiled here are small herbaceous sub–shrubs, usually no more than 3' tall by 3' wide. The leaves are deeply lobed to parted. Developing from leaf axils, the long stalks support 5–petaled perfect flowers.

Geranium caespitosum, usually the sparser of the two, is covered by a fine pubescence. The leaves are 5–parted, with each part being divided into 3 lobes. The flowers are composed of 5 disk–arranged purple to pink petals.

Geranium richardsonii's leaves are 2"–5" wide and distinctly lobed with 3–7 divisions. The flowers are somewhat glandular and white to pale pink. The purple veins that develop from each petal's base, radiating towards the tip, are striking when examined closely.

Distribution
Geranium caespitosum is found throughout the inter–mountain West where it commonly frequents Ponderosa pine forests. G. richardsonii has a wider range – both the western mountain and Pacific states host the plant. This species is found at higher elevations and/or associated with mixed conifer/Aspen forests. Both plants prefer woodland margins/forest openings rather than heavy shade.

Chemistry
Geranium (general): phenolic acids: quinic acid, shikimic acid, neochlorogenic acid, chlorogenic acid, ellagic acid; galloylglucoses; ellagitannins; flavonoids: quercetin, myricetin, kaempferol, malvidin.

Medicinal Uses
As a root medicine, Geranium is similar in use to Alumroot, Bistort, Saxifrage, or nearly any other tannin–based plant. Use the tea as a daily oral

rinse if plagued by spongy and bleeding gums[41]. Gargle with it for the short–term relief of a sore throat, especially if the oral tissues are pallid and lax. The isotonic nasal wash is well used in chronic sinusitis, particularly if there is copious mucus discharge.

Like other tannin–containing plants, Geranium is an intestinal binder. Drink the root tea in simple cases of diarrhea. The addition of aromatic herbs such as Monarda or Field mint will be of use if there is accompanying spasm. Used solely or in combination, Geranium will decrease evacuation time, allowing the stool to more fully form. This combination (with Monarda) is also fair in addressing bacterial/protozoal (Giardia/Entamoeba) intestinal infections, though Simaruba and Barberry family plants are typically stronger.

The root tea or tincture is inconsistent when applied to nausea and gastritis. Some find it relieving; others find it unsettling. Start with a small amount. If there is improvement, proceed with a larger dosage.

Use the room temperature tea as a soothing sitz bath for vaginal–area irritations (Geranium is moderately inhibiting to Trichomonas vaginalis). This preparation is also well used as a postpartum toner. It will lessen any passive hemorrhaging and soothe abraded tissues.

As a field poultice Geranium comes in handy if in need of a topical preparation for mild burns, insect bites and stings, and other skin inflammations. Related preparations (wash, fomentation, or the dried powdered root) can be used in a similar fashion.

Indications
- » Sores/Ulcerations, mouth/gum (gargle)
- » Pharyngitis (gargle)
- » Sinusitis, chronic (nasal wash)
- » Diarrhea/Loose stools
- » Nausea/Gastritis
- » Vaginal irritation (external)
- » As a postpartum tonic (external)
- » Insect stings/bites/Rashes (external)

---

41 Poorly healing and easily traumatized tissues often point to a simple nutritional deficiency. Before using herbs to remedy these types of problems first try supplementation with vitamin C, related flavonoids, and essential fatty acids. Even drinking the fresh juice of one or two lemons daily may be enough to make a difference.

Collection

Gather the narrow taproots. Usually cream–pinkish internally, judge a root's potency by chewing on a fresh piece. If astringent, then it will make a good medicine.

If unfamiliar with Geranium and its collection in conifer–Aspen zones, wait until flower development to be certain of its identification – basal leaf growth of Aconite and Larkspur (internally toxic) appear like Geranium.

A less serious point of confusion: most gardeners call plants of the Pelargonium genus, Geranium. Pelargonium includes Scented geranium, Rose geranium, Citrus geranium, etc. Although belonging to the same family, true Geranium and Pelargonium are different plants. No harm will come if Pelargonium is used internally in lieu of Geranium. It essentially is a weaker medicinal analog.

Preparations/Dosage

» Decoction: 4–6 oz. 2–3 times daily
» FPT/DPT (50% alcohol, 10% glycerin): 30–60 drops 2–3 times daily
» Wash/Fomentation/Sitz bath: as needed

Cautions

There is little to be concerned of when using Geranium. It belongs to a family virtually free of toxic plants (at least in North America). Sensitive individuals may experience gastrointestinal and/or renal irritation when using larger amounts long–term – no different than if drinking too much Black/Green tea. During pregnancy keep Geranium use to several days to one week or so at a time.

Goldenrod
Asteraceae/Sunflower Family

Solidago L.
Giant goldenrod, Rocky mountain goldenrod, Western goldenrod, etc.

Solidago spp.

Description
A variable plant with dozens of species throughout the West, Goldenrod is a perennial herb of varying height: from a foot or so to person size. The leaves are simple (generally lance–shaped and linear) and entire or toothed. The yellow inflorescence contains both disk and ray flower types. From simple spikes to spreading arrangements that curl sickle–like, Goldenrod derives its common name from its flowering characteristics. Many species are thicket–forming, arising from extensive subsurface mat–like rhizome networks.

Distribution
Most species of Goldenrod prefer dry and open forests, meadows, and full–sun forest margins. Drier streamsides, draw edges, and ditches are other common places for the plant. Solidago is a circumpolar genus. In the West, except for some Southwestern regions, it's a common plant.

Chemistry
Phenolics: chlorogenic acid, rutin, hyperoside, isoqueritrin, quercitrin; sesquiterpenes; diterpenes; saponins.

Medicinal Uses
One of the main medicinal species of Goldenrod is Solidago canadensis (more of biotype, rather than a specific species), a plant common to the Northeast and northern Midwest. Fortunately, Goldenrod as a group is chemically homogenous (at least the phenolics) with little variation from species to species. In theory, they are all interchangeable; however, the taller species that are somewhat aromatic when crushed will make the best medicines.

Use Goldenrod tea if plagued by chronic nephritis, or more specifically, non–septic autoimmune–related kidney inflammation. More appropriate in long–standing and subacute cases, Goldenrod subtly reduces nephron inflammation. Regular use of the tea improves the filtering ability of compromised nephrons, often lessening high levels of prctein, leukocytes, and erythrocytes in the urine. Don't expect lost kidney function to return, but if plagued by low–level autoimmune/constitutional impairment of the area, Goldenrod will likely do some good. Moreover, it is indicated for difficult to resolve lumbar sensitivity, painful urination, and mucus discharge from related stone or infection involvements.

The hot tea of Goldenrod is a reliable diaphoretic. Here the plant's stimulating sub–aromatics are more noticeable: they reliably promote sweating, particularly if the fever is mid–range and dry.

Indications
» Kidney inflammation, chronic
» Urinary tract inflammation, chronic
» Fever, as a diaphoretic

Collection
Clip the herbage, either in flower or not, when the leaves are new and healthy. Dry it well spaced or placed loosely in a paper bag. Garble the leaves (and flowers) from the stems. Discard the stems and store the garbled material for tea. If aromatic, the roots/rhizomes too can be dried for tea.

Preparations/Dosage
» Infusion: 4–6 oz. 2–3 times daily

Cautions
Goldenrod pollen is a common allergen. If sensitive to the plant, gather the leaf material prior to flowering.

Green Gentian
Gentianaceae/Gentian Family

Frasera speciosa

Frasera speciosa Dougl. ex Griseb. *(Swertia radiata)*
Deer's ears, Elkweed, Monument plant, Cebadilla

Description
A fascinating plant, Green gentian is said to be biannual; however, most are in fact perennial, and for those not growing in optimal conditions, decades can pass before they produce a flowering stalk. Like Agave, once the plant flowers, it dies.

Green gentian is comprised of a large rosette–funnel of obovate to oblanceolate leaves, some reaching 1'–1½' in length. One or more years is needed to pass for the central 3'–8' flowering stalk to develop. Leaf whorls are uniformly spaced at increments along the stalk. The flowers develop in narrow panicles in leaf/stalk junctures. They are 4–lobed, light green, and purple spotted. The fruit is a lobed capsule containing ⅛" long, flat, brown seeds.

Distribution
Look to meadow openings in Aspen–conifer forests throughout the interior western states: from southern Washington, east to Montana and western South Dakota, Green gentian spans south to California, Arizona, New Mexico, and western Texas.

Chemistry
Frasera (general): flavonoids; iridoid and secoiridoid glycosides; sterols; triterpenoids; xanthonoids.

Medicinal Uses
Like many Gentian family plants, Green gentian affects more than just gastric secretion; it also has sway over the intestinal, hepatic, and biliary systems. For dyspepsia/indigestion drink several ounces of the tea or the tincture diluted in water, especially if increased water intake throughout the day does not remedy the situation. The plant increases an array of gut–intestinal secretory components necessary for proper food breakdown and assimilation (and elimination). When mixed with a aromatic carminative

such as Field mint or Monarda, Green gentian will more reliably stimulant surface vasodilation (more blood equals more activity, resulting in a more capable digestive environment).

Consider Green gentian a good therapy for the restoration of proper digestive response after gastrointestinal sickness. Post feeding tube intervention, anorexia nervosa, or even self–induced gastrointestinal deficiencies from a very limited pure diet (orthorexia) are several indications for Green gentian. Taken 5–10 minutes before meals, Green gentian's bitter tonic activity will serve as a digestive training herb.

Green gentian's effect on the liver/gallbladder regions are secondary; however, they align well with its stimulatory nature. As an augmentor of bile synthesis and release, constipation and intestinal stasis from poor secretory response are often improved. In fact, Green gentian can be thought of as a 'pre–laxative': try it before resorting to other directly laxative herbs – Senna, Aloe, Buckthorn, etc.

Borderline type–2 diabetics and hyperglycemics will find Green gentian helpful via its mild blood sugar lowering effects. The tea taken before meals likely influences the liver's role in circulating blood sugar levels, and therefore provides a small but still noticeable lowering effect. For most though, losing excess weight, increasing exercise, and reducing simple carbohydrate intake will have the greatest impact on the situation.

Indications
» Dyspepsia, asecretory
» As a digestive training aid
» Deficiency, hepatic/biliary
» Constipation, mild
» Hyperglycemia

Collection
The plant's stout daikon–like forked tap root can reach depths of three–plus feet. Considering this, most collectors prefer to unearth several smaller plants as opposed to one large plant. The leaf growth gives some (but not always) indication of the root's size.

Green gentian's leaf material is at most half–strength compared to the root, but it is nearly effortless to collect. Grab a leaf by its top and snip with pruners at its base. 6–10 leaves is often enough for 8 ounces of tincture – but a larger drop dose will be needed to match the root's potency.

Preparations

Chop the roots into small pieces. At this point they can be tinctured fresh or dried for later use. I suggest using the tea or dry plant tincture if there is existing liver tenderness. Drying removes some of the root's harshness (see Cautions). I've had at least one collection mold when drying due to the root's high water content. I recommend using a dehydrator.

Dosage

» FPT/DPT (50% alcohol) of root: 20–40 drops 2–3 times daily
» Root decoction/Cold infusion: 3–6 ounces 2–3 times daily

Cautions

Sensitive individuals may experience liver tenderness with fresh root preparations: for some it will be an energetic chologogue/laxative. Dried root preparations are well tolerated and usually problem free. Do not use any part if there is an active liver inflammation or a gallbladder/duct blockage, though suffers of chronic liver inflammation (long-standing hepatitis, cirrhosis, chemical exposure, etc., may see some betterment with the plant). Small sub-laxative doses are acceptable during pregnancy.

Grindelia

Asteraceae/Sunflower Family

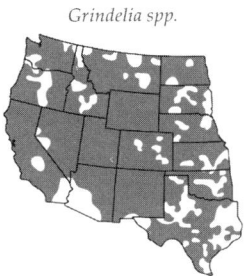

Grindelia spp.

Grindelia squarrosa (Pursh) Dunal
Gumweed, Curlycup gumweed

Grindelia nuda Alph. Wood
Curlytop gumweed

Description

As a biannual or short lived perennial, Grindelia squarrosa stands 1'–3' tall. Older plants are typically multi-stemmed; younger ones may only have a single stem, but both have many-branched tops. The leaf blades are usually toothed (but on occasion they are entire) and oblong to oblanceolate. They are about 2–4 times longer than broad. The flower heads are sticky with resin and composed of sizeable involucres with spreading or recurved phyllaries. Mature flower heads have 25–40 ray florets. Nearly identical in appearance is G. nuda[42]. The only difference it presents is an absence of ray florets. Its flowers are composed of only disk florets.

Distribution
Disturbed soils, roadsides, and open grassy areas are places to find Grindelia squarrosa. Throughout three-fourths of the country, its range is extensive. From California, it is found to Texas, north to Wyoming and further into Canada, finally east to mid and northeastern states. It is absent from most of Southeast.

Grindelia nuda is found throughout the southwestern region of the country. From California, it ranges to the Four Corner states, Texas, Oklahoma, Missouri, and Kansas.

Chemistry
For related Grindelia robusta: essential oils: α-pinene, camphene, β-pinene, p-cimene, limonene, γ-terpinene, cis-pinen-2-ol, p-cymene, terpinolene, α-campholenal, nopinone, camphor, trans-pinocarveol, pinocarvone, isoborneol, borneol, p-cymen-8-ol, terpinen-4-ol, myrtenal, methyl chavicol, myrtenol, verbenone, trans-carveol, cis-carveol, carvone, perilla aldehyde, (e)-anethole, bornyl acetate, δ-elemene, α-cubebene, α-copaene, α-humulene, γ-muurolene, germacrene d, β-selinene, bornyl isovalerate, γ-cadinene, δ-cadinene, germacrene-b, spathulenol, humulene-oxide, t-cadinol, β-eudesmol, calamenol; flavonoids: kaempferol, quercetagetin, quercetin; phenolic acids.

Medicinal Uses
Jesuit Priests along the California Coast first became interested in Grindelia after observing local Indians collect and utilize the plant for various ailments. Over the following centuries, continued experimentation and study led to several Grindelia species becoming official in the United States Pharmacopeia and National Formulary where they remained until the early/mid 1900s.

Long recognized as a lung medicine, Grindelia is useful for a number of chronic to subacute conditions. Indications for the plant are bronchitis with a sense of airway constriction, raw and irritated pectoral membranes, and dry cough. Through the plant's aromatics, bronchial membranes are

---

42 Some classification treatments consider G. nuda not a distinct species, but rather a type of G. squarrosa found in the Southwest.

moistened and microbes are inhibited. Grindelia is usually expectorating in activity. However, in certain situations it can lessen bronchial secretion. Bronchorrhoea in the weakened and aged, due to chronic infection or general lowered vitality, will respond well to the plant.

For those whom suffer from asthma, or at least asthmatic-like breathing as a constitutional tendency, Grindelia will be helpful. The same indicators previously mentioned for the plant's use apply here: constriction, labored breathing, and dry cough or membranes. In these people, Grindelia will ease breathing and be found opening to the lungs. Used solely or combined with Ligusticum, emphysema sufferers should also note a subtle change in tissue oxygenation.

Smoked alone, or with Lobelia and/or Henbane, Grindelia has a prompt opening effect on the spasmodic constriction of an asthma attack. This is not a healing approach, but rather one that gives symptomatic results in acute situations.

Often the case with many aromatic expectorants, the kidneys, bladder, and urethra are all influenced by Grindelia's antimicrobial volatiles. Use it in long-standing chronic infections where irritation, with or without mucus discharge, is the main symptom.

Grindelia's best kept secret is its healing activity on Poison ivy rashes. A century and a half ago, a lotion made by diluting the fluidextract with water (or the fresh plant poultice) was considered a nearly fool-proof application for the condition. Today it still preforms. Apply the ointment to old, poorly healing ulcers, or to any skin condition where repair of the epithelium is necessary. Chronic eczema also responds well to the plant's external application.

Indications
- Bronchitis, with a dry cough
- Bronchitis/Bronchorrhea, chronic
- Asthma, with bronchial irritation
- Urinary tract infection/irritation, chronic
- Poison ivy rash (external)
- Ulcers, skin, chronic (external)
- Eczema, chronic (external)

Collection
Both the flowers and leaves are gathered. However, the strongest medicine comes from the immature flower heads. They are prime when covered with resin in the early/mid–summer.

Preparations/Dosage
» FPT/DPT (70% alcohol): 20–50 drops 2–3 times daily
» Fluidextract: 10–15 drops 2–3 times daily
» Eternal preparations: as needed

Cautions
Due to Grindelia's influence of the bronchial and renal areas, some irritation may be seen with over use. Keep internal dosages low during pregnancy and while nursing.

Grindelia squarrosa/nuda is a known selenium accumulator[43]. For internal uses, I believe there is little to fear from alcoholic preparations (as opposed to animals grazing the whole plant).

Hawthorn
Rosaceae/Rose Family

Crataegus erythropoda Ashe
Cerro hawthorn

Crataegus rivularis Nutt.
River hawthorn

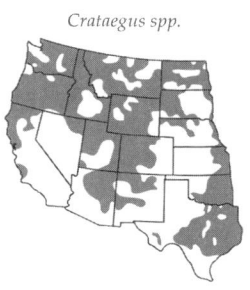

Crataegus spp.

Description
Growing to be a large bush to small tree, both species (and most others) are outfitted with stout thorns. Hawthorn's leaf structure is variable: Crataegus erythropoda has an ovate leaf blade that is slightly less than twice as long as wide. Its leaf serrations are non–uniform. C. rivularis's leaves are twice as long as wide, more or less elliptic, and are also irregularly serrated. Both plants have 5–petaled, white to pinkish flowers, which form in branch end

---

43 Problems have been reported for livestock when grazing on Grindelia growing in high–selenium soils (much of Colorado, central Nevada, Montana, North Dakota, and coastal–southern California).

corymbs. The mature fruit is red (usually) to purple, large pea–sized, seed filled, mealy, and semi–sweet.

Distribution
Crataegus erythropoda ranges from northern Arizona and New Mexico to eastern Colorado, southeastern Utah, and Wyoming. C. rivularis has a more expansive western range. Common to most interior western states, the plant is found from Montana to Arizona, New Mexico, and Texas. In certain areas, their ranges overlap. Both species are found along mid–mountain streams and creeks.

Chemistry
Flavonoids: hyperoside, vitexin; procyanidins.

Medicinal Uses
With almost no cardiovascular ailment uninfluenced by Hawthorn, the plant's broad application is impressive. The reason the plant affects so many heart issues is because nearly every problem can be benefited when the organ is coaxed to function more efficiently.

Hawthorn particularly affects the coronary artery and muscle fibers of the heart. Because it subtly increases coronary artery blood flow, heart tissue nutrition and oxygenation are augmented. Due to this influence, even the small vessel networks within the heart are positively affected. The tea or tincture's effect is particularly noticeable if the heart or related vascular tissue has been damaged from ischemia or infraction.

One of Hawthorn signature indications is weak and devitalized heart action due to cardiovascular disease. Vascular dynamics (blood movement) are affected positively: similar to Garlic, peripheral vascular resistance is decreased. With Hawthorn, blood literally passes through the vessels with less drag. This results in a more efficient cardiovascular environment.

Partly due to Hawthorn's flavonoid portion, its net effect is cardio-protective. Specifically, in states of blood/oxygen deficiency, it increases cell death tolerance while improving myocardial performance. Hawthorn protects and preserves cell membranes, which ultimately diminishes and wards against heart damage.

The plant's influence on the heart beat is positively inotropic, yet negatively chronotropic: the force of the heart's contraction is increased while the rate is decreased. The organ's activity steadies and becomes more efficient.

Because of this, its application is worthwhile in most arrhythmia disturbances, or erratic action of the heart. Additionally, if the heart is under exaggerated sympathetic influence, usually the rate is slowed with Hawthorn. Likewise, if the organ is stressed from disease or hypertension, the heart rate too will decease to a healthier level.

Due to Hawthorn's increase in blood delivery to the heart, and its influence of the myocardium, incidence of angina pectoris and associated shortness of breath, discomfort, and chest oppression are reduced. I have observed significant results with both mitral and aortic valve regurgitations: the plant's effect is not so much on the malformed valve, but rather on the heart's ability of compensation. It is impressive to see an individual's cardiac output scored at stage III before Hawthorn, then stage II while drinking 24 oz. of tea daily, with no adjunctive pharmaceutical treatment. Of course Hawthorn has limits. I have observed the plant having little effect on other valve situations and on SA/AV node disturbances.

High blood pressure (as a symptom of arteriosclerosis or valve/structural problems) is often reduced (10–20%). Both systolic and diastolic readings are influenced, and heart rates during Hawthorn supplementation usually fall approximately 10% as well. These indicators point to a reduced workload; exercise tolerance and anaerobic threshold increase, indicating the heart can do more with less stress on the myocardium.

Some secondary problems associated with cardiovascular disease, or just plain and simple old hearts, are benefited by Hawthorn: pulmonary edema, edema of the extremities, and even chronic indigestion due to vascular deficiency are bettered to varying degrees; however, depending on the issue's severity, often stronger heart herbs (Convallaria or Dogbane for instance) will be needed.

Whether suffering from atherosclerosis or wishing to prevent the condition, Hawthorn is one of the best herbal remedies we have. Its vascular protective effects have direct influence on arterial wall elasticity and health. Cell membrane permeability, adhesion, leukocyte activity, and other inflammatory factors are positively influenced by Hawthorn.

The fresh plant tincture of the fruit has a marked effect on emotional states associated with grief and loss. To varying degrees, gloom, heartache, and depression are lifted. It is not uncommon for those whom have suffered a severe loss to have physical symptoms of heart distress, such as palpitation, oppression, pain, and shortness of breath. In conventional circles this symptom set is referred to as takotsubo cardiomyopathy, stress cardiomyopathy, or 'broken heart syndrome' – a temporary period of heart distress that includes myocardial enlargement and irregular/inefficient activity caused by stress hormones. Hawthorn will lighten the emotions, as well as counter related physical symptoms.

Lastly, due to Hawthorn's significant flavonoid content, it will be supportive of varicose conditions. Like Rose hips, under its influence tissue permeability will decrease, resulting in improved venous return and overall performance. For this purpose, take Hawthorn if suffering from venous problems in conjunction with cardiovascular issues. If there is no underlying heart problem then try Rose hips, for Hawthorn's cardiovascular effects are unneeded.

Indications
» Arrhythmia
» Tachycardia
» Angina pectoris
» Regurgitation, valvular
» Hypertension
» Atherosclerosis
» Stress cardiomyopathy
» Varicosities

Collection
The leaves, flowers, and berries are all medicinally active, though the berries are longest in traditional use (I also prefer the fruit over the other parts). Collect the young leaves and flowers (equal proportions) in the spring and the ripe berries in late summer.

Preparations
Hawthorn lends itself to most preparations. The recent fresh plant tincture has the most profound emotional effect.

Dosage
» FPT/DPT (60% alcohol): 30–60 drops 2–3 times daily
» Berry/Leaf/Flower infusion: 4–8 oz. 2–3 times daily

Cautions

Heart pharmaceutical dosing may need to be adjusted if used in conjunction with Hawthorn, otherwise there is little to no caution associated with its use.

Hedeoma
Lamiaceae/Mint Family

Hedeoma spp.

Hedeoma Pers.
False pennyroyal, Mock pennyroyal, Western pennyroyal

Description
Hedeoma is a small, herbaceous annual or perennial with pubescent and aromatic foliage. Its opposite leaves are linear to lanceolate, often entire, but sometimes toothed. Both the calyx and corolla are tubular, 2–lipped, and 5–lobed. Most species have purple to blue flowers; several are almost white.

Distribution
Except for Washington, Idaho, most of Oregon and California, and much of Nevada, Hedeoma is a common western plant. Most species are found throughout New Mexico and Texas, around mountain–woodlands (below alpine but above desert elevations), hillsides, and next to draws and gullies. Hedeoma drummondii is one of the wider ranging species.

Chemistry
Volatiles for Hedeoma drummondii: α–pinene, β–pinene, camphene, myrcene, limonene, menthone, isomenthone, 4–terpineol, isopulegone, menthol, pulegone, borneol.

Medicinal Uses
Like other native pulegone–containing herbs (Monardella and Poliomintha), consider Hedeoma a weaker medicinal version of true Pennyroyal (Mentha pulegium). Much of its physiological effect, at least on the female reproductive system, is due to its volatile oil element.

One of Hedeoma oblongifolia's (Poléo chino or Nana–pennyroyal) historical uses (other species are similar) among isolated mountain–dwelling Spanish New Mexicans, was as a stimulating emmenagogue. Drink the hot tea or tincture in hot water when menses is slow to start, particularly if there is associated pelvic cramping with an overall sense of regional congestion (it combines well with Yellow pond lily). If a hot compress helps, it is likely that Hedeoma will as well.

Try a stout cup of tea if there is stomach bloating with indigestion. Most find it soothing via its expelling effect on trapped gas and mild anesthetic effect on the stomach lining.

The hot tea is a diaphoretic. Drink a cup or two if trying to break a dry, mild to moderate fever. Taking a hot bath and keeping warm in bed will further assist the body's natural infection–fighting process (an elevated temperate is not a disease symptom but rather the body's response to foreign invaders). Diaphoretic herbs essentially speed up what the body is already attempting on its own.

A Hedeoma wash is mildly antiseptic towards a range of bacteria and fungi. The essential oil of Hedeoma applied topically, diluted in equal portions of olive oil, will have the strongest antimicrobial effect.

Indications
- Menstruation, slowed, with regional congestion
- Indigestion with gas and bloating
- Fever, dry, mild to moderate temperature
- As a mild antiseptic (external)

Collection
Hedeoma is time consuming to collect, not because the process is inherently difficult, but because one leafing stem weighs about the same as *one* blade of grass. If a dense bunch is stumbled upon, consider yourself lucky. Gather the top half of leafing/flowering stems.

Preparations/Dosage
- FPT/DPT (50% alcohol): 30–60 drops 2–3 times daily
- Infusion: 4–6 oz. 2–3 times daily
- Essential oil: 1–2 drops 2–3 times daily
- Spirit: 10–20 drops 2–3 times daily
- External preparations: as needed

Cautions

Do not use Hedeoma during pregnancy or large amounts while nursing. 1–2 drops of the essential oil is a fine replacement for a dose of tincture or a cup of tea, but more may irritate the kidneys.

Henbane

Solanaceae/Nightshade Family

Hyoscyamus niger L.
Black henbane, Common henbane, Hairy henbane, Stinking roger

Description

An herbaceous annual or biannual, Henbane stands several feet high at maturity. The entire plant is viscid–glandular (and odiferous) with varying length hair. Depending on growing locale/variant some specimens are sparsely pubescent and others are notably hairy. The leaves are sessile and sharply lobed to sinuate. The flower's 5 petals are united and funnel–form. Visually striking, they are yellow–cream with purple veins. The capsules are pitcher–shaped and hold many small brown seeds.

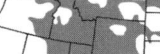

Hyoscyamus niger

Distribution

An Old World native, waif to sometimes invasive plant, Henbane's core area is Idaho, Montana, and Wyoming. In these states and surrounding areas, it's often listed as a noxious weed. Henbane is almost always found in once–disturbed soils such as old fields, pastures, and roadsides.

Chemistry

Tropane alkaloids: anisodamine, hyoscyamine, scopolamine; pyrrolidine alkaloid: cuscohygrine.

Medicinal Uses

Known to herbal doctors of the past as a plant not to be trifled with, Henbane joins Datura and Belladonna as an alkaloid–rich drug–herb capable of providing decisive symptomatic relief for several troubling issues. Rich in tropane alkaloids, nearly all of Henbane's effects are due to its anticholinergic influence of the peripheral and central nervous systems.

Henbane's safest and most reliable utilization is its topical application to most things painful and swollen. The ointment or liniment are fine preparations for pain relief from contusions, bruises, and blows. It's an effective choice as a post–workout martial–arts liniment. For arthritic joints, chronic neuralgias, and headache pain try a warm fomentation made with the strongly brewed tea. A liniment–soaked cloth can be applied as well to the same problems if the warmth of the fomentation is contraindicated. Upon availability of the fresh plant, the juice from the crushed leaf (or a fresh leaf poultice) too can be topically applied for similar issues. A suppository made with equal parts of Henbane and Sweet clover oil makes a successful hemorrhoid treatment. 1–2 drops (no more) of the tincture, as an ear drop, is an effective earache treatment.

Henbane's internal use is not caution free, but if approached with sensibility, the herb will provide relief for a number of spasmolytic problems. To proceed safely, for an average–weighted adult start with 5–10 drops of the tincture in a little water as a beginning dose. For sensitive individuals one internal dose will be adequate; for others, several may be needed. Once the first dose is imbibed, wait 20 minutes and monitor yourself for a lessening of symptoms. Continue with a second dose of 5–10 drops only if needed and no toxic symptoms have developed (see Cautions). Continue with a third if need be, though any more than three 10 drop doses in a span of an hour will most likely produce several unwanted side effects.

Spastic diarrhea, in cases of food poisoning, irritable bowel syndrome, and even herbicide/insecticide exposure, will lessen with Henbane. It should be especially considered if emptying has become exhausting and evacuations are water–like.

Consider Henbane for the relief of motion/sea sickness, other forms of nausea, and vomiting, especially dry–heaves, where the offending contents have already been voided.

Menstrual cramps and ovarian pain will be calmed, and too, if a menstrual–type headache has developed during this phase of the cycle, then Henbane will be of use. Yellow pond lily or Western peony (or Cramp bark/Black haw) should be employed first; however, if they are found ineffective, try Henbane.

For spasmodic coughing and asthmatic constriction, Henbane is quieting and opening, though if there is excessive mucus (humid asthma) Datura (similar cautions) is more specific. Even in wintertime (or allergy–induced) bronchitis where the cough is dry, irritative, and barking, it will bring relief (Henbane was once used as a bronchial sedative in pertussis/whooping cough). For these issues, it combines well with Wild cherry.

The urinary tract (kidneys, bladder, ureters, and urethra) is another area that is influenced by Henbane. Used in the past for constriction, pain, and spasm, usually due to stone passage, its wisest application these days is to irritation, congestion, and frequent urination (or the urge to urinate without much urine).

As a central nervous system sedative, I am hesitant to recommend it, as there are so many other effective herbal sedatives that lack the risk of Henbane. However, with herbs like this one (drug–herb), where there is a greater potential for toxicity, there exists also a greater certainly of action. Using the same dosing schedule as outlined earlier, take Henbane before bed if suffering from insomnia dependent on mental agitation or tissue irritation, especially if the already–mentioned issues are inhibiting sleep. Be careful though, along with unwanted physical symptoms, larger doses of Henbane before bed may cause negative dreams and alternating feelings of depression/paranoia – see Cautions.

Indications
- » Parasympathetic/cholinergic functions, to suppress
- » Pain/Inflammation/Swelling (external)
- » Diarrhea/Spasm, intestinal
- » Nausea/Vomiting
- » Cramps, uterine/ovarian
- » Cough, with constriction/irritation
- » Spasm/Constriction/Irritation, urinary tract
- » Insomnia, with agitation and tissue irritation

Collection
The entire plant is active – the stems are the least potent and seeds the most. The leaves and flowering/budding tops are the traditional articles of the old drug trade and the dosage recommendation of 5–10 drops of the tincture pertains to these parts. Some accounts state that the seeds are 10 times more potent than the other parts...use the seeds at your own risk. Prune the leafing–flowering tops and dry them normally for wash, fomentation, or dried plant tincture preparations, or tincture the tops fresh.

Preparations

As opposed to infusing the herb for tea and having potencies vary from brew to brew, the tincture is more consistent in potency and therefore better suited for internal use (each new tincture batch should be tested to dial–in its potency – some will be 3 drops per does, others 5 or 10).

A sensible approach to the tincture's storage (and dispensing) is its dilution. For instance, if the fresh plant tincture (which contains approximately 80% alcohol) is diluted with 10 parts of an alcohol (80%)/water (20%) solution, then 50 drops (½ teaspoon) would equal 5 drops of the base tincture. This is not an uncommon practice for high–potency tinctures. The increased per–dose volume/dilution serves as an extra safety feature.

Topical preparations, particularly headache applications, if applied long enough, will cause systemic effects. If subtle vision changes, 'spaced–out' feelings, and mouth dryness manifest, it's best to remove the preparation.

Dosage

» FPT/DPT (50% alcohol): 5–10 drops 1–3 times a day
» External preparations: 1–3 times a day

Cautions

Henbane's effects are dose–dependent. Small amounts (as recommended) are generally sedative on muscular/nerve fibers. Larger amounts act as stimulants to the same areas. For instance, low/high internal dosage is the difference between antispasmodic and spasmodic; between slowed heart rate and raised; between sedation and agitation; between relaxation and constriction. Henbane is not an herb that produces more of the same as the dosage increases. In many cases, it causes the opposite.

Do not use Henbane during pregnancy or while breast feeding (if ingested during this time, some of the plant's tropane alkaloids will be passed to the baby via the mother's milk). Henbane users should be generally healthy and preferably not taking pharmaceuticals, but especially drugs related to seizures, muscle spasms, incontinence, depression/anxiety, mental illness, Parkinson's, and dementia/Alzheimer's.

Dry mouth, heat flush sensations, pupil dilation, altered audio–visual perceptions and heart rate (usually slowed) are several low–level overdose reactions to be aware of. Large overdose (the accidental ingestion of a quarter–ounce or more of the tincture) may result in temporary paralysis, convulsions, gastroenteritis, fever, tachycardia, arrhythmia, memory loss, hallucinations, and psychotic behavior. With the ingestion of very large amounts, death occurs (rarely) due to respiratory paralysis.

It should be clear that Henbane is a drug masquerading as an herb. Approach it with the prudence it deserves. It's not an herb to have in proximity of foolish or ignorant people. KEEP HENBANE OUT OF THE REACH OF CHILDREN.

Hollyhock
Malvaceae/Mallow Family

Alcea rosea

Alcea rosea L. *(Althaea rosea)*
Common hollyhock

Description
A large herbaceous perennial, Hollyhock develops a stout central stem which produces many large, alternating, serrate, lobed leaves. Both the leaves and stem are covered by short appressed hairs. The showy flower spike is comprised of numerous, large, 5–petaled flowers. Depending on cultivar they are various shades of pink, red, purple to yellow and white. The disk–shaped capsules contain many seeds.

Distribution
Hollyhock is thought to be native to southwestern China; however, wild plants appear to be nonexistent or lacking, making the plant's place of origin more estimation than fact. Today, Hollyhock is found either cultivated or feral almost worldwide. In America, it does best in temperate regions (common throughout the mountain states) as a planted ornamental. In this context, it is common and widespread. As an occasional escapee, it is encountered infrequently.

Chemistry
Malvaceae general: various polysaccharides (pectin, mucilage, and starch), namely arabinogalactans; tannins; anthocyanins/anthocyanidins.

Medicinal Uses

Marshmallow's lesser known counterpart, Hollyhock, influences the lungs, urinary tract, skin, and immunity. Users find benefit from the tea for beginning stage bronchitis when the lungs and throat feel hot and irritated. Relatedly, due to its reduction of tissue irritation and bronchial inflammation, most find it soothing if there is an unproductive cough. Combined with an antimicrobial herb such as White sage, Eucalyptus, or Monarda, Hollyhock also makes as excellent sore throat gargle.

Due to Hollyhock's polysaccharide content, it provides a mild immunological boast to the bronchial area. The plant's immunologic mucilages (mainly arabinogalactan and other related compounds) serve to heighten lung immunity by stimulating alveolar macrophages (dust cells). This in turn makes the bronchial region more resilient and active, particularly if there is an infection.

Urethral and bladder irritation responds well to Hollyhock. Urinary tract tissues are soothed with the plant's use; however, if there is an active infection, the situation will be better addressed with the addition of an appropriate urinary tract antibacterial herb such as Uva–ursi or Juniper. Occasionally suffers of interstitial cystitis or poorly defined chronic bladder irritation will find some relief with regular use of the tea.

Hollyhock makes an excellent emollient poultice. Its overall soothing and softening influence is useful in reducing injury swelling, bringing abscesses to a head, and urging splinters to slowly gravitate to the skin's surface. The powdered leaf also is used as a base material for poultice combinations.

Indications

» Bronchitis, with an irritative cough
» As a general cold/flu tea with lung involvement
» Irritation, urinary tract
» As a soothing poultice

Collection

Collect Hollyhock's herbaceous portions in the spring or summer when its growth is full and new. Both leaves and flowers are active. The roots are gathered year–round. Before drying them for tea, discard the woody parts.

Preparations
To prepare the poultice, slowly stir enough hot water into the dried and powdered herb/root so a pudding–like consistency is obtained. Place this glob in several folds of cheesecloth or flannel and then apply it to the affected area (after it has sufficiently cooled – but is still warm). Cover it with a warm damp towel. Repeat the process as needed.

Dosage
» Infusion (cold or standard): 4–8 oz. 2–3 times daily
» Poultice: as needed

Cautions
There are no cautions for normal usage.

Hops
Cannabaceae/Hemp Family

Humulus lupulus var. neomexicanus

Humulus lupulus var. neomexicanus A. Nelson & Cockerell
Western hops

Description
Like its cultivated European relative (var. lupulus), Hops is a perennial twining vine. Oppositely arranged, its leaves are coarse, serrated, palmate, and 3–7 parted. The upper surfaces are very rough; the lower sides are distinctly yellow–gland dotted. The small male flowers are 5–parted and held in loose panicles. The female flowers are borne in pairs and surrounded by numerous persistent bracts that when mature, appear cone or catkin–like. Like the leaves, they are gland dotted (base of cone bracts) and hang interspersed throughout the foliage. The entire plant, especially the female flowers, is aromatic.

Distribution
Hops' range stretches from Montana south to Arizona, New Mexico, and western Texas. It's mostly a plant of the middle to upper mountains, where it grows along drainages climbing over support shrubs. Lacking these, it

appears as a leafy ground cover, vining over dry streambed rocks or mountainside scree.

Chemistry

For Humulus lupulus var. lupulus (var. neomexicanus similar): terpenes: β–caryophyllene, farnesene, humulene, myrcene; bitter acids: α–acids: humulone, cohumulone, adhumulone; β–acids: lupulone, colupulone, adlupulone; chalcones: xanthohumol, isoxanthohumol, desmethylxanthohumol, prenylnaringenin; flavonol glycosides: kaempferol, quercetin, quercitrin, rutin; catechins: catechin gallate, epicatechin gallate.

Medicinal Uses

The medicinal uses of native North American varieties[44] are patterned after European Hops. Although potency differences likely exist, this variance can be reduced by collection timing: the more bitter, aromatic, and sticky the strobiles, the more analogous medicinal uses will be.

As an age–old sedative, Hops' use is broadly indicated by central nervous system excitability. Use it to allay sleeplessness, insomnia, and nervous tension (particularly for women if associated with perimenopausal complaints). Some find its sedative qualities similar to Valerian's, particularly if dried (upon drying lupamaric and lupulinic acids are converted to isovaleric acid). Hops also combines well with Valerian.

Belonging to a family known for its hormonal–like influences, traditional lore suggests that female collectors often started menses early after several days of stobiles gathering. Relatedly, Hops is thought to diminish estrogen deficiency complaints, such as perimenopausal issues (hot flashes, irritability, sleeplessness, irregular menorrhea etc.) But, the problem with relying upon Hops for relief of these varying issues is that there is little predictability in exactly how or to what degree Hops' estrogenic compounds interact with hormonal receptors sites. Do they inhibit, compete, or replace innate estrogen, and for how long? However much we wish this herb to have a clear effect on the matter – it does not.

For young men/teens of nervous/excitable temperament, whom are obsessively preoccupied (more so than usual) by sexual thoughts and excessive wet dreams (nocturnal emission), Hops is worth a try. It best reduces

---

44 Aside from var. neomexicanus profiled here, var. lupuloides and var. pubescens are the two other native varieties. Just as useful, they are found in more eastern parts of the country.

this tendency when there is associated mental irritability and possibly genital or bladder irritation. For males Hops tends to be an anaphrodisiac; for women, especially if estrogen-deficient, Hops will be a mild aphrodisiac. It is a sensible premise that Hops' effect here is due to some combined hormonal-nervous system influence.

As an aromatic bitter, those whom suffer from asecretory indigestion, especially if triggered by stress, will benefit from Hops. Taken before meals it stimulates mouth and gut secretions, both essential to proper food digestion and assimilation. It's also worth noting that Hops tends to reduce gastric ulcer formation. Its antibacterial volatile oil content, which is inhibiting to Helicobacter pylori, is likely responsible for this.

Effective against an array of gram-positive bacteria (some strains of Micrococcus, Staphylococcus, Mycobacterium, and Streptomycetes) and fungi (Candida albicans, Trichophyton, Fusarium, and Mucor strains), use Hops as an antibacterial/antifungal wash for cuts, scrapes, and as a general disinfectant. In lieu of the strobiles, the leaves made into a tea or powder are also well applied to these infections.

Hops can be utilized as three related but distinct parts. They are as follows: strobiles (female flowers or the 'hops'), foliage, and resin glands (known as lupulinum or lupulin). The female flowers, certainly the best known part, contain the most balanced mix of attributes. They are equally sedative, stomachic, and antimicrobial. One drawback to flower use is its bulkiness: 1 ounce in weight seems to take up about 8 oz. of space. Hops foliage, primarily composed of leaf material, is less sedative, but still stomachic and antibacterial. Lastly lupulinum, the dislodged resin glands found on the strobile and leaf: this yellowish powder is most noticeable at the bottom of the bagged or jarred flowers. In all medicinal aspects, the isolated resin glands are the strongest part of Hops.

Indications

- » Insomnia
- » Nervousness/Anxiety
- » Perimenopausal complaints
- » As an anaphrodisiac (men)
- » Gastritis/Indigestion
- » Ulcer, gastric
- » Cuts/Scrapes (external)

Collection

The female strobiles mature mid to late summer. They'll be sticky and aromatic when ready to collect. The foliage is gathered from male and/or female plants. Hops' resin glands are sifted from the dried foliage and flowers. Put the dried herb/flowers in a plastic bag or jar and shake the container vigorously. Collect the yellowish sediment at the container's bottom, then prepare it as indicated below.

Preparations

All parts of Hops tend to degrade quickly after drying. Optimally, use the dried material within 6 months of collection. Prepare the resin gland powder as a dry plant tincture. This part/preparation will be the strongest sedative. The fresh plant tincture of the flowers is subtler yet broad in effect. It is best suited for everyday use.

Dosage

- » FPT/DPT of flowers/foliage (60% alcohol): 30–60 drops 2–3 times daily
- » Fluidextract of flowers/foliage: 10–20 drops 2–3 times daily
- » DPT of resin glands (70% alcohol): 20–40 drops 2–3 times daily
- » Flower/Foliage infusion: 3–6 oz. 2–3 times daily

Cautions

Its occasional use during pregnancy or while nursing is not a problem; however, consistent use (or mega doses) should be avoided during these times. Although the plant's estrogenic qualities are minor, there's really no way of knowing how the plant combines with a complex mother/baby chemistry.

Other Uses

For some a Hops' pillow, made with the flowers, can be nearly miraculous at producing sleep. This is likely the best first–try method for people whom may be repulsed by Hops' bitter taste or skittish of herbs in general. The plant's aromatics are likely responsible for the pillow's effect.

Hoptree
Rutaceae/Rue Family

Ptelea crenulata, trifoliata

Ptelea crenulata Greene
California hoptree

Ptelea trifoliata L.
Wafer ash, Wingseed, Shrubby trefoil, Prairie grub

Description
Hoptree grows to be a small tree to large shrub. Its plum–colored bark is in distinct contrast to its bright green trifoliate leaves. Depending on species/subspecies, they are shiny to hairy and when crushed emit a pleasant citrus–like scent. The flowers are 4–petaled, greenish–white, and fragrant. Hoptree's fruit are flat and each is surrounded by a straw–colored ovoid wing.

Distribution
Ptelea crenulata, the more limited in distribution of the two species, is found mainly throughout northern–central California among woodland and scrub vegetation. P. trifoliata, often divided into four separate subspecies, is wide–ranging. From Arizona and Utah, it extends to Minnesota, Florida, Maine, and Canada. Rocky streamsides, hillsides, and ravine sides are common sites for the plant.

Chemistry
Ptelea trifoliata: furanocoumarins: bergapten, isopimpinellin, imperatorin; quinoline alkaloids: isopteleforine, ptelefolidine, ptelefoline, ptelefructine, ptelefolidone, o–methylptelefolonium; volatile oils.

Medicinal Uses
Half of what Hoptree is useful for can be discerned by its unmistakable aromatic citrus–like scent. The other half of the plant's therapeutic influence is gleaned once a leaf is tasted: bitter. Mainly an herbal medicine for the gastrointestinal tract, use the tea or tincture for problems of gastric deficiency and weakness. Stimulating to gastric/intestinal secretions and blood movement in these tissues, Hoptree best fits issues of chronic gastrointestinal

sluggishness. A cup of tea or dose of tincture diluted in a little water before meals will stimulate the area so food is better digested. Assimilation and nutrient absorption within the small intestine are also augmented. The plant is well-applied towards area constitutional deficiencies. It also has use in reestablishing normal gastrointestinal patterns if recovering from regional surgery, transitioning back to solid food, or even when reestablishing a regular eating pattern after an acute anorectic episode.

In the late 1800s it was reported that Hoptree contained berberine. This report is suspect since (to my knowledge) the report has not been duplicated. Nevertheless, Hoptree combines well with true berberine-containing herbs such as Oregongrape, Barberry, or Coptis for gastrointestinal microbial complaints (food poisoning). It accents these stronger antimicrobials with its aromatic-carminative qualities, which most find settling to residual nausea. However, some people find this combination just too bitter and actually nausea-promoting. If this is the case, substitute 10 drops of Monarda spirt (or 60 drops of the tincture) for Hoptree. Silk tassel too can be added if spastic diarrhea is a symptom.

As an anthelmintic, combine Hoptree with Sagebrush (as a 1:1 combination or the tincture added to Sagebrush tea). 3-4 cups of tea a day for initial pinworm and roundworm infestations is a basic plan; however, for advanced infections pharmaceutical antiparasitic treatment may be necessary.

Sufferers of bronchial constriction and shortened breathing (non-emergency), whether related to asthma or environmental/allergic reaction, often see an opening effect with Hoptree. It's unknown whether it is inflammation-reducing or directly antispasmodic; either way the herb's application here has historical precedence.

Indications
» Deficiency, gastrointestinal
» Indigestion/Dyspepsia, chronic
» As a recovery herb, post gastrointestinal trauma
» Food poisoning, as a mild antimicrobial/carminative
» Infection, pinworm/roundworm
» Bronchial constriction, asthma-like

Collection
Both the leaves/immature fruit and root bark are active. The leaves are the simplest to gather: grasp a leafing bunch at its branch end and snip. Along

with this part's ease of collection, the plant's pleasant citrus–like aromatics become quite apparent when the leaves are handled. For root bark collection, I recommend digging a number of smaller trees – sapling sized.

Too bad Hoptree does not taste like it smells. Bitter! For the would-be essential oil distiller, this is a plant of significant potential. Since its bitterness is less associated with its aromatic fraction, the essential oil will be more aromatic carminative and less bitter stimulation.

Preparations/Dosage
- » FPT/DPT (65% alcohol): 20–40 drops 2–3 times daily
- » Infusion: 2–4 oz. 2–3 times daily
- » Spirit: 5–10 drops 2–3 times daily

Cautions
Skin rashes have been reported with heavy internal use. It's possible that this has a connection to the plant's furanocoumarin content (or another constituent group). Pregnant or breast feeding mothers and babies should forgo Hoptree's use – it's a chemically complex plant (with affiliations to Rue/Ruta).

Other Uses
I've had good results with topically applying the spirit as an insect repellent (mosquitoes). Its effect seems to only last an hour or so, making semi–frequent reapplication necessary. It's possible that the spirit's/essential oil's performance will be better if used as part of a formula (with Citronella for instance).

Per an 1879 issue of The Gardener's Chronicle, German settlers in Texas around 1860 began to use Ptelea fruit as an occasional replacement for Hops in beer brewing (which then lead to one of the tree's main common names).

Horsetail
Equisetaceae/Horsetail Family

Equisetum arvense L. *(Equisetum boreale, E. calderi, E. saxicola)*
Common horsetail, Canutillo

Equisetum arvense

Description
Like other Equisetum species, Horsetail emerges from underground spreading rhizomes. Arising in early spring, the fertile stems are topped by spore filled cones. They are flesh–colored and 6"–1' tall. Developing shortly after, the infertile stems have numerous whorls of small jointed branchlets. They appear as upturned cylindrical feather dusters.

Distribution
Horsetail is common throughout much of the West. Look for it along streams, in moist soils, and in drainage areas.

Chemistry
Flavonoids: chlorogenic acid, kaempferol, dihydrokaempferol, hydroxycinnamic acid, equisetumpyrone, quercetin, protogenkwanin, gossypetin, luteolin, apigenin, protoapigenin, genkwanin, naringenin; silicic acid, silica, calcium, potassium, phosphorus.

Medicinal Uses
Mainly a urinary tract medicine, Horsetail is used to diminish bladder/renal irritability. Soothing to painful urination, internal preparations are both diuretic and lithotropic. As a daily tea, kidney stone formation is reduced through the plant's ability of increasing urine volume.

Although its mechanism of action is not completely understood, Horsetail lessens passive hemorrhaging. Use it if there is blood in the urine from physical injury or gastrointestinal bleeding from minor ulceration. Internal preparations may even be useful if there is blood–tinged sputum from a severe cough.

Topically and internally, Horsetail facilitates wound healing and tissue repair. This is mainly due to its flavonoid, silica, and silicic acid contents. Use the plant to strengthen the hair, nails, skin and connective tissues. It also makes a good tea for fortifying bones, whether damaged by injury or weakened from osteoporosis.

Indications
- Urination, painful
- Kidney stones, as a preventative
- Hemorrhaging, passive
- Ulceration, gastrointestinal
- Weakened hair, nails, skin, bones, and connective tissues
- Wounds (external and internal)

Collection
Horsetail has the highest quercetin quantities in its new spring growth – approximately 50% of its total flavonoid content. As spring changes to summer, the plant's quercetin quickly diminishes.

Clip the stems at their bases and use them fresh (juice) or dry. After drying, the stems are easily garbled into 1"–2" sections for storage.

Preparations/Dosage
- Fresh juice: ½–1 oz. 2–3 times daily
- Herb infusion: 2–4 oz. 2–3 times daily
- Poultice: as needed

Cautions
Do not collect and use the plant around contaminated areas: when exposed to common agricultural chemicals, Horsetail has been known to produce several toxic compounds. In addition, excessive quantities of the tea or juice may irritate the kidneys.

Hound's Tongue
Boraginaceae/Borage Family

Cynoglossum officinale L.
Gypsyflower

Cynoglossum officinale

Description
A biannual herb, Hound's tongue's first year of growth is composed of a floppy basal clutch of oblanceolate leaves, with each leaf resembling a panting 'hound's tongue'. Like the rest of the plant, they are sub–glandular and musky scented. Its second year of growth is mostly stem oriented. The stem leaves are acute, sessile, and pubescent (the stem too). The small flowers are purplish–red and form in cymes. The seeds are ovoid, flattened, bristly, and stick to clothing once dried.

Distribution
Common throughout the interior western states, look for this European native in disturbed soils: roadsides, field sides, and forest edges. Most states list the plant as a noxious weed as it can be invasive in pastures and fields (and sicken grazing animals).

Chemistry
Allantoin; pyrrolizidine alkaloids: trachelanthamine, viridiflorine, rinderine, echinatine, 3'–acetylechinatine, amabiline, 7–angeloylheliotridine, heliosupine.

Medicinal Uses
Hounds's tongue is a topically applied vulnerary, essentially identical in use to Comfrey. Due to its allantoin concentration, it is best used as a mender of wounds, ulcerations, and cuts. Additionally, it excels as a burn dressing and healer of residual tissue disruption from bites, stings, and outbreaks.

Not to be used internally, Hound's tongue contains a number of hepatotoxic pyrrolizidine alkaloids, often in concentrations higher than Russian comfrey. Grazing animals usually avoid the fresh plant, but if enough of it is accidentally included in hay, it can cause poisonings.

Indications
» Wounds/Ulcers/Burns/Bites (external)

Collection
The entire plant is active, but the large first year leaves lend themselves best to collection and preparation. Use the herbaceous material fresh (poultice) or dry for oil, salve, or ointment preparations.

Preparations/Dosage
» Topical preparation: as needed

Cautions
There are no cautions for external use. Do not use Hound's tongue internally.

Juniper
Cupressaceae/Cypress Family

Juniperus communis L. *(Juniperus canadensis)*
Common juniper

Juniperus communis

Description
An evergreen, low–growing shrub (rarely a small tree), Juniper tends to be laterally spreading in growth. Lance-shaped and needle–like, the leaves are whitish above and dark–green beneath. The blue–black berries take 2 seasons to fully ripen. They are fleshy, sweet, pungent, and contain 1–3 small, hard seeds.

Distribution
Considered to be the most widespread species, Juniper communis is found worldwide throughout the Northern Hemisphere. In the West, it is encountered at montane elevations. Nearly all parts of the Rocky Mountains (and outlier chains) commonly support the plant.

Chemistry
Prominent volatiles include: α–pinene, β–pinene, sabinene, myrcene, δ–2–carene, α–phellandrene, β–phellandrene, δ–3–carene, limonene, bornyl

acetate, (e)–caryophyllene, α–humulene, α–muurolene, germacrene a, germacrene d, germacrene d–4–ol, γ–cadinene, δ–cadinene, α–cadinol.

Medicinal Uses

Few medicinal plants have been used as long and for the same issues by geographically disconnected groups of people, as Juniper. Nearly universally agreed upon, Juniper's main area of effect is the urinary tract. As a stimulant to the area, it works best to alleviate subacute/chronic urinary tract irritability and discomfort. Use it in chronic cystitis and painful urination accompanied by mucus in the urine. Although alcoholic preparations tend to extract Juniper's volatile constituents more completely, the leaf/berry tea is useful too as a urinary antiseptic (both fungal and bacterial strains are inhibited). Small amounts of the tea are also useful in addressing low–grade, on and off again nephritis, particularly if used in formula.

Due to Juniper's aromatics, it tends to be a carminative of moderate strength. Several ounces of the tea or 30–40 drops of the tincture can lessen stomach bloating and cramping. Topical preparations are helpful in resolving long–standing episodes of eczema and psoriasis. Through the plant's interesting mix of antiinflammatory qualities and stimulating aromatics, it often is the right plant for long–standing problems of the urinary tract and skin.

Indications
» Infection, urinary tract, chronic
» Nephritis, chronic
» Dyspepsia, with bloating
» Eczema/Psoriasis (external)

Collection
Collect the leaves and/or fruit alone or together. Both parts are equally potent. Dry them normally.

Preparations
For internal use, Juniper's essential oil fraction can be prepared as a spirit or the essential oil can be added to ointment and oil bases.

Dosage
» Leaf/Berry infusion: 4–6 ounces 2–3 times daily

- » FPT/DPT (75% alcohol): 30–40 drops 2–3 times daily
- » Spirit: 10–20 drops 2–3 times daily
- » Ointment/Oil/Salve: as needed

Cautions
Small amounts of Juniper are fine during pregnancy. However, it's contraindicated as an everyday herb – the plant's volatiles may prove too uterine stimulating to be used safely. Do not use it internally if plagued by acute kidney inflammation.

Other Uses
The berries are traditionally used in flavoring gin.

Larkspur
Ranunculaceae/Buttercup Family

Delphinium spp.

Delphinium L.
Lark's claw, Knight's spur

Description
The majority of Larkspur species are perennial and have tuberous roots. Their growth is vertical and either single or multi–stemmed. The taller species, which concern us here, often reach heights of 3'–4'. The leaves are mostly basal and are 3–7 lobed with each lobe often compounded. Larkspur's flower is its most unique feature. It is comprised of five sepals and four petals patterned in a very distinctive claw–spur arrangement. The flower color can be pink to white, but most species are blue to purple. The seed capsules are 3–parted (mostly) and contain many small grey to brown–black seeds.

Distribution
Fond of clearings, forest margins, and meadows, Larkspur is mainly found in full–sun environments. With approximately seventy species native to America, the majority are found in the West with California hosting the greatest number of any one state.

Chemistry
Diterpene and norditerpene alkaloids.

Medicinal Uses
Delphinium ajacis and D. staphisagria (Stavesacre) were the two official species (European natives) once used as topical insecticides – mainly to kill head lice. Even though North American plants never became official medicines, due to constituent similarities, local species should be similarly effective.

For the treatment of head lice, apply the tincture generously to the hair and scalp, yet away from the eyes (the use of a shower cap will help). After 30 minutes rinse the area thoroughly. After drying the hair with a towel use a 'lice comb' to remove the nits. Repeat this whole process again in 7–10 days.

This is a baseline approach. The timing/duration used here is not much different than that of over–the–counter permethrin–based treatments. Additional applications, or a longer per–dosage exposure may be necessary for total eradication. For children, dilute the tincture with equal amounts of a 90% alcohol/10% water solution before applying (see Cautions).

Try Larkspur seed tincture in a spray bottle as an insecticide on non–edible/non–medicinal plants. Rivaling commercial agents, its potential here is significant.

Indications
» Infestation, head lice (external)

Collection
Gather the seed capsules of tall species when they are just beginning to split open. Place both the stems and capsules in a box or paper bag. Once dry, knock the seed capsules or garble them to release the seeds. Sift and discard any capsule or stem part. In lieu of hand gathering, the seed of Delphinium ajacis is commercially available. It is sold through ornamental garden seed catalogs and the like.

Preparations
A high percentage of alcohol is needed to extract the necessary components from the seed. Water preparations of the seed (strong tea) will be found lacking in strength.

Dosage

» DPT (90% alcohol, 1:10) as a scalp/hair wash

Cautions

Before the arrival of modern over–the–counter lice treatments, Larkspur[45] based soaks/shampoos were some of the main treatments. However, the problem then with Larkspur, as today, was its potential toxicity. Dizziness, changes in heart activity/respiration, and other nervous system symptoms were reported with its external use (though usually only with long exposures). It is a superb insecticide, but one that is somewhat toxic, not only to lice, but people too. Would I use it or apply it to a family member if afflicted by lice? Probably not. There is really nothing to be gained by using Larkspur as a lice treatment considering that OTC treatments are relatively safe and effective.

That being said, if for whatever reason (possibly pyrethrin/permethrin–resistant head lice, which is becoming more common) the reader decides to go forward with Larkspur, there are a number of things to keep in mind. Firstly, I caution against women using Larkspur during pregnancy or while breast–feeding. Be extremely careful with its application to children: dilute the tincture with equal parts of a water–alcohol mixture before applying. Additionally, monitor them for changes in respiration, light–headedness, or anything out of the ordinary, and be sure to rinse the tincture from the hair/scalp thoroughly after 30 minutes. Keep it away from the eyes, and lastly, Larkspur is for external use only.

---

45   Larkspur is chemically similar to Aconite (Aconitum) – a related plant medicine/poison that is little used today due to toxicity dangers. Additionally, pharmaceuticals used today for what Aconite was used for (inflammatory cardiovascular complaints/tachycardia) provide a much better risk–to–reward ratio.

Ligusticum
Apiaceae/Carrot Family

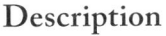
Ligusticum porteri

Ligusticum porteri Coult. & Rose
Bear root, Chuchupate, Colorado cough root, Mountain lovage, Oshá, Porter's lovage, Raíz de cochino

Description
Ligusticum is a substantial Carrot family perennial. Standing between 2'–4', the plant has stout stems and is leafy with large and finely–divided foliage. The leaf blades are between 6" to 12" long. The individual leaflets are ovate and incised. The white flower clusters form in umbels above the body of the plant. The mature fruit are oblong, slightly flattened to cylindrical, and ribbed. Ligusticum's roots are strongly aromatic and have hairy crowns.

Because there are a number of botanically related and similarly appearing poisonous plants (Poison hemlock), obtaining a positive identification before collection cannot be stressed more. If identifying Ligusticum for the first time it is optimal to have the assistance of someone familiar with the plant or at the very least, several field guides to assist in identification. Do not let eagerness and excitement override thoroughness. Mistakes made with Poison hemlock (or Water hemlock) could be fatal. Conioselinum scopulorum (Hemlock parsley) is another related plant that is often confused with Ligusticum. Fortunately, Conioselinum is not poisonous, but it's not particularly medicinal either.

Distribution
Ligusticum ranges from Wyoming, Nevada, Utah, and Colorado, south through Arizona, New Mexico, and into Mexico. Look to the mountains, where Aspen and conifers are prolific. It is typically not found in the shade of a dense tree canopy, but in the open on slopes and above streamsides. The plant is a prolific seeder and takes easily to logged and burnt areas.

Chemistry
Phthalides: diligustilide, riligustilide, z–ligustilide, tokinolide b; furanocoumarins; monoterpenes.

Medicinal Uses

Ligusticum was well-known among the majority of southwestern (and northern Mexican) American Indian tribes (Apache, Hopi, Paiute, and Tarahumara for instance). It commanded an above-average degree of respect because of its effectiveness and maintained potency once dried. These factors also helped to make it a durable and sought-after regional trade item.

For the respiratory tract, the plant loosens lodged phlegm in beginning-stage bronchitis when the lungs feel hot and dry, or inversely, in respiratory afflictions that have left the lungs tired and lax. Relatedly, take it when there is a non-productive dry cough, usually at the start (or end) of a respiratory infection. Even the simplistic blanket-approach of using the plant from first to last cough, will likely give benefit. The plant's array of aromatics is antibacterial as well as antiviral.

Influenza sufferers will notice a marked improvement after taking the herb even for just a day. Not only is it directly inhibiting to various influenza strains, Ligusticum is helpful in lessening a number of secondary flu symptoms such as fever, nausea, and aches and pains. Its diaphoretic effects are best employed when the skin is dry and the fever low to moderate.

Alone, or combined with Yerba mansa (Anemopsis californica), Ligusticum makes a decent sore throat gargle. For strep throat, it combines well with Stillingia and/or White sage. Its anodyne qualities lessen pain and sensitivity. Singers and orators will too benefit from Ligusticum's anesthetic effect on stressed vocal chords. In these cases, it is optimally combined with Yerba mansa and/or Jack-in-the-pulpit.

Like other aromatic Carrot family plants, Ligusticum serves as a decent carminative. The tea or tincture is quieting to gas pains. Fullness and bloating are diminished. Even colicy babies can be given a teaspoon or so of the tea.

Like a mild Angelica in effect, some women will find the plant mildly stimulating to menses. Associated cramping also tends to lessen. It is best used when menses is sluggish or late due to a cold/flu/or stress.

Indications

» Bronchitis with a non-productive cough
» Flu with cough and fever
» Pharyngitis
» Vocal cords, stressed

Collection

Begin digging a foot or two away from the stems, giving attention to the tap roots which may travel laterally as well as vertically. The roots mangle/shred easily and are strongly aromatic – if not, then recheck and make sure the proper plant is being harvested. The foliage is of little medicinal value, but can be eaten raw or cooked for its mild carrot–parsley flavor.

Many of the populations throughout the Southwest are isolated, scarce, and exist in remnant stands[46]. The Sky Island populations of southern Arizona and New Mexico are particularly fragile and should not be picked. Further north within its core range (Rockies) Ligusticum is stable and exists in substantial stands.

Several common sense gathering practices can be followed in order to keep populations intact. 1. Gather only a couple of plants from each stand. 2. Do not collect the largest plants of the group. 3. Leave the plants that are fruit bearing.

Preparations

Wash the roots thoroughly. If drying Ligusticum, split the crown and tap roots length–wise, as to expose larger areas to the drying effects of air.

Dosage

» FPT/DPT (70% alcohol): 30–60 drops 2–3 times daily
» Root infusion (cold or standard): 4–6 oz. 2–3 times daily
» Syrup: 1 teaspoon 3–4 times daily

Cautions

Do not take Ligusticum while pregnant due to the plant's vascular influence of the reproductive area. Like many medicinal plants, some of Ligusticum's constituents will be transferred through breast milk to a nursing baby. For nursing babies with a respiratory infection, having the mother take the plant is an effective way to dose the baby.

---

46 One trend that has taken shape lately is the distillation of Ligusticum roots for their essential oil content. Given the plant's already fragile existence (in the Southwest) and that the essential oil has no significant medicinal advantage over whole plant preparations, this practice is unfortunate. It's one thing to distill herbaceous portions of non–threatened plants. But to use this process on the roots of a potentially threatened plant? The practice is shortsighted and overly–damaging to the species.

Ligusticum's small furanocoumarin content should not cause any sun–sensitivity problem; however, if taking pharmaceuticals that have photosensitizing side effects, the combination may be problematic.

Other Uses
Ligusticum roots seem to be a sort of catnip for bears. Their attraction to them may be a cause for concern to some who are collecting the plant in bear country (I don't recommend keeping the roots your tent!). Even polar bears, who are outside of Ligusticum's range, take to the root as if it is in their genetic disposition[47]. I cannot vouch for this, but whereas bears are attracted to the root, rattlesnakes are supposedly repelled by it.

Lomatium
Apiaceae/Carrot Family

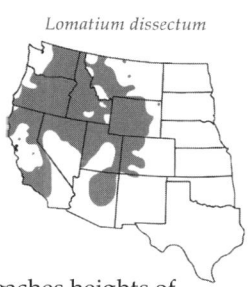

Lomatium dissectum

Lomatium dissectum (Nutt.) Mathias & Constance
(*Ferula dissecta, Leptotaenia dissecta*)
Biscuit root, Cough root, Desert parley, Indian balsam

Description
A stout–stemmed perennial, Lomatium commonly reaches heights of 2'–3', though larger plants are not uncommon when conditions are prime. The fern–like leaf blades are triangular in outline, ternate, then 2–4 times pinnate. They have thickened petiole sheaths, with the upper stem leaves being smaller than the lower leaves. The small yellow to purple petaled flowers form in umbels. The ½" long fruit are oblong to oval and when crushed are aromatic. Freshly sliced, the thickened roots weep a milky exudate and are also aromatic.

Distribution
Western Canada, Montana to New Mexico, west to the Pacific Coast states, Lomatium has a fairly wide distribution. Arid semi–desert foothills, scrublands, and openings are common growing spots.

---

47 Ethnobotanist Shawn Sigstedt has conducted some interesting research on bear–Ligusticum interactions. He has documented a number of bear species' attraction to the root.

Chemistry

Coumarins; fatty acids: linolenic acid, palmitic acid; tetronic acids; volatile oils: α–bisabolol, β–caryophyllene, cuparene, limonene, longifolene, (E)–2–methyl–3–octen–5–yne, β–myrcene, (E)–β–ocimene, β–phellandrene.

Medicinal Uses

Lomatium belongs to a tier of important aromatic–balsamic plant medicines. Like closely related Ligusticum, the plant has a long history of indigenous use. It can basically be said: whomever lived around the plant and knew of it, principally employed the root towards wintertime lung distresses.

As a bronchial stimulant/expectorant and area–specific antimicrobial/antiviral agent, its influence is significant if used with propriety and sensibility. Most forms of bronchitis respond well to Lomatium, but it will especially be helpful if expectoration is difficult and additional infectious symptoms present themselves: gastrointestinal disarray, body aches, and fever.

For related pharyngitis and laryngitis, especially if swollen lymph nodes are part of the symptom picture, a tincture–in–water solution gargled throughout the day will come in handy. Though not as anesthetic as Ligusticum, small frequent doses work best for these throat–oriented maladies. Whether it's common wintertime bronchitis, related throat issues, or the flu, simply start taking Lomatium at the onset of symptoms and continue several days after becoming symptom free.

In present–day herbal circles the re–telling of Dr. Ernst T. Krebs' observations of the Washoe Indians of western Nevada/eastern California whom used Lomatium during the Spanish Flu Epidemic is standard fare. He reported (Bulletin of the Nevada State Board of Health, 1920) that the mortality rates were much higher in the surrounding non–Lomatium Indian communities compared to the Lomatium–using Washoe tribe (no or very few deaths). Even though I view this kind of one–off anecdotal report with some healthy skepticism (there's also a conflict of interest – Dr. Krebs did go on to formulate and sell a Lomatium–based patent remedy called Balsamea), his observation is in alignment with the plant's traditional use.

Lomatium is usually found by individuals with dry skin and an elevated temperature to be moderately to strongly diaphoretic – no surprise considering the plant's chemical and botanical affiliations. Its warming and skin dilating influences are often needed anyway considering the bronchial situations Lomatium best addresses. Additionally, Lomatium is a mild

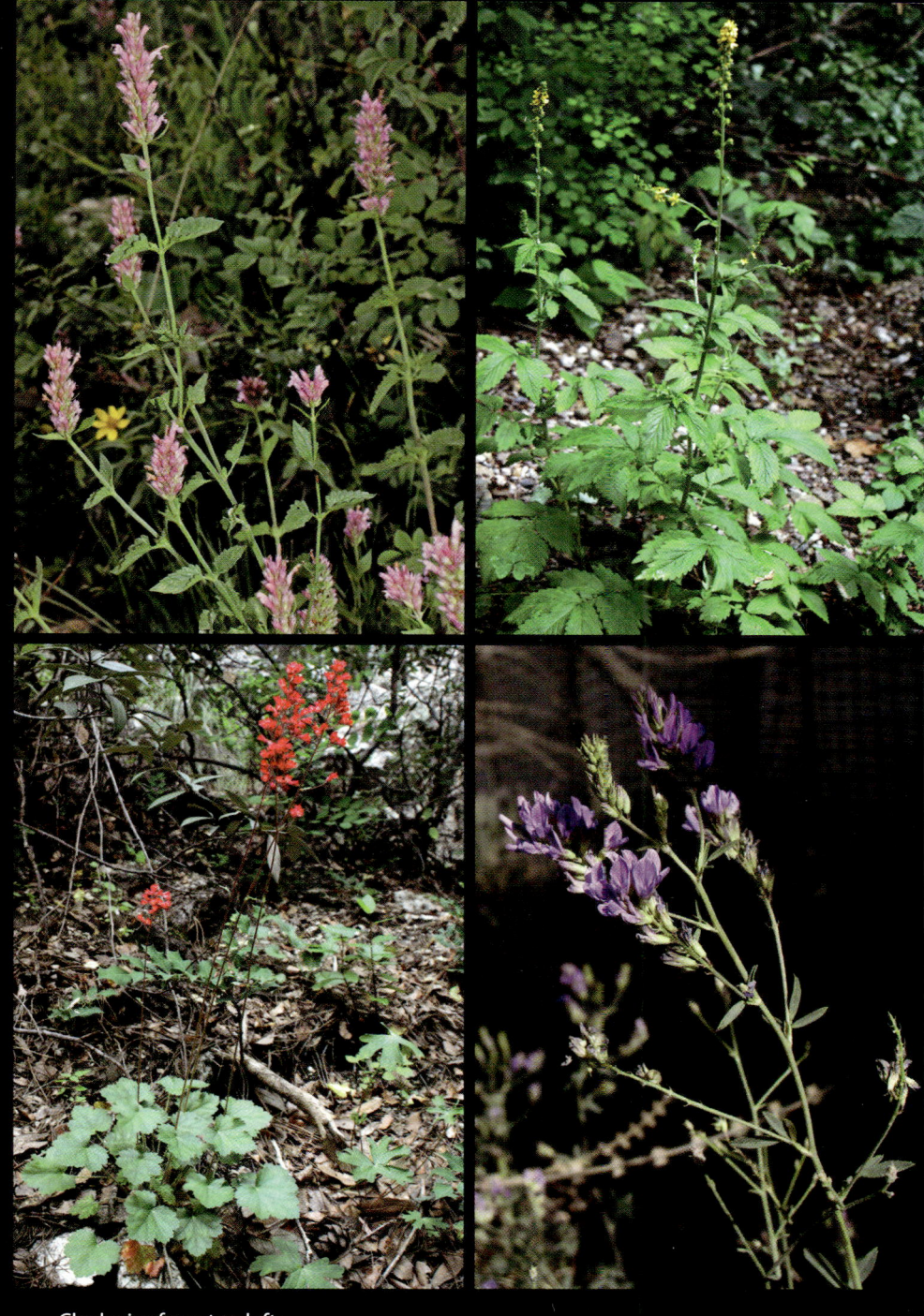

Clockwise from top left:
1. Agastache (*Agastache pallidiflora*); 2. Agrimony (*Agrimonia striata*); 3. Alfalfa (*Medicago sativa*); 4. Alumroot (*Heuchera sanguinea*).

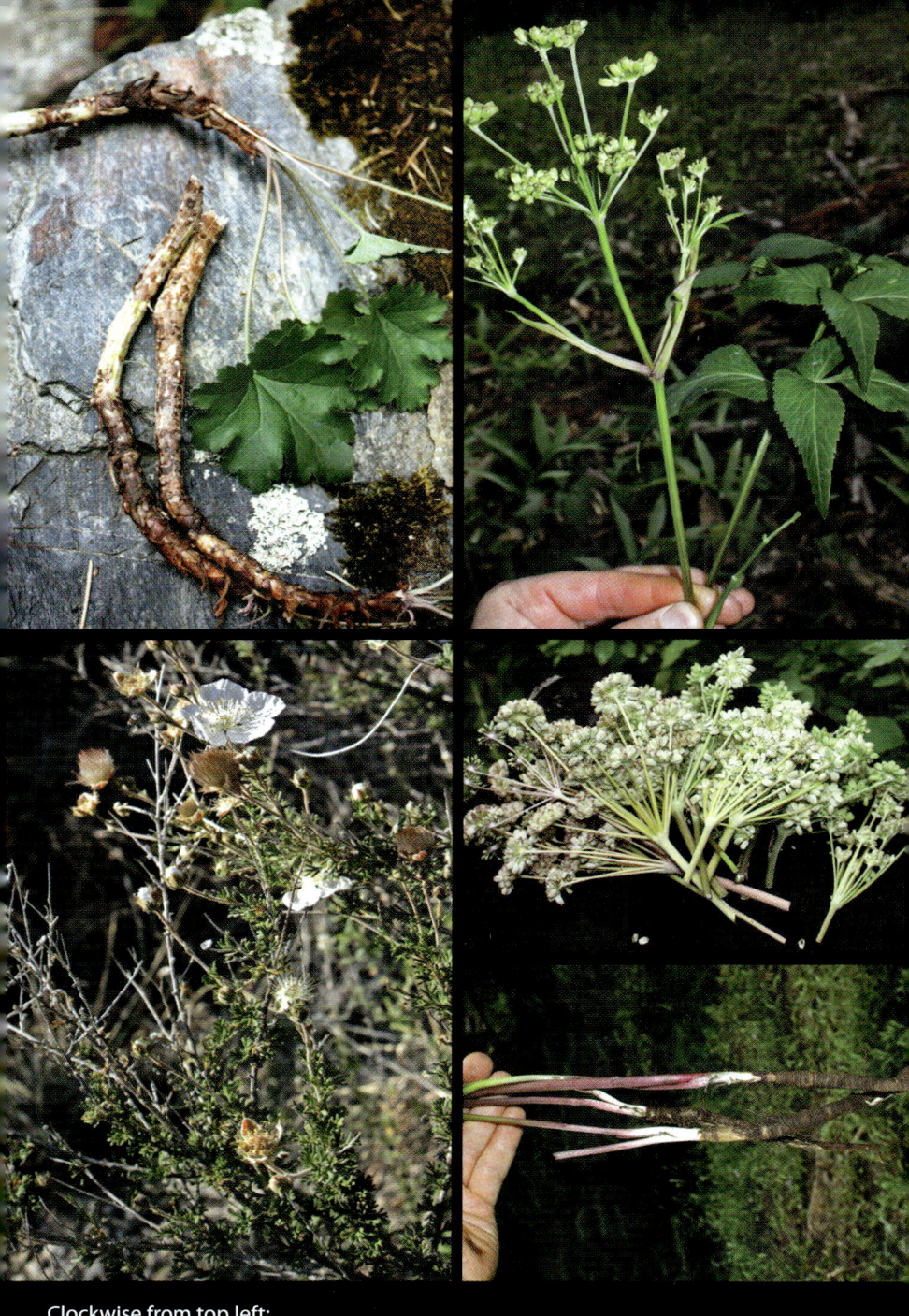

Clockwise from top left:
5. Alumroot (*Heuchera sanguinea*); 6. Angelica (*Angelica pinnata*); 7. Angelica (*Angelica pinnata*); 8. Angelica (*Angelica pinnata*); 9. Apache plume (*Fallugia paradoxa*)

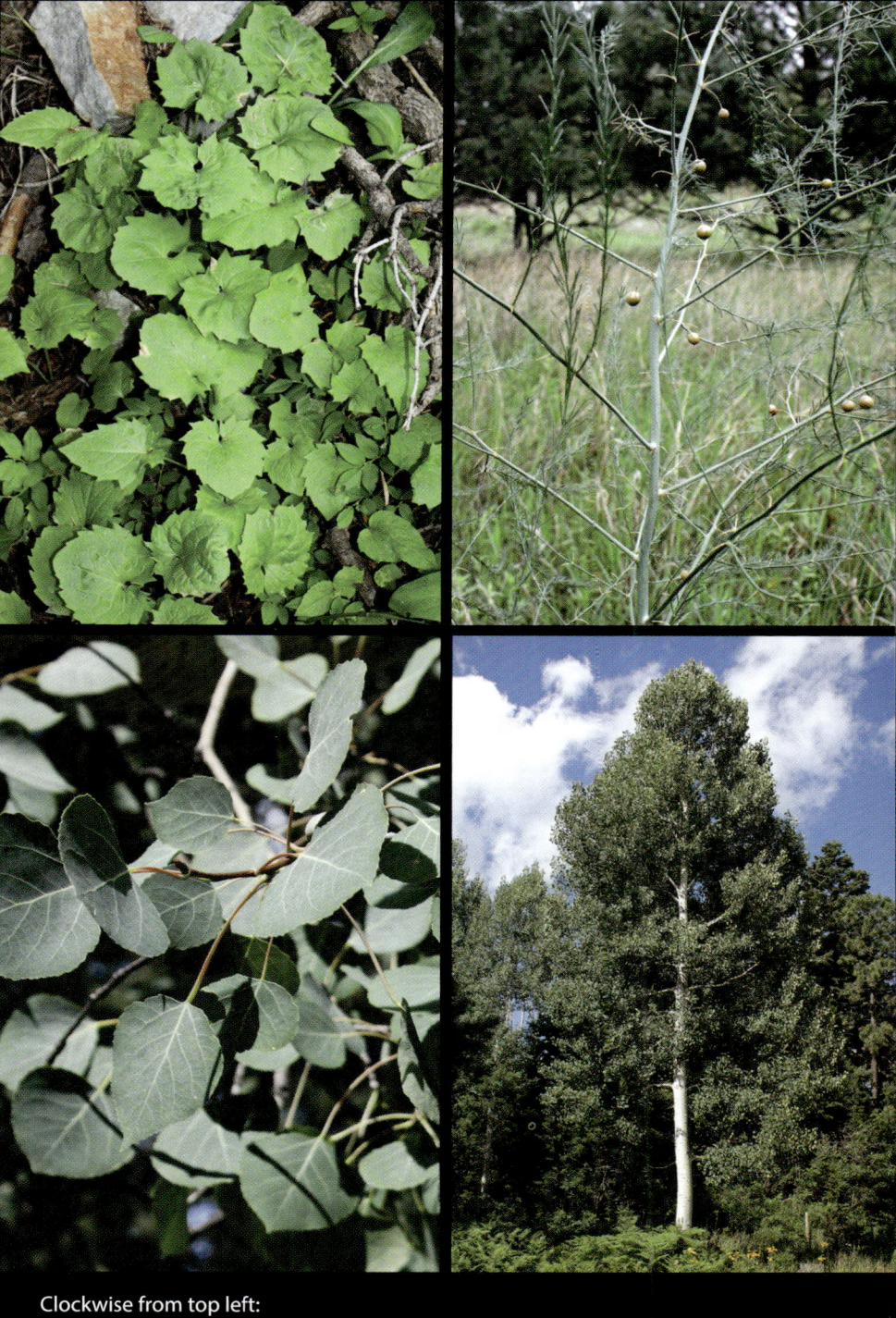

Clockwise from top left:
10. Arnica (*Arnica cordifolia*); 11. Asparagus (*Asparagus officinalis*); 12. Aspen (*Populus tremuloides*); 13. Aspen (*Populus tremuloides*).

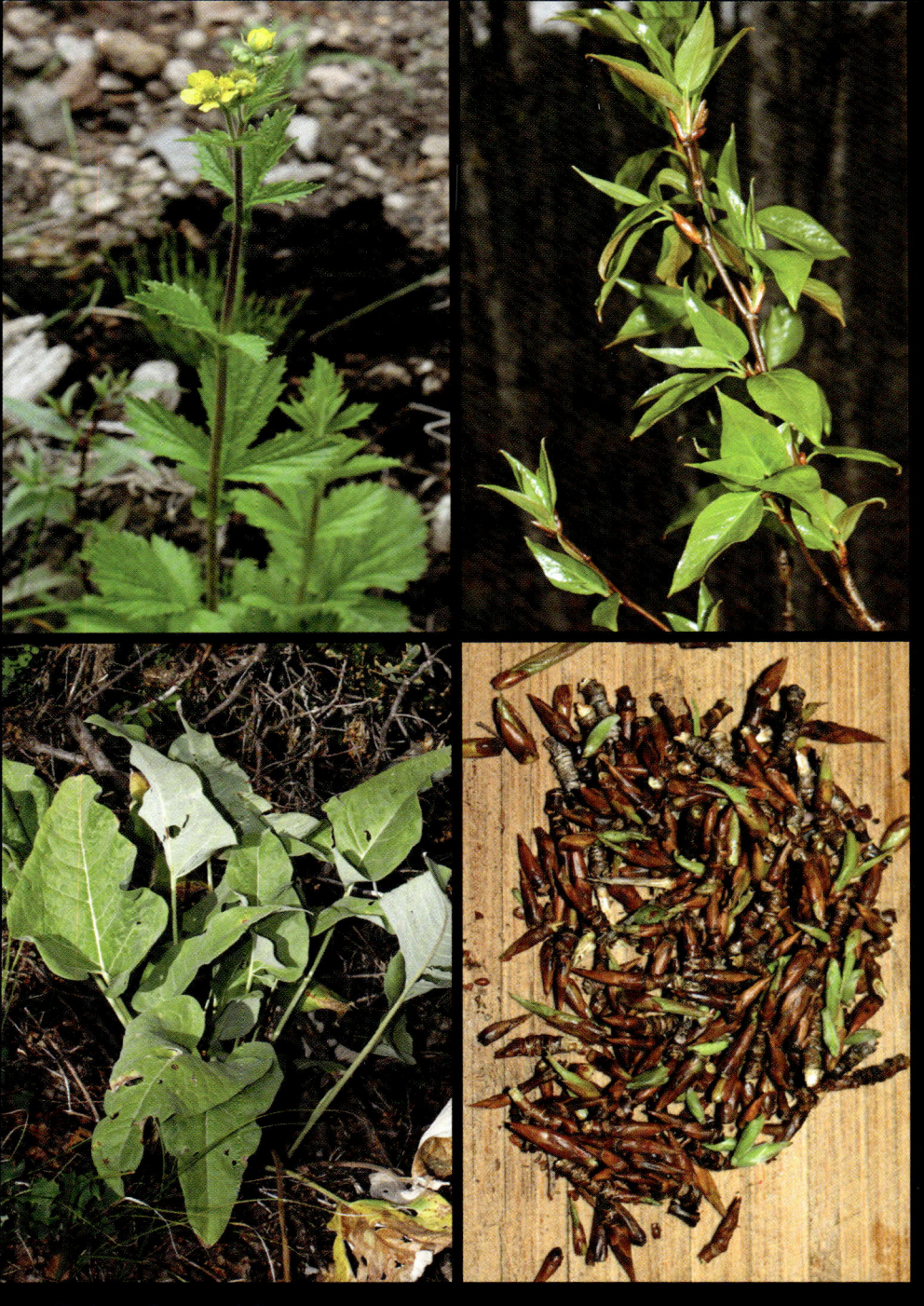

Clockwise from top left:
14. Avens (*Geum macrophyllum var. perincisum)*; 15. Balsam poplar (*Populus balsamifera*);
16. Balsam poplar (*Populus balsamifera*); 17. Balsamroot (*Balsamorhiza sagittata*).

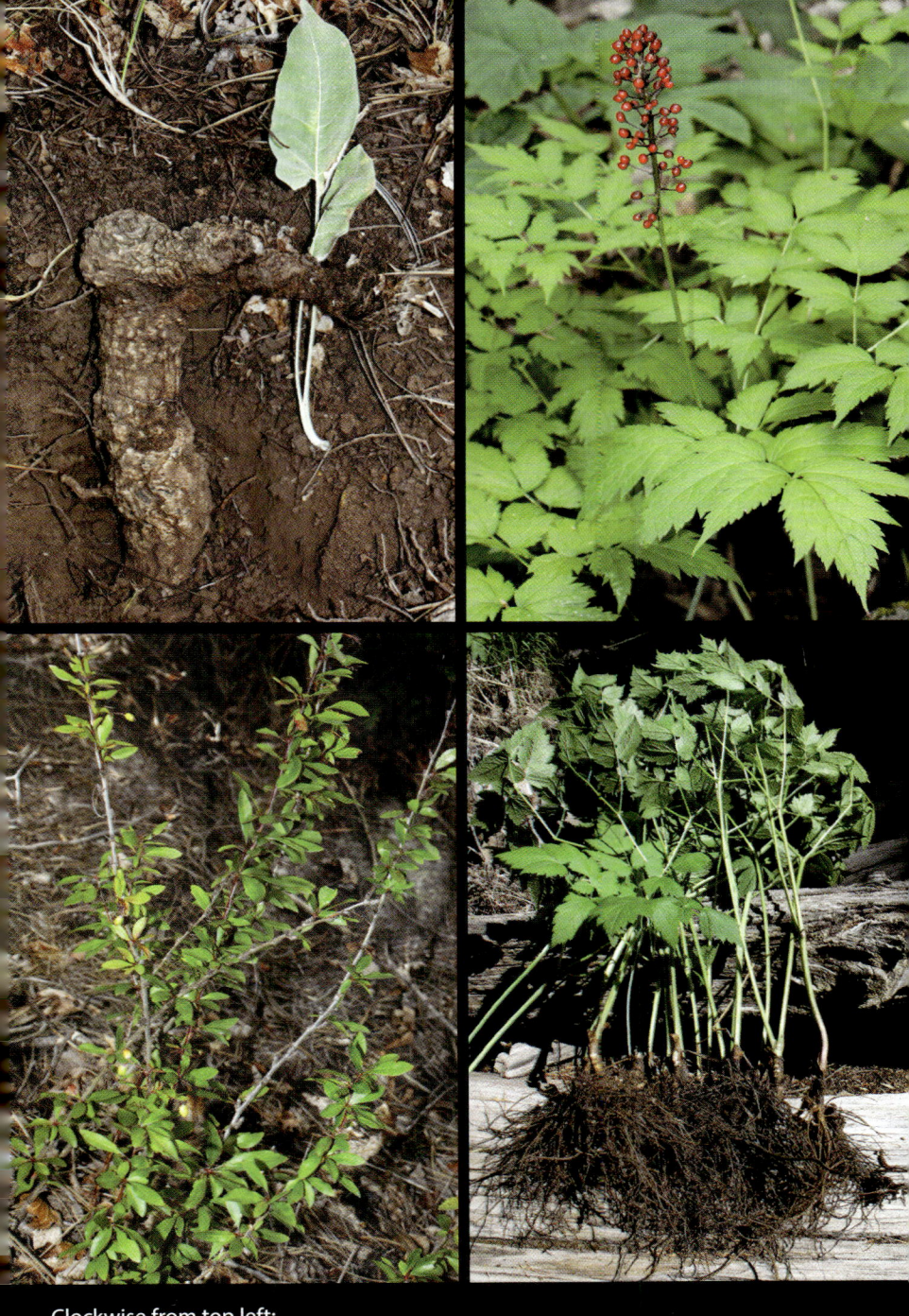

Clockwise from top left:
18. Balsamroot (*Balsamorhiza sagittata*); 19. Baneberry (*Actaea rubra*); 20. Baneberry

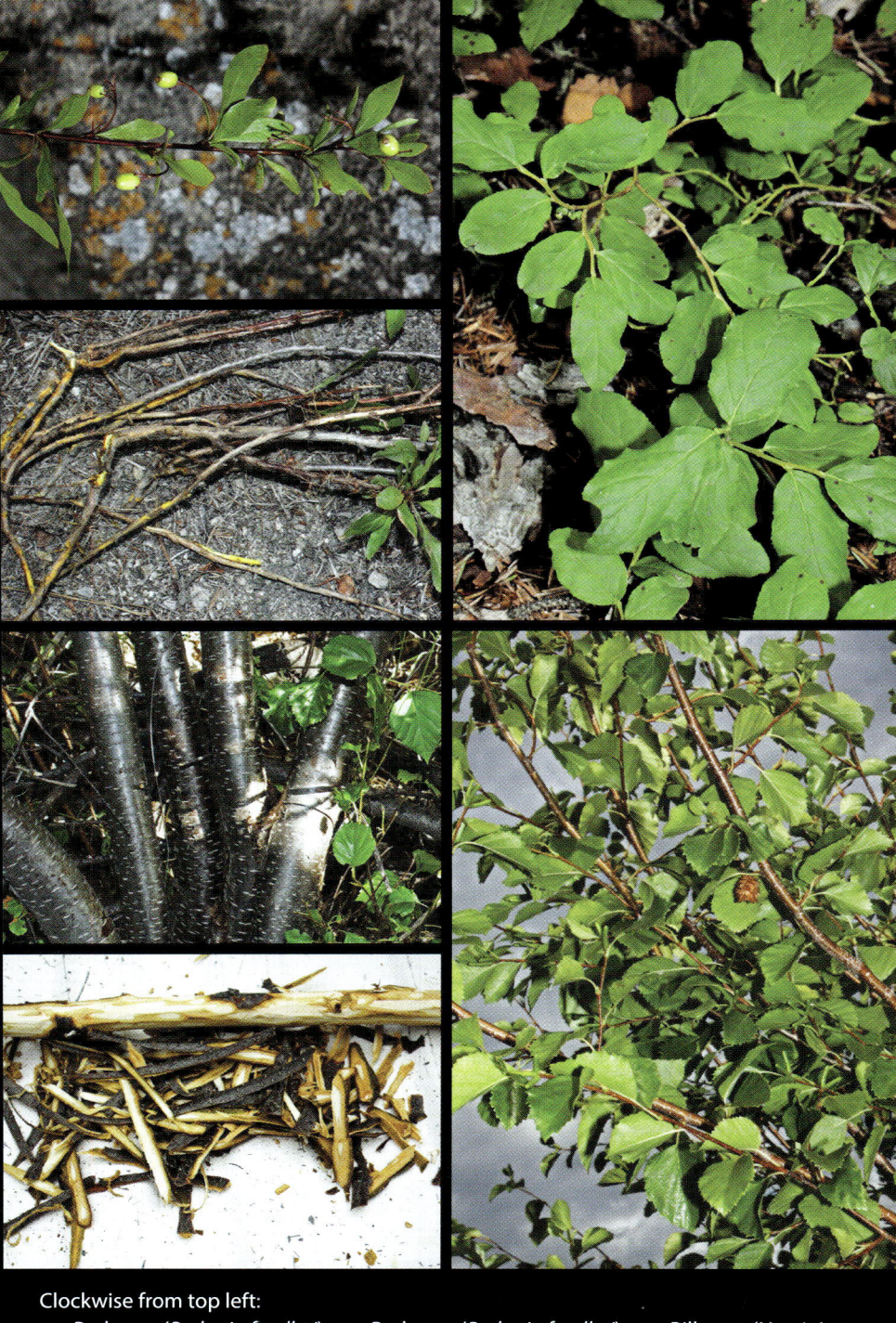

Clockwise from top left:
22. Barberry (*Berberis fendleri*); 23. Barberry (*Berberis fendleri*); 24. Bilberry (*Vaccinium myrtillus*); 25. Birch (*Betula occidentalis*); 26. Birch (*Betula occidentalis*); 27. Birch (*Betula occidentalis*).

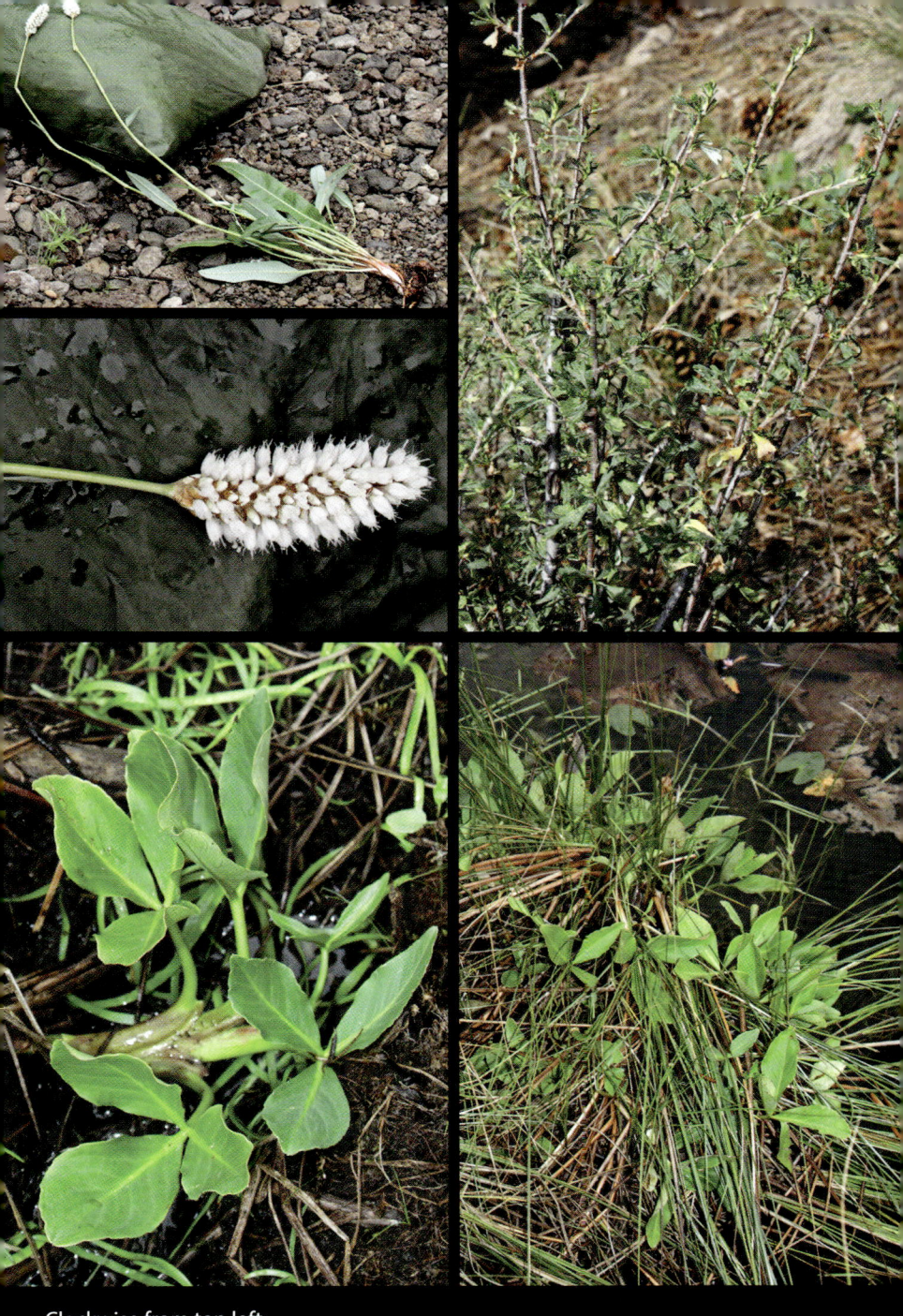

Clockwise from top left:
28. Bistort (*Bistorta bistortoides*); 29. Bistort (*Bistorta bistortoides*); 30. Bitterbrush (*Purshia tridentata*); 31. Bogbean (*Menyanthes trifoliata*); 32. Bogbean (*Menyanthes trifoliata*)

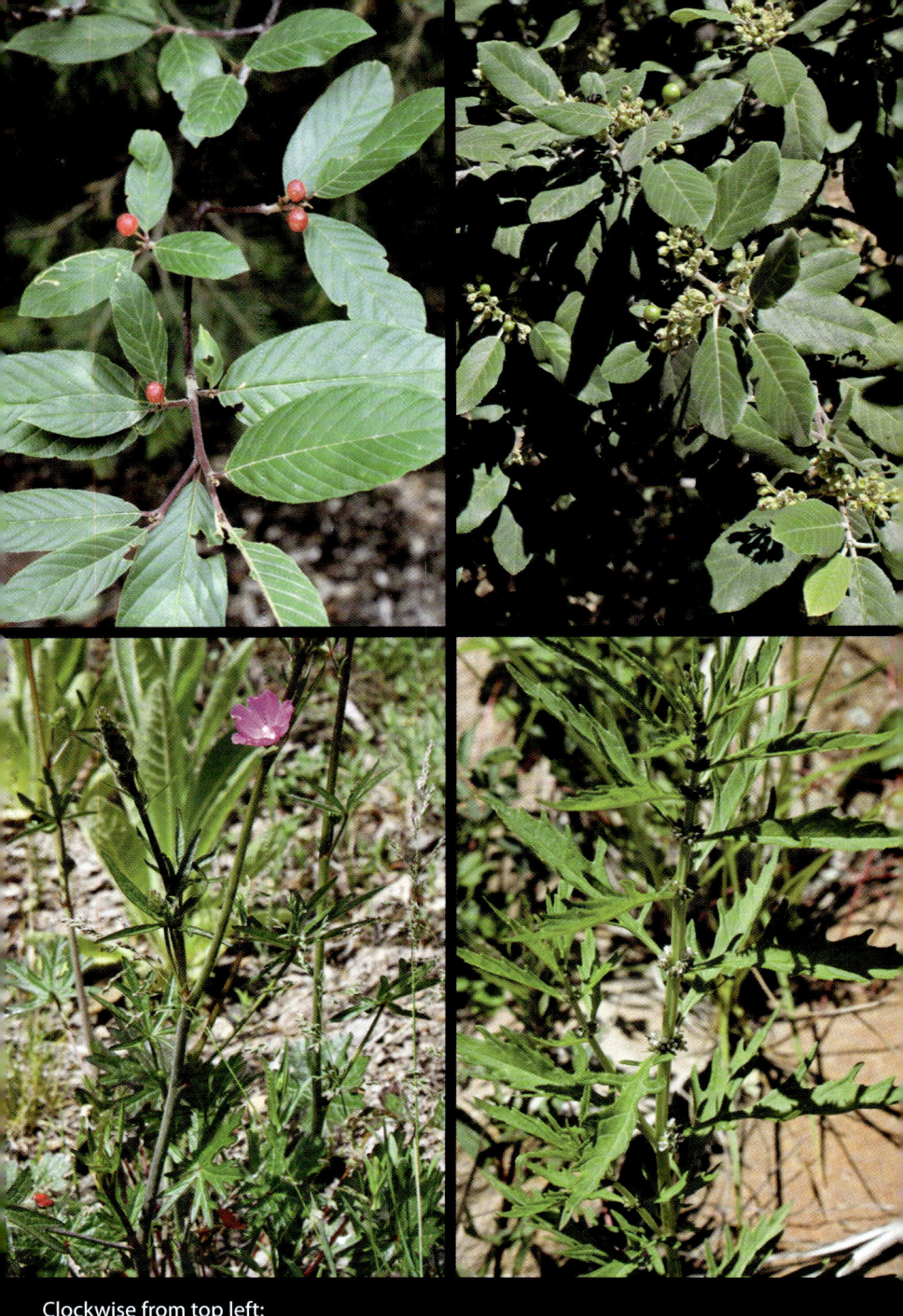

Clockwise from top left:
33. Buckthorn (*Rhamnus betulifolia*); 34. Buckthorn (*Rhamnus californica*); 35. Bugleweed (*Lycopus americanus*); 36. Checker mallow (*Sidalcea neomexicana*)

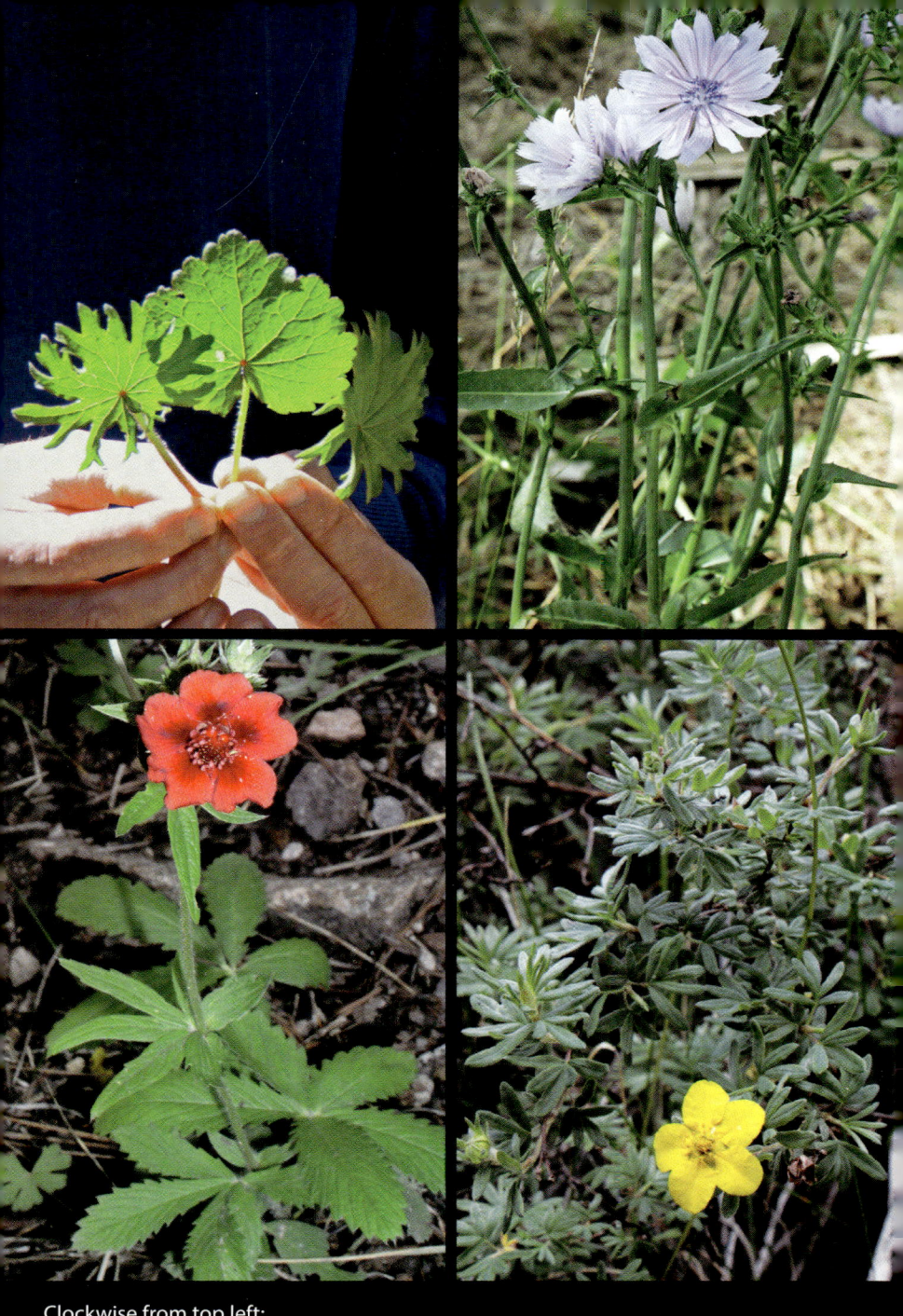

Clockwise from top left:
37. Checker mallow (*Sidalcea neomexicana*); 38. Chicory (*Cichorium intybus*); 39. Cinquefoil (*Potentilla fruticosa*); 40. Cinquefoil (*Potentilla thurberi*)

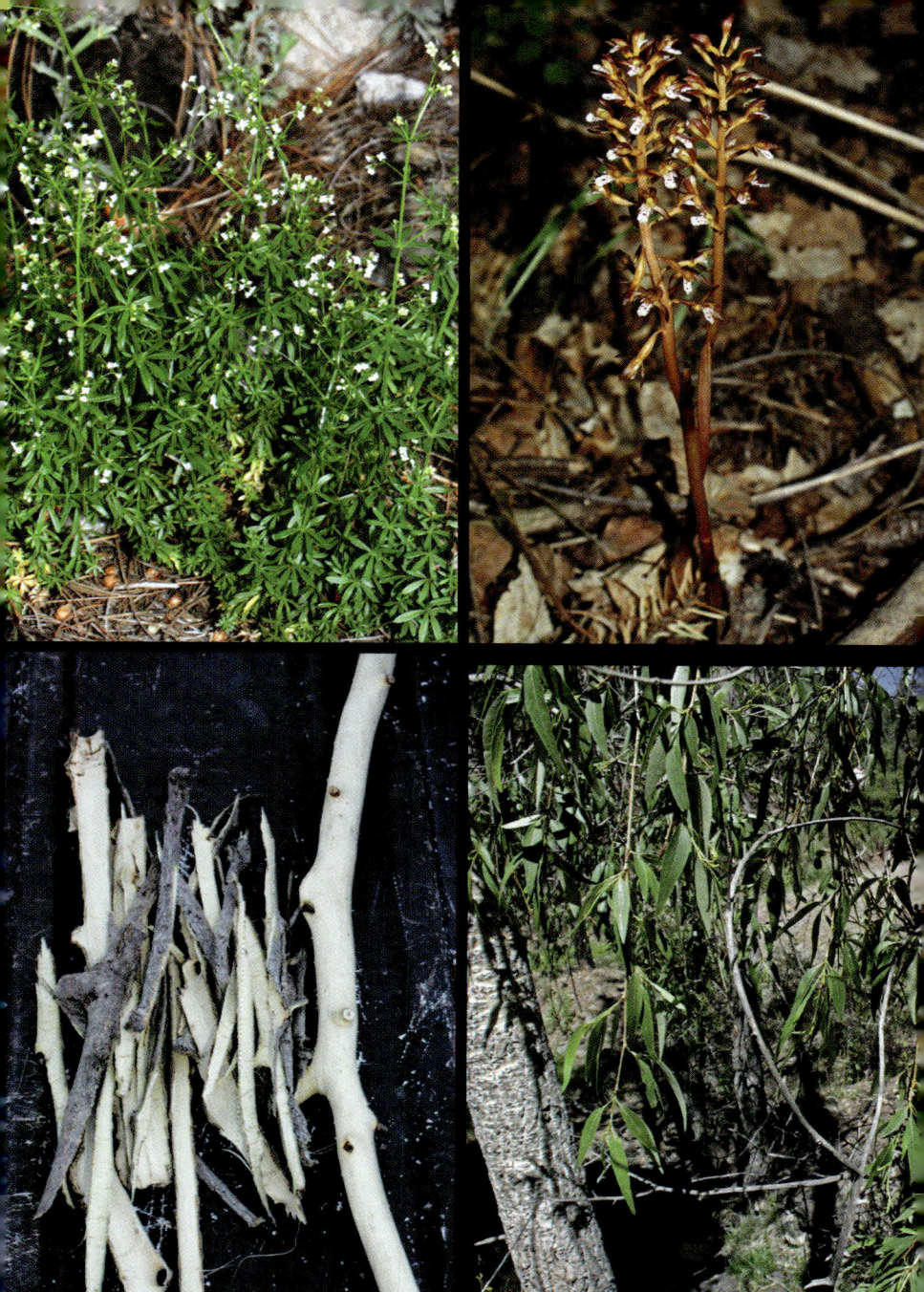

Clockwise from top left:
41. Cleavers (*Galium aparine*); 42. Coral root (*Corallorhiza maculata*) 43. Cottonwood (*Populus angustifolia*); 44. Cottonwood (*Populus angustifolia*)

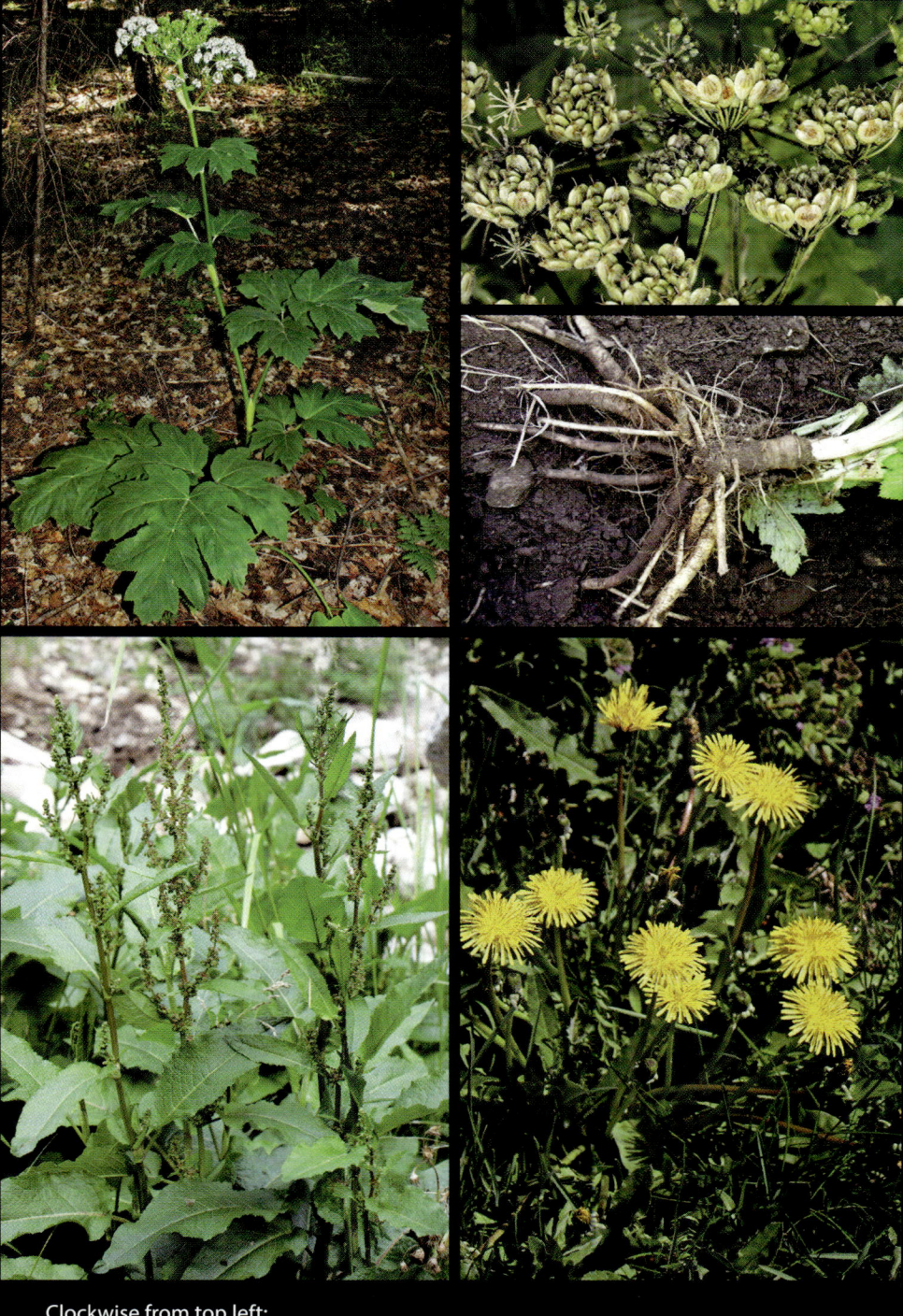

Clockwise from top left:
45. Cow parsnip (*Heracleum maximum*); 46. Cow parsnip (*Heracleum maximum*); 47. Cow parsnip (*Heracleum maximum*); 48. Dandelion (*Taraxacum officinale*); 49. Dock (*Rumex obtusifolius*).

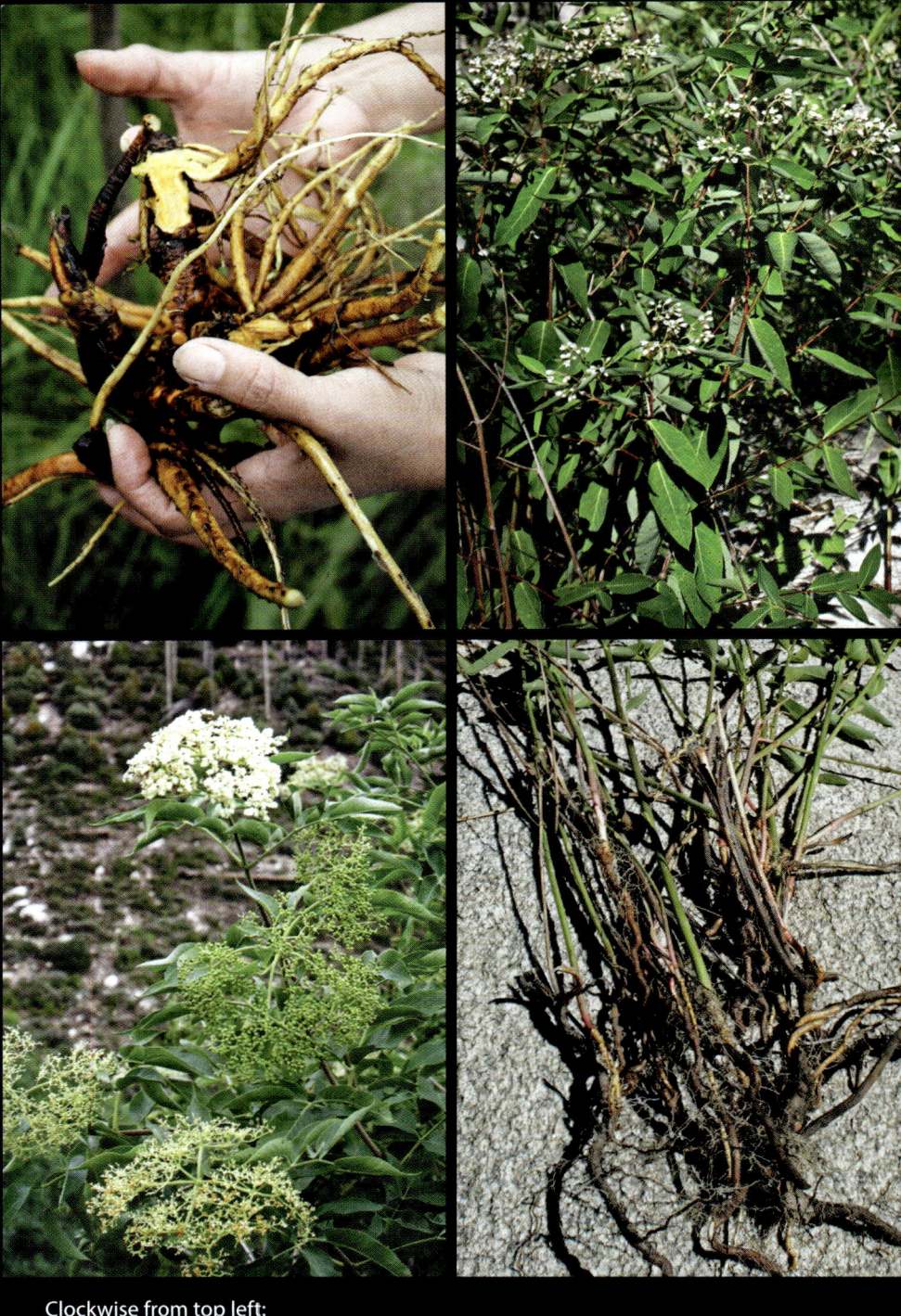

Clockwise from top left:
50. Dock (*Rumex crispus*); 51. Dogbane (*Apocynum cannabinum*); 52. Dogbane (*Apocynum cannabinum*); 53. Elder (*Sambucus cerulea*).

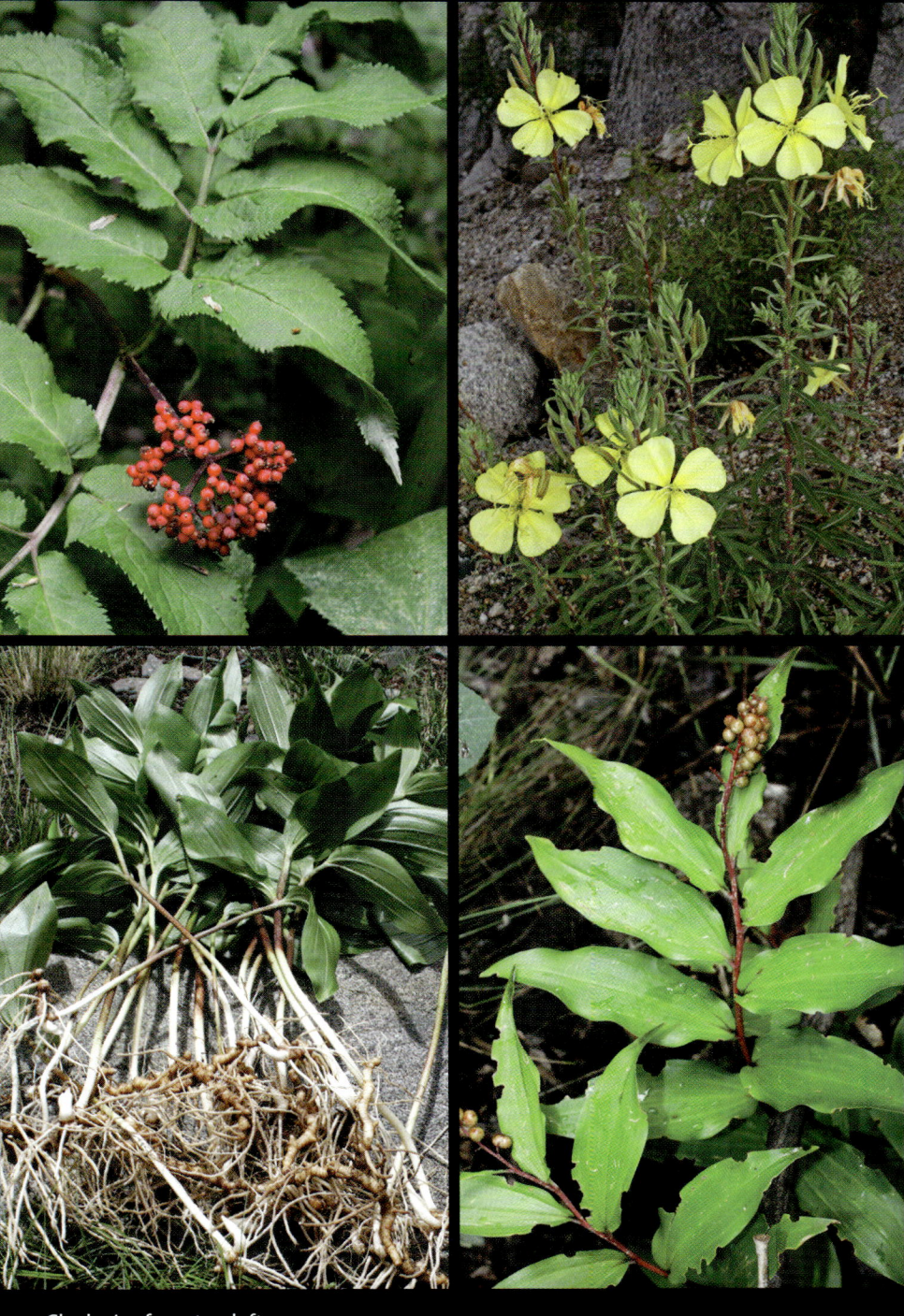

Clockwise from top left:
54. Elder (*Sambucus microbotrys*); 55. Evening primrose (*Oenothera elata*); 56. False Solomon's seal (*Maianthemum racemosum*); 57. False Sclomon's seal (*Maianthemum racemosum*).

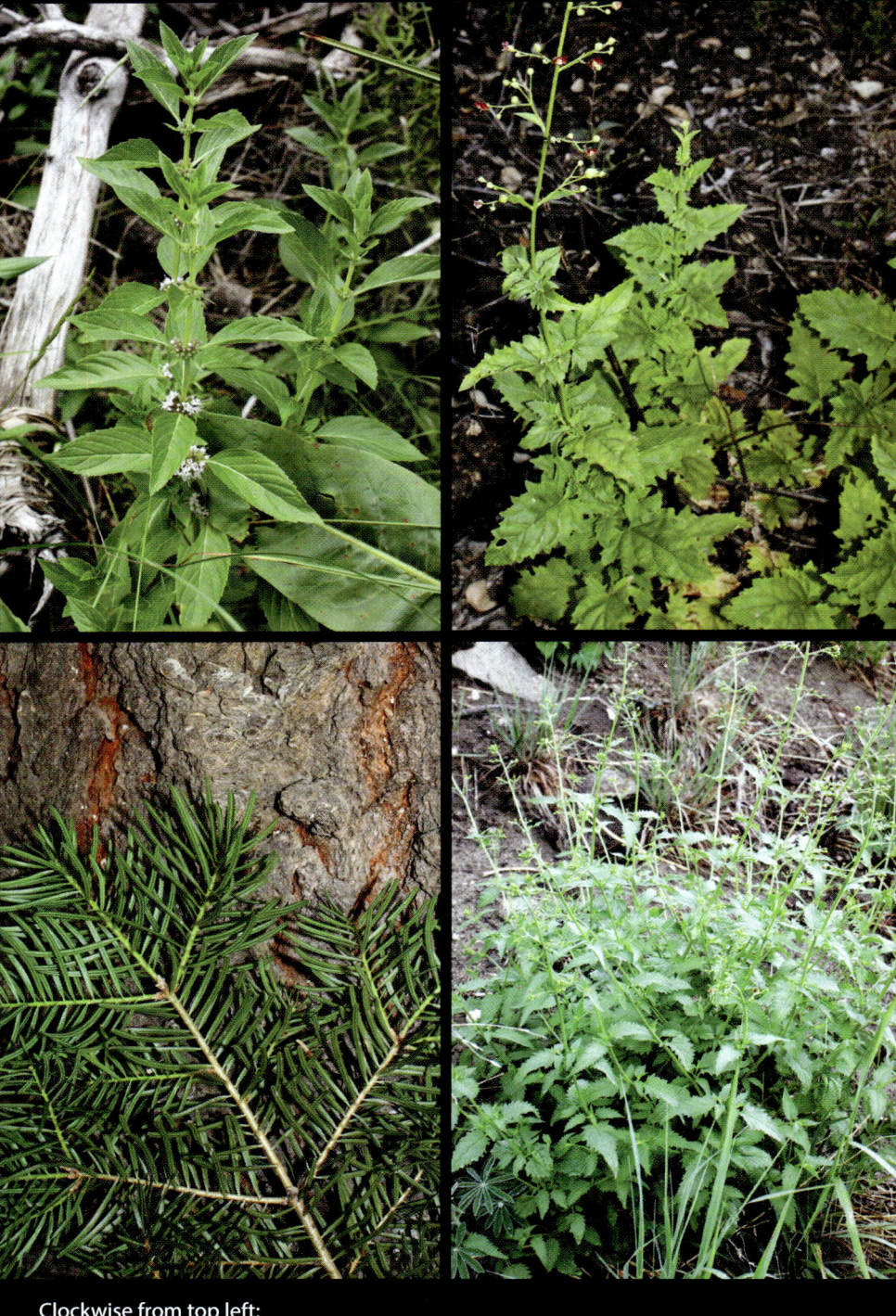

Clockwise from top left:
58. Field mint (*Mentha arvensis*); 59. Figwort (*Scrophularia californica*); 60. Figwort (*Scrophularia parviflora*); 61. Fir (*Abies concolor*).

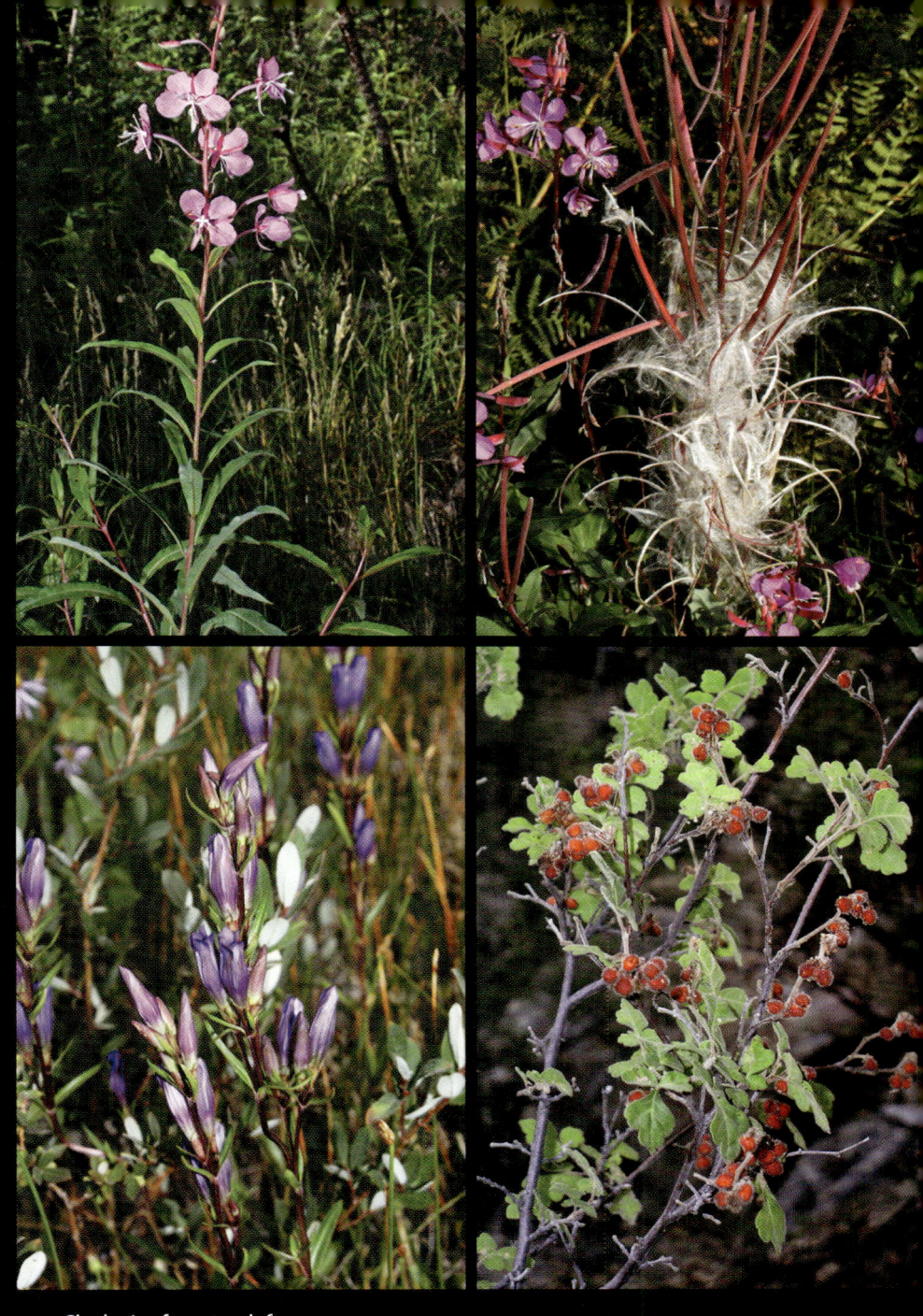

Clockwise from top left:
62. Fireweed (*Chamerion angustifolium*); 63. Fireweed (*Chamerion angustifolium*); 64. Fragrant sumac (*Rhus aromatica*); 65. Gentian (*Gentiana affinis*).

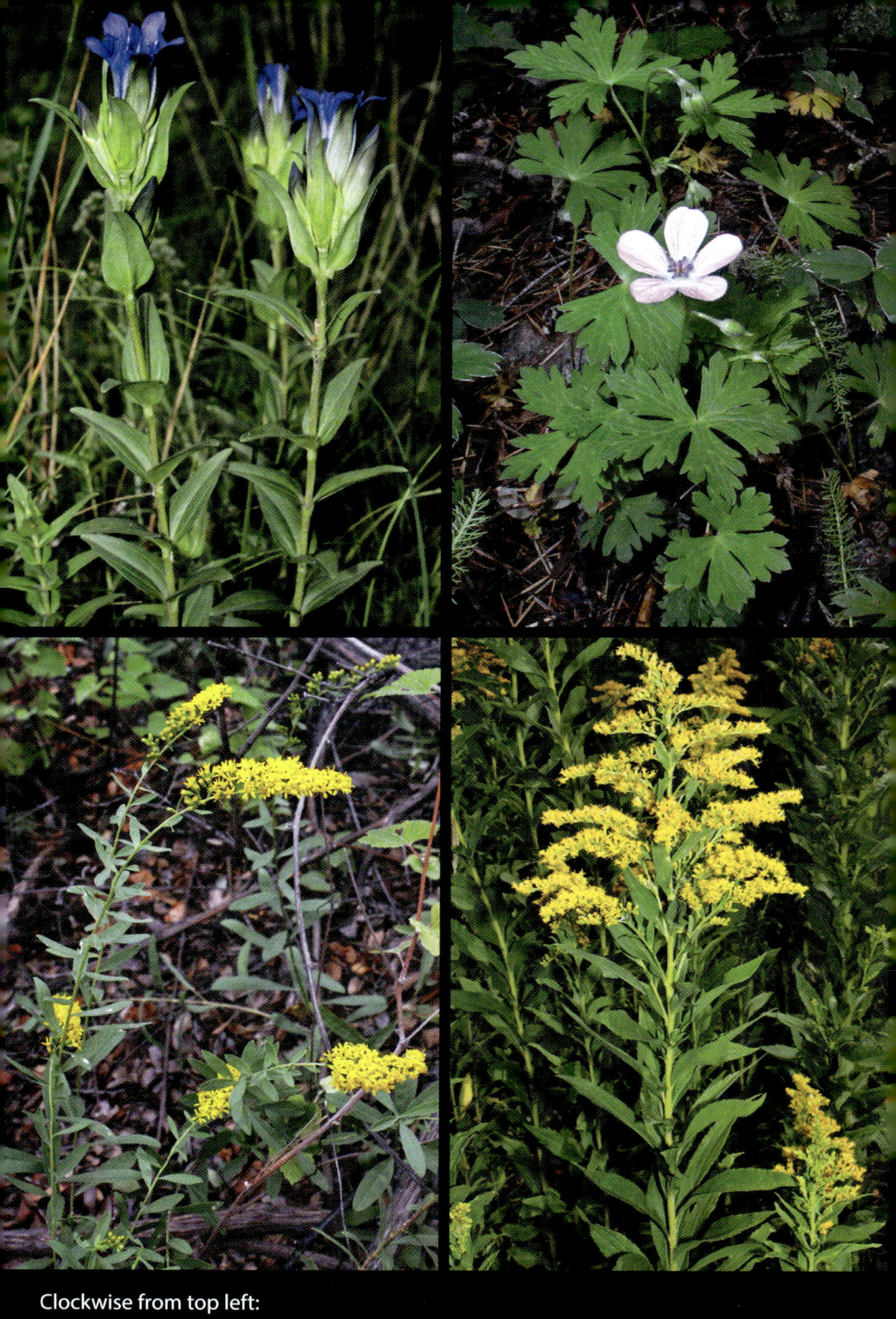

Clockwise from top left:
66. Gentian (*Gentiana parryi*); 67. Geranium (*Geranium richardsonii*); 68. Goldenrod

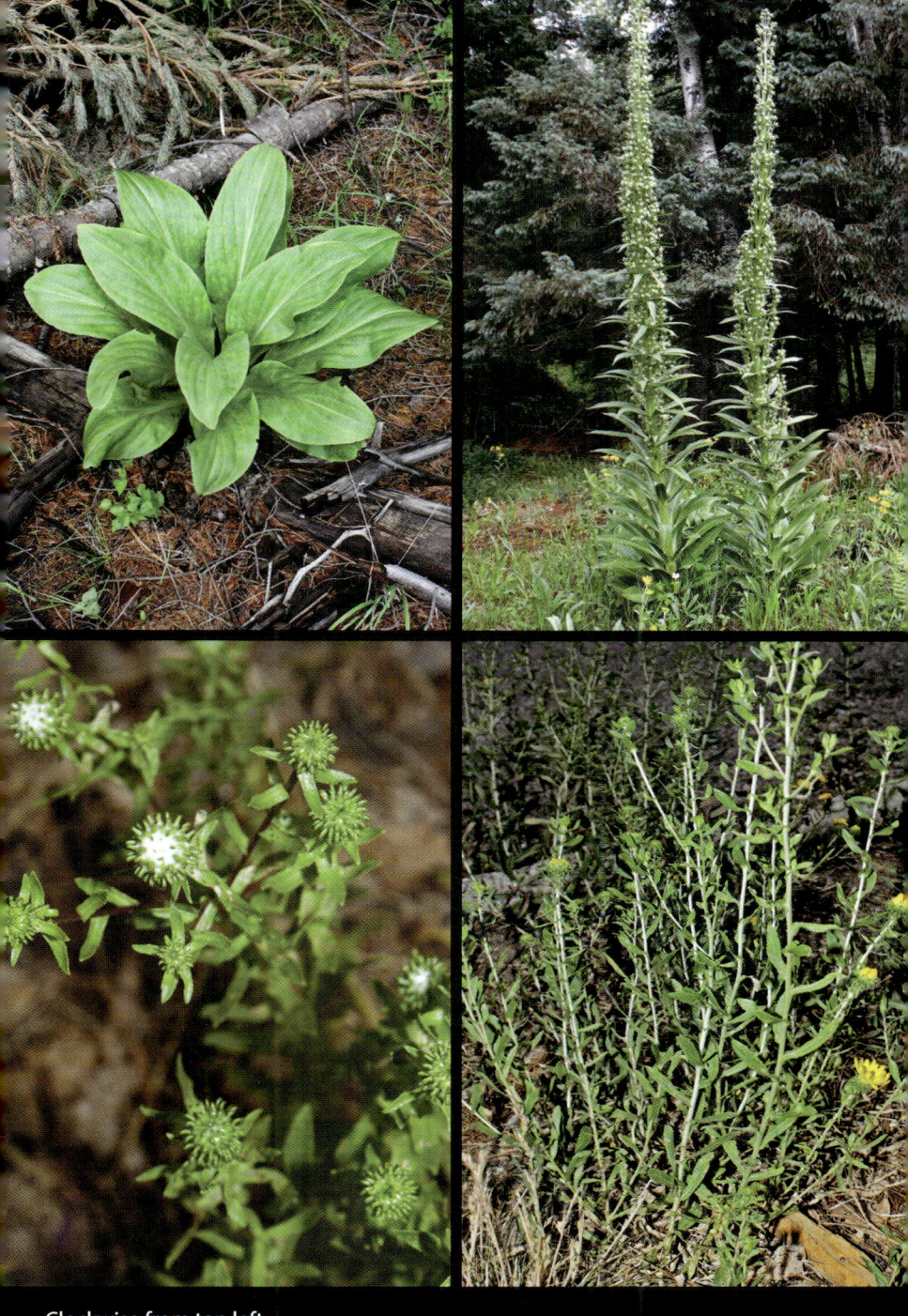

Clockwise from top left:
70. Green gentian (*Frasera speciosa*); 71. Green gentian (*Frasera speciosa*); 72. Grindelia (*Grindelia squarrosa*); 73. Grindelia (*Grindelia squarrosa*)

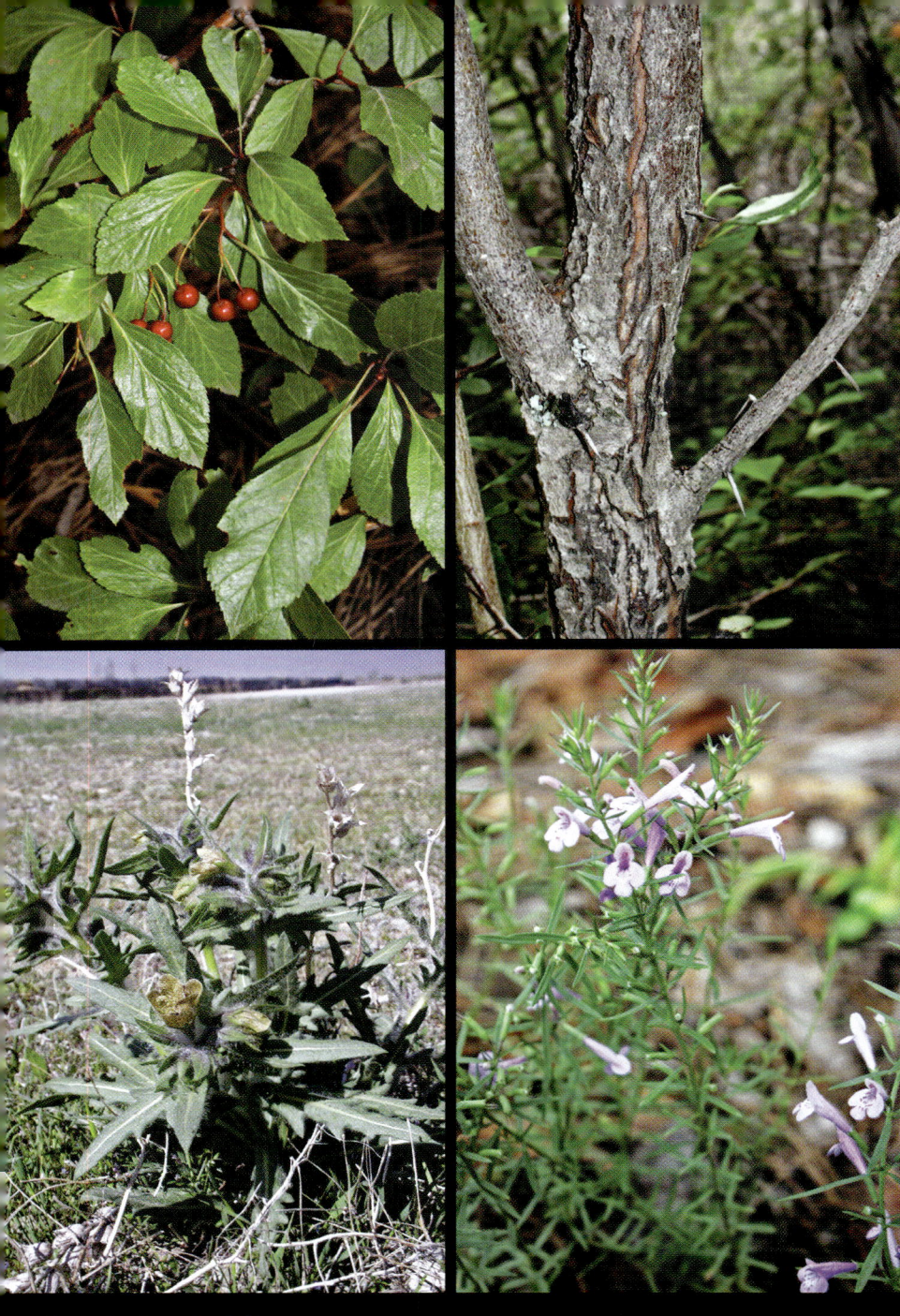

Clockwise from top left:
74. Hawthorn (*Crataegus rivularis*); 75. Hawthorn (*Crataegus rivularis*); 76. Hedeoma

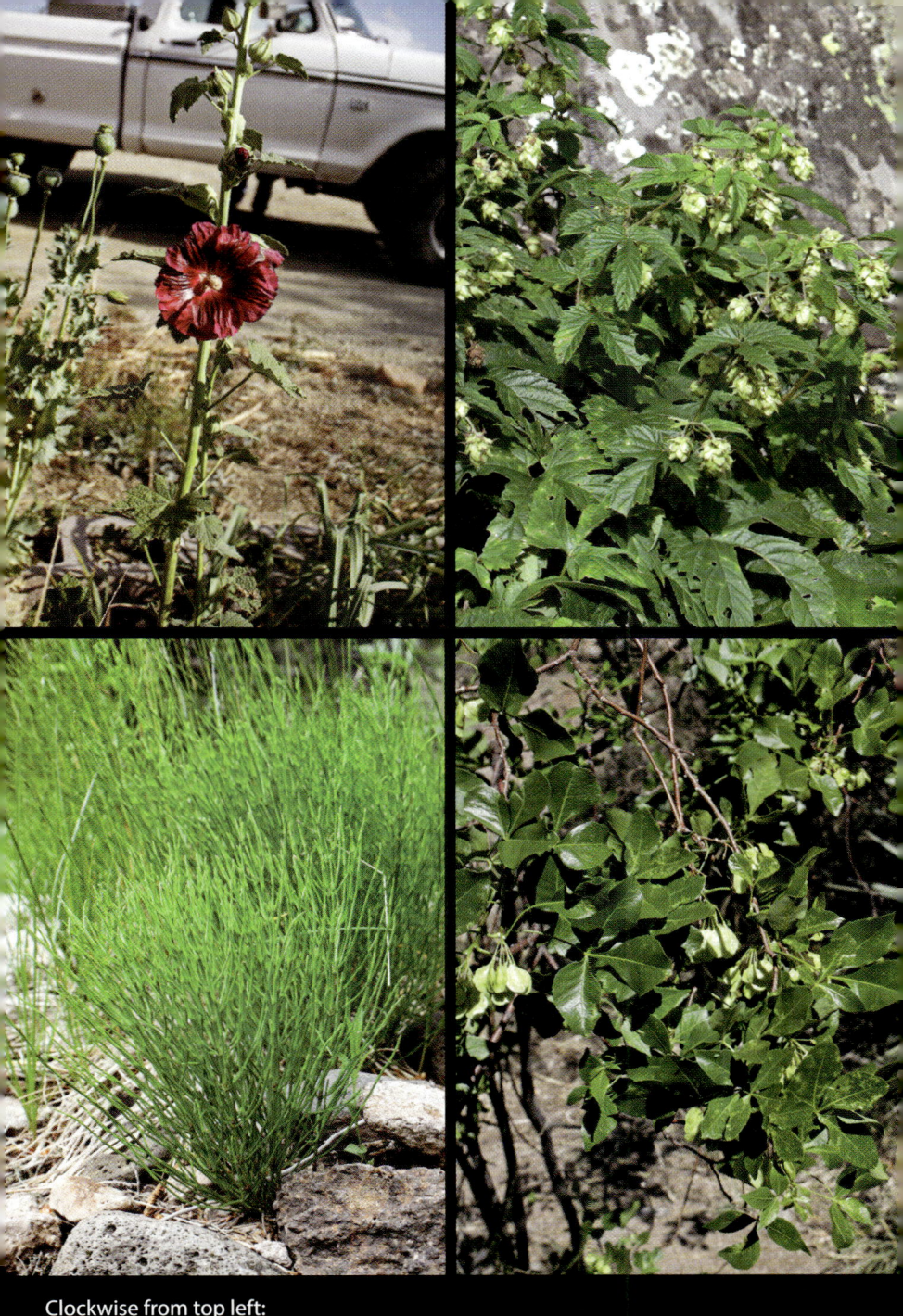

Clockwise from top left:
78. Hollyhock (*Althea rosea*); 79. Hops (*Humulus neomexicanus*); 80. Hoptree (*Ptelea trifoliata*); 81. Horsetail (*Equisetum arvense*)

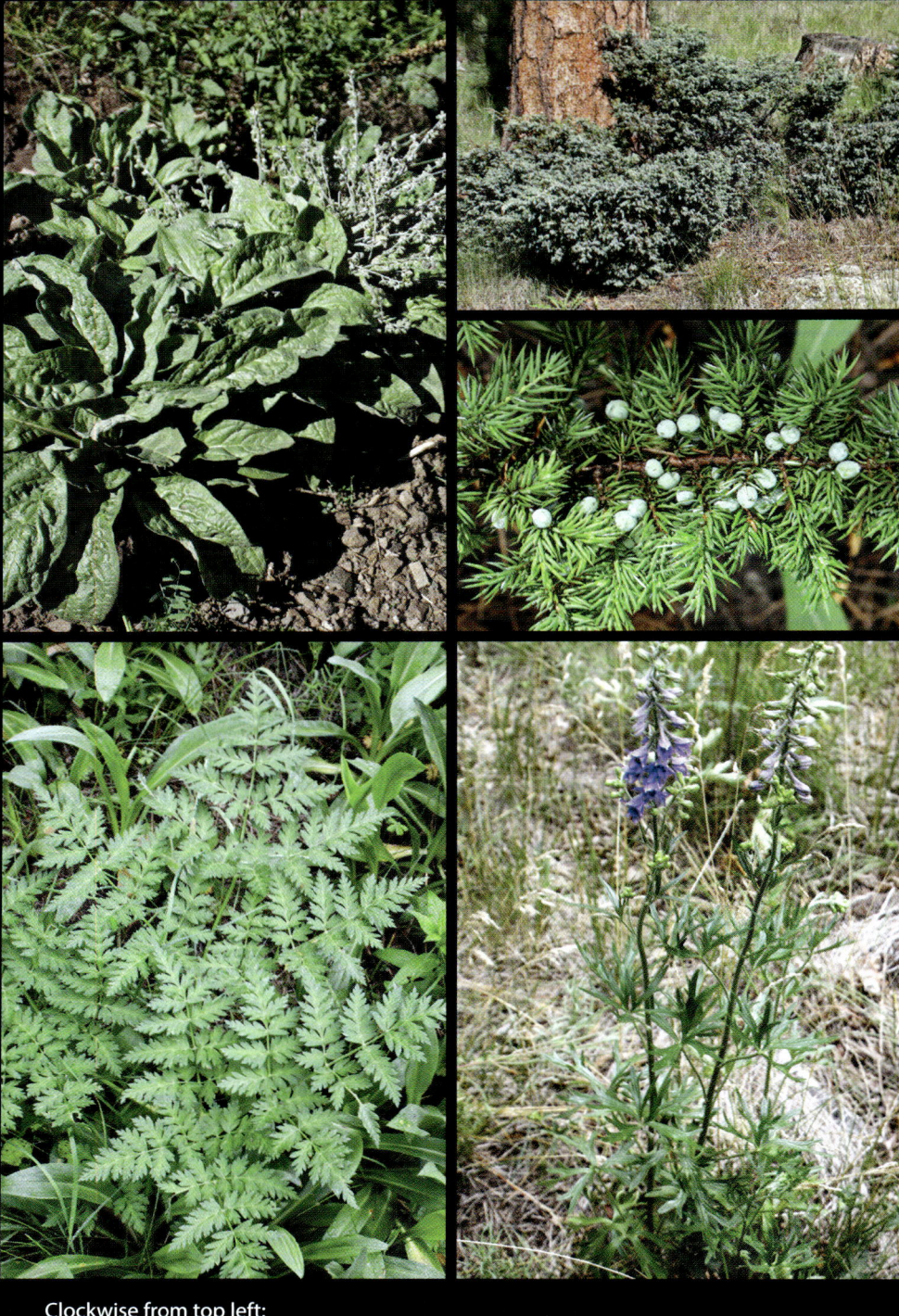

Clockwise from top left:
82. Hound's tongue (*Cynoglossum officinale*); 83. Juniper (*Juniperus communis*); 84. Juniper (*Juniperus communis*); 85. Larkspur (*Delphinium geraniifolium*); 86. Ligusticum (*Ligusticum porteri*).

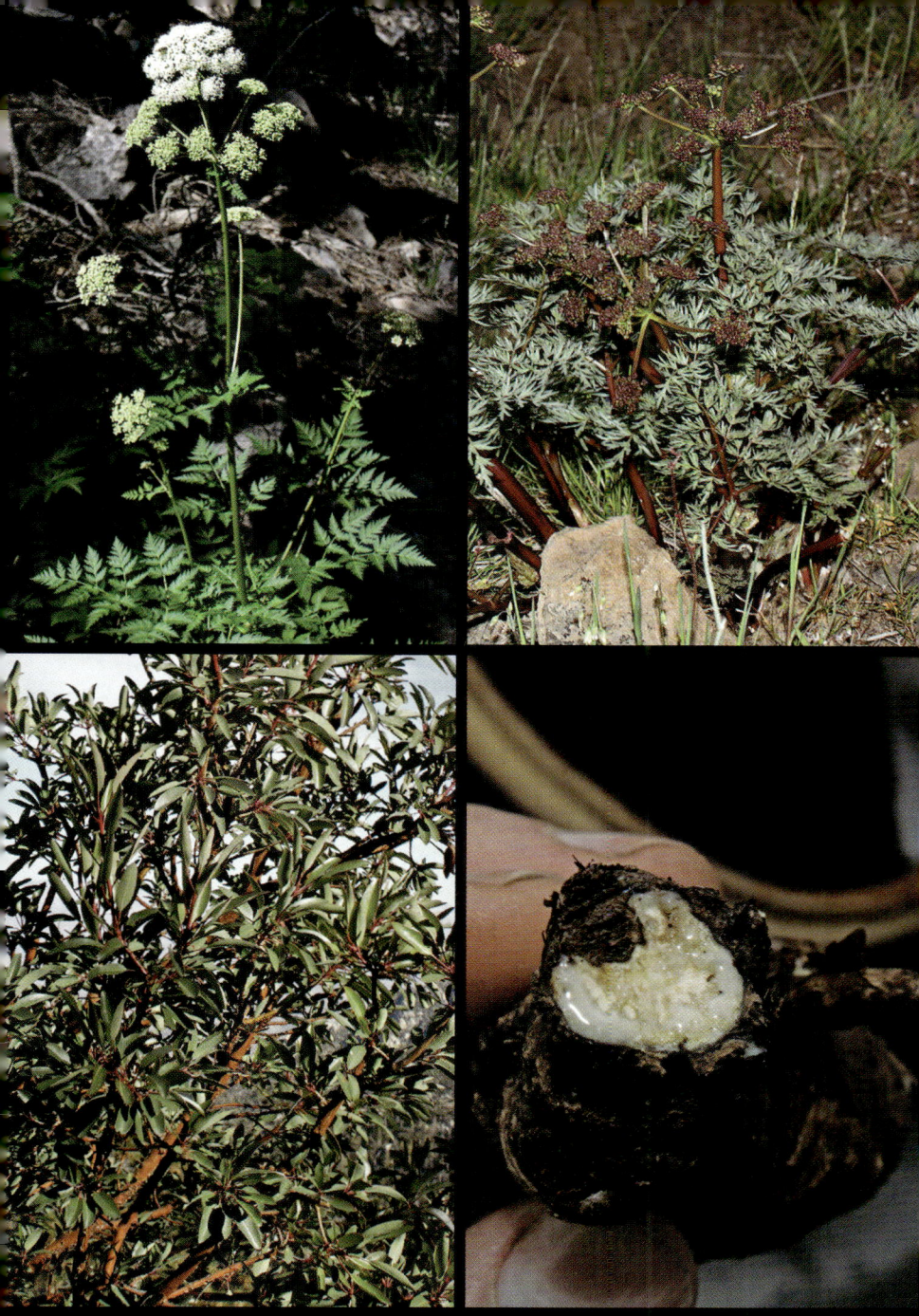

Clockwise from top left:
87. Ligusticum (*Ligusticum porteri*); 88. Lomatium (*Lomatium dissectum*); 89. Lomatium

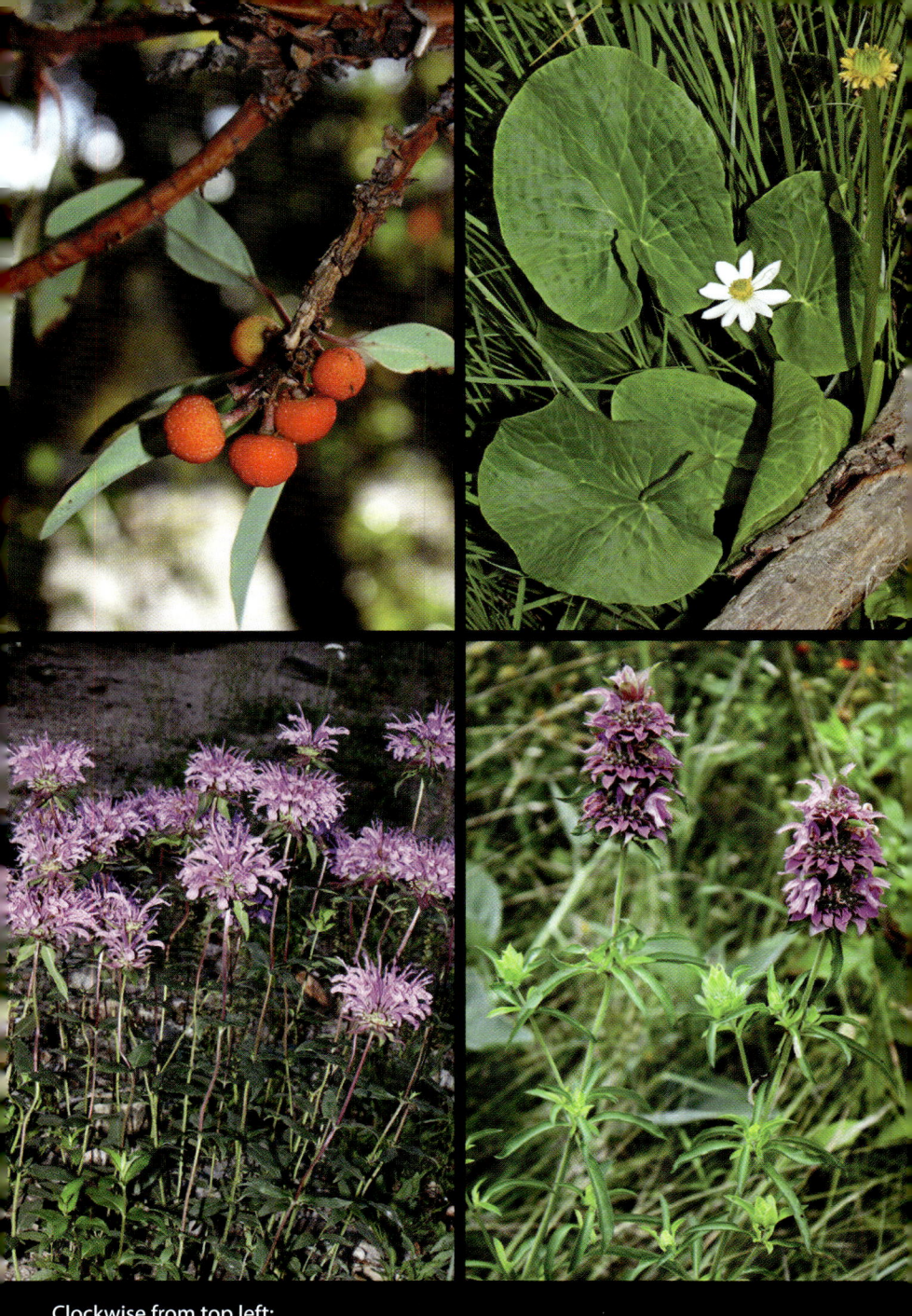

Clockwise from top left:
91. Madrone (*Arbutus arizonica*); 92. Marsh marigold (*Caltha leptosepala*); 93. Monarda (*Monarda citriodora*); 94. Monarda (*Monarda fistulosa*)

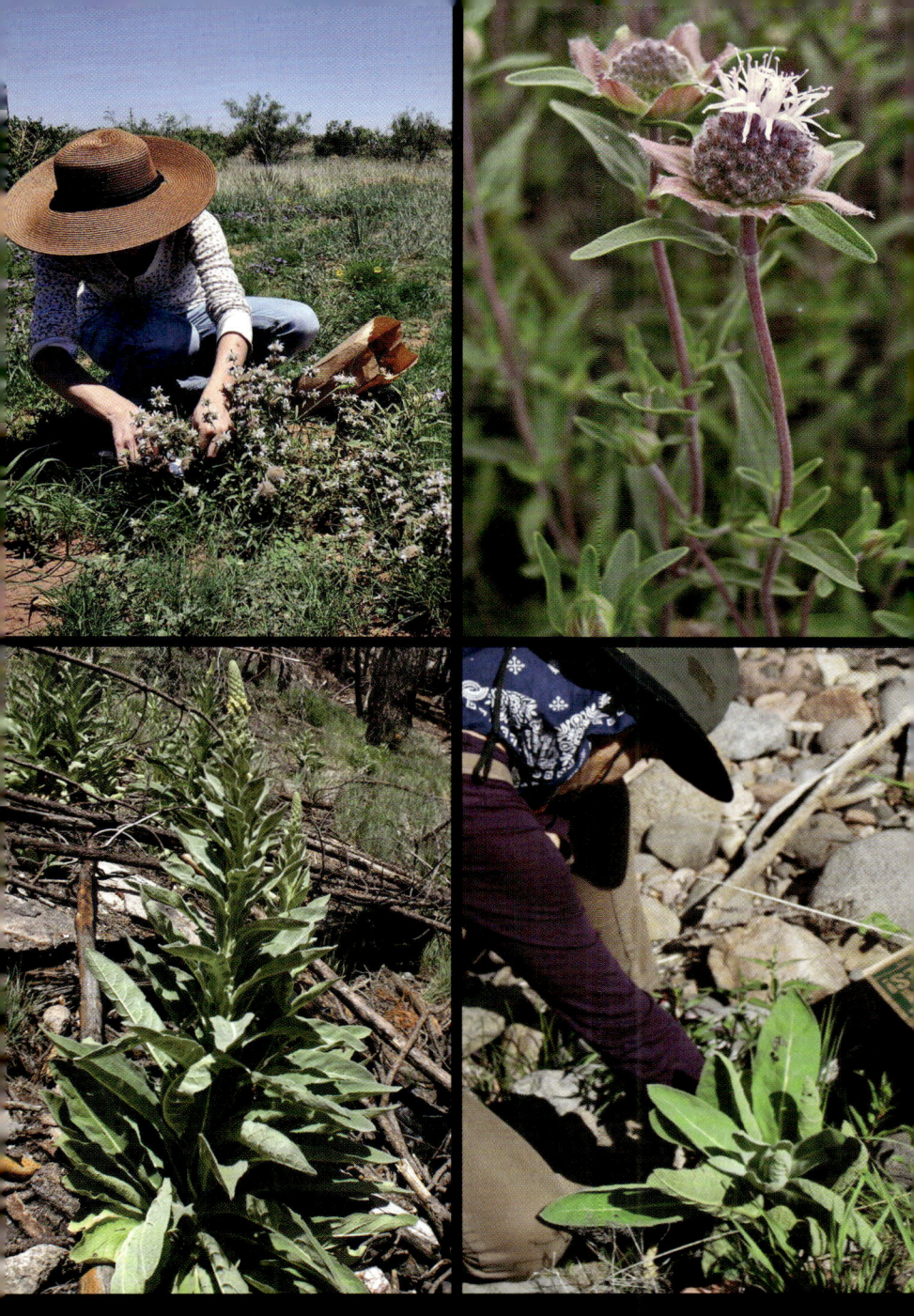

Clockwise from top left:
95. Monarda (*Monarda pectinata*); 96. Monardella (*Monardella odoratissima*); 97. Mullein (*Verbascum thapsus*); 98. Mullein (*Verbascum thapsus*)

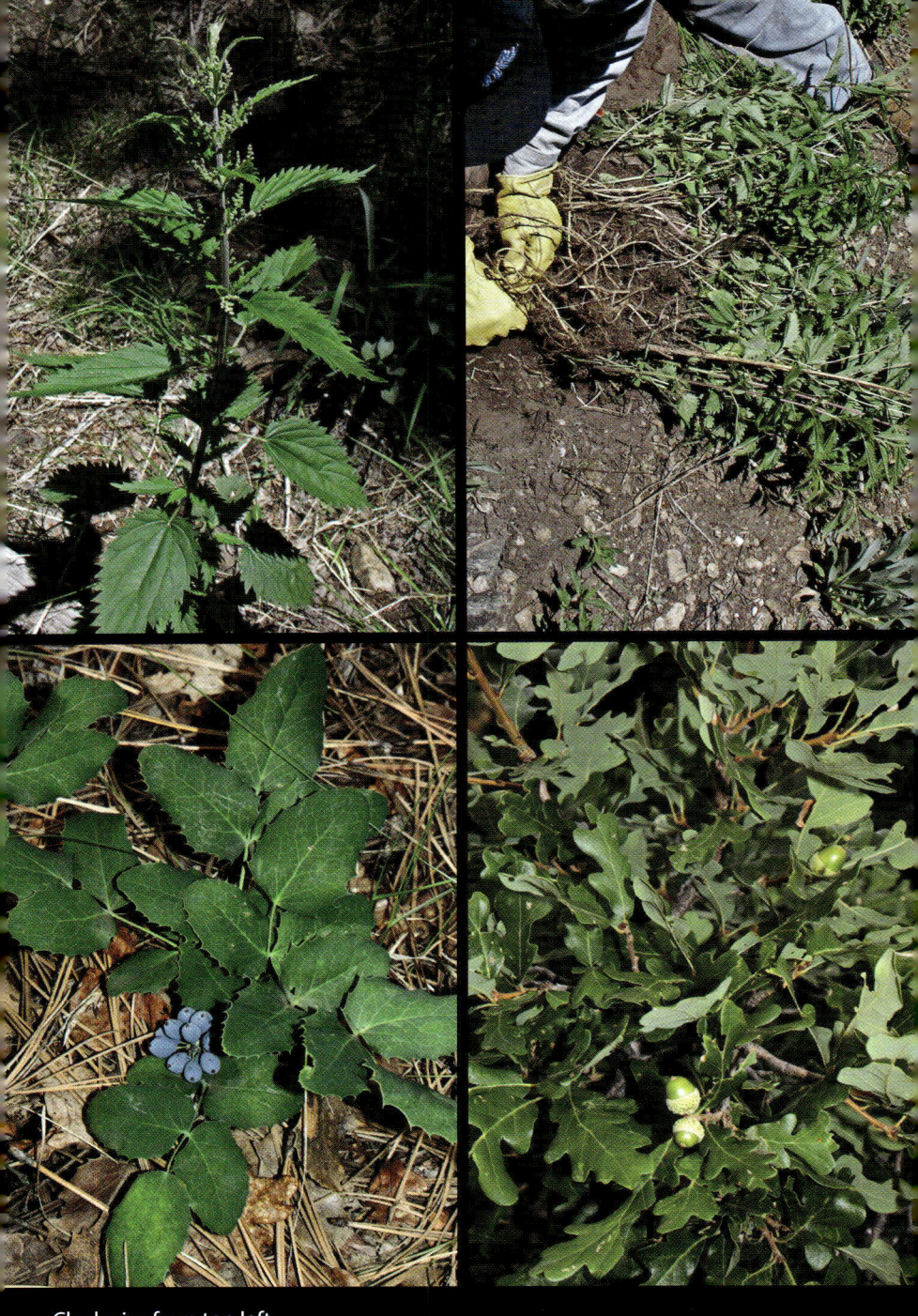

Clockwise from top left:
99. Nettle (*Urtica dioica subsp. gracilis*); 100. Nettle (*Urtica dioica subsp. gracilis*); 101. Oak

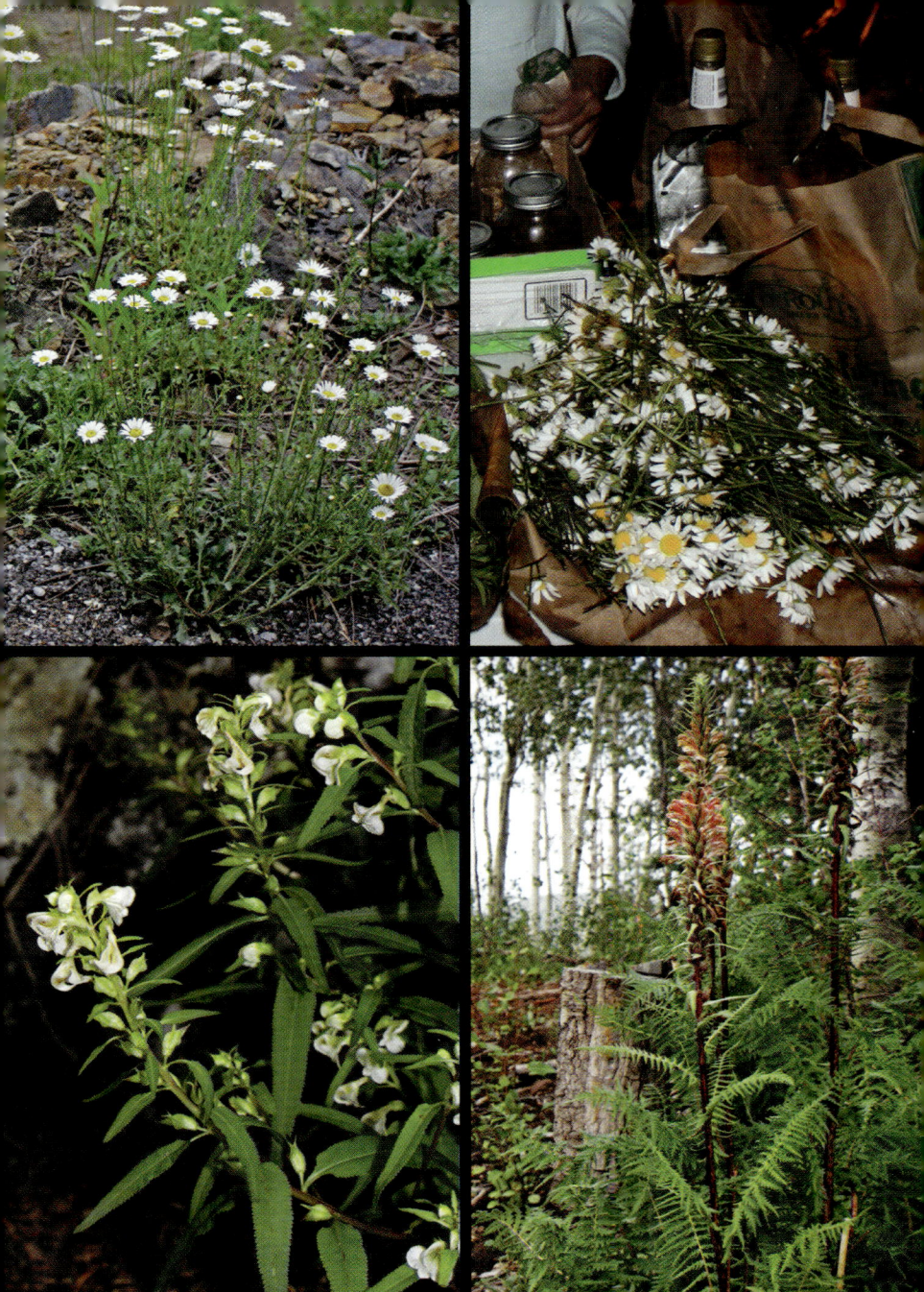

Clockwise from top left:
103. Ox–eye daisy (*Leucanthemum vulgare*); 104. Ox–eye daisy (*Leucanthemum vulgare*); 105. Pedicularis (*Pedicularis procera*); 106. Pedicularis (*Pedicularis racemosa*)

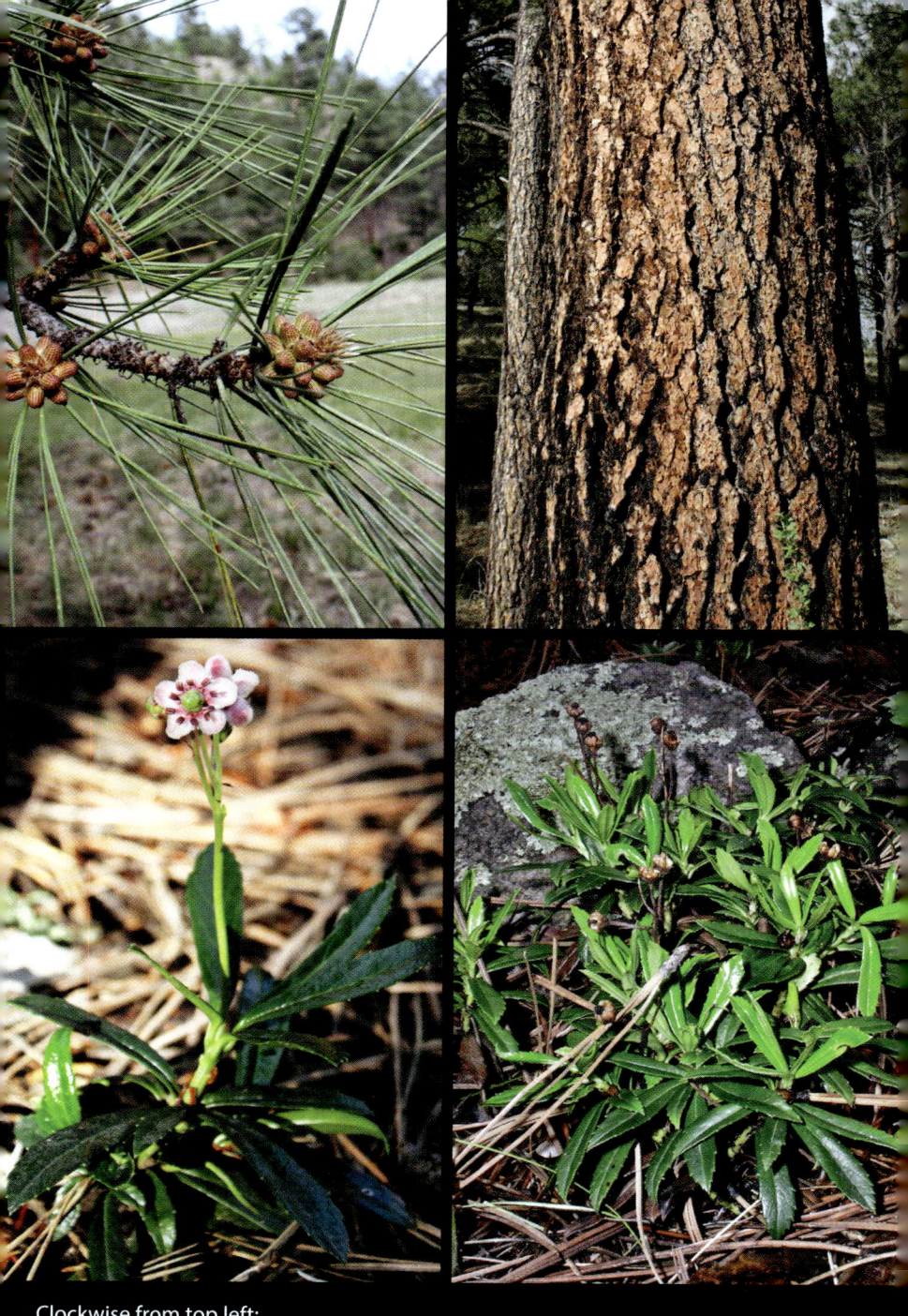

Clockwise from top left:
107. Pine (*Pinus ponderosa*); 108. Pine (*Pinus ponderosa*); 109. Pipsissewa (*Chimaphila umbellata*); 110. Pipsissewa (*Chimaphila umbellata*).

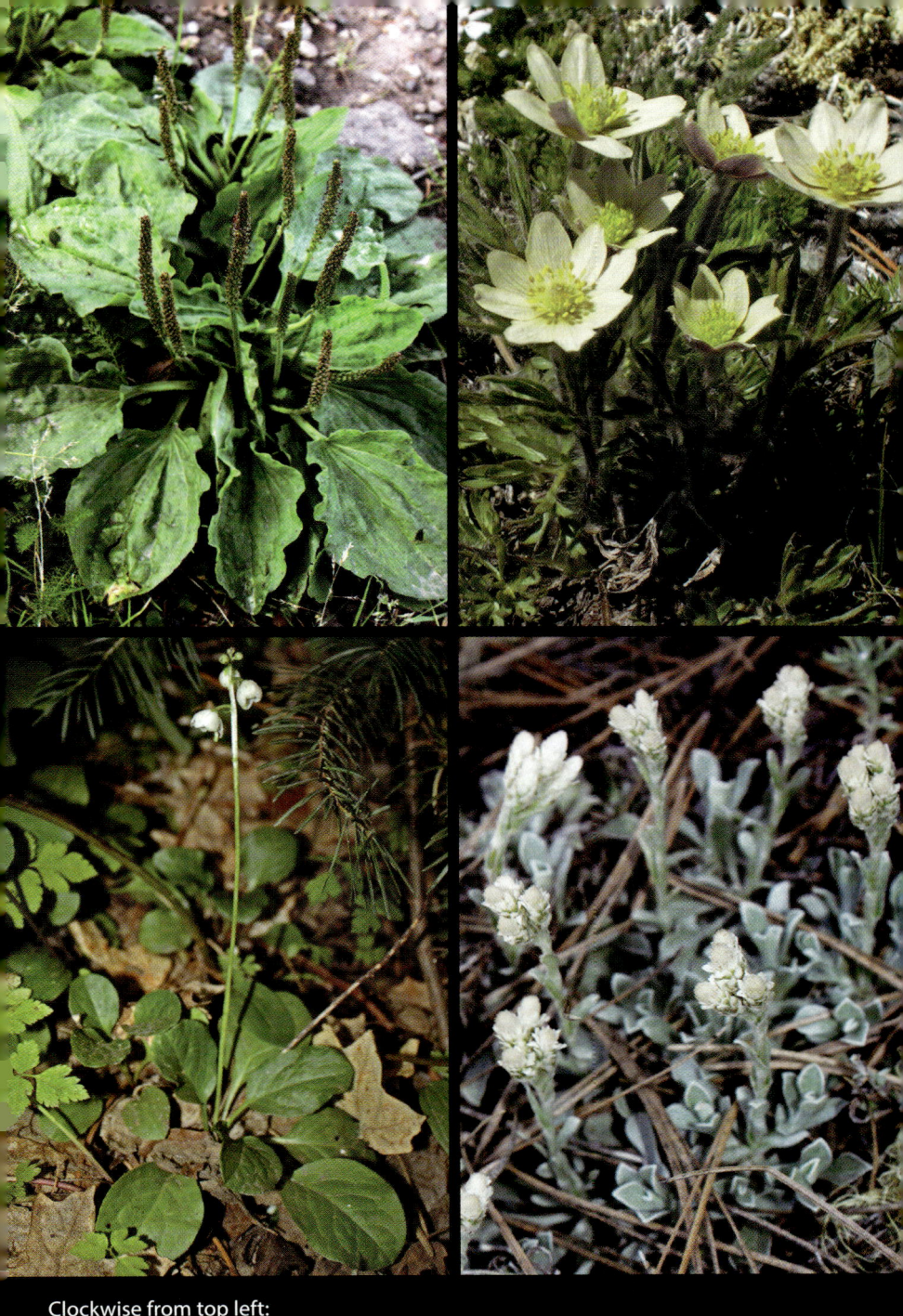

Clockwise from top left:
111. Plantain (*Plantago major*); 112. Pulsatilla (*Pulsatilla occidentalis*); 113. Pussytoes (*Antennaria parvifolia*); 114. Pyrola (*Pyrola elliptica*)

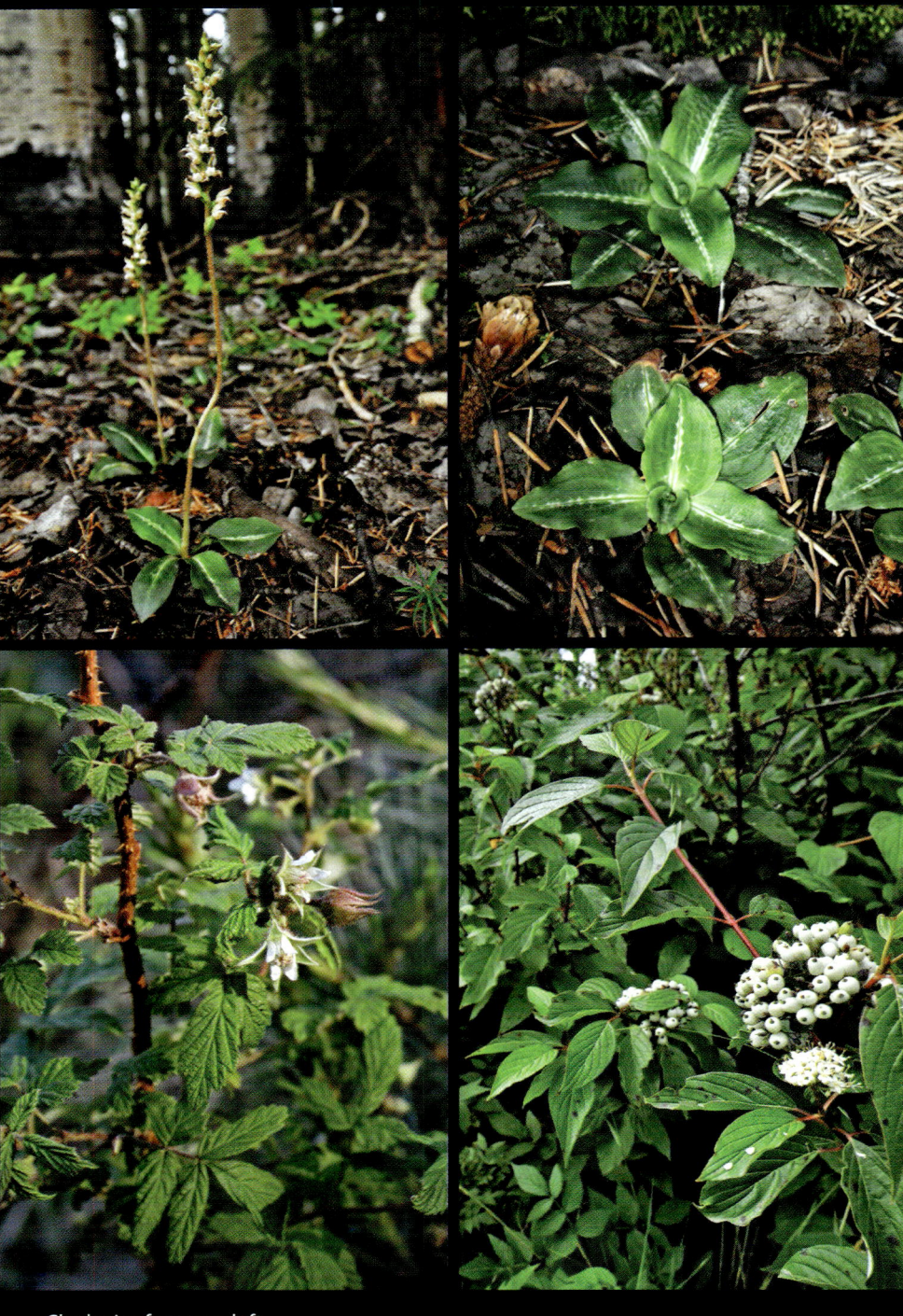

Clockwise from top left:
115. Rattlesnake plantain (*Goodyera oblongifolia*); 116. Rattlesnake plantain (*Goodyera oblongifolia*); 117. Red osier dogwood (*Cornus sericea*); 118. Red raspberry (*Rubus idaeus* var. *strigosus*).

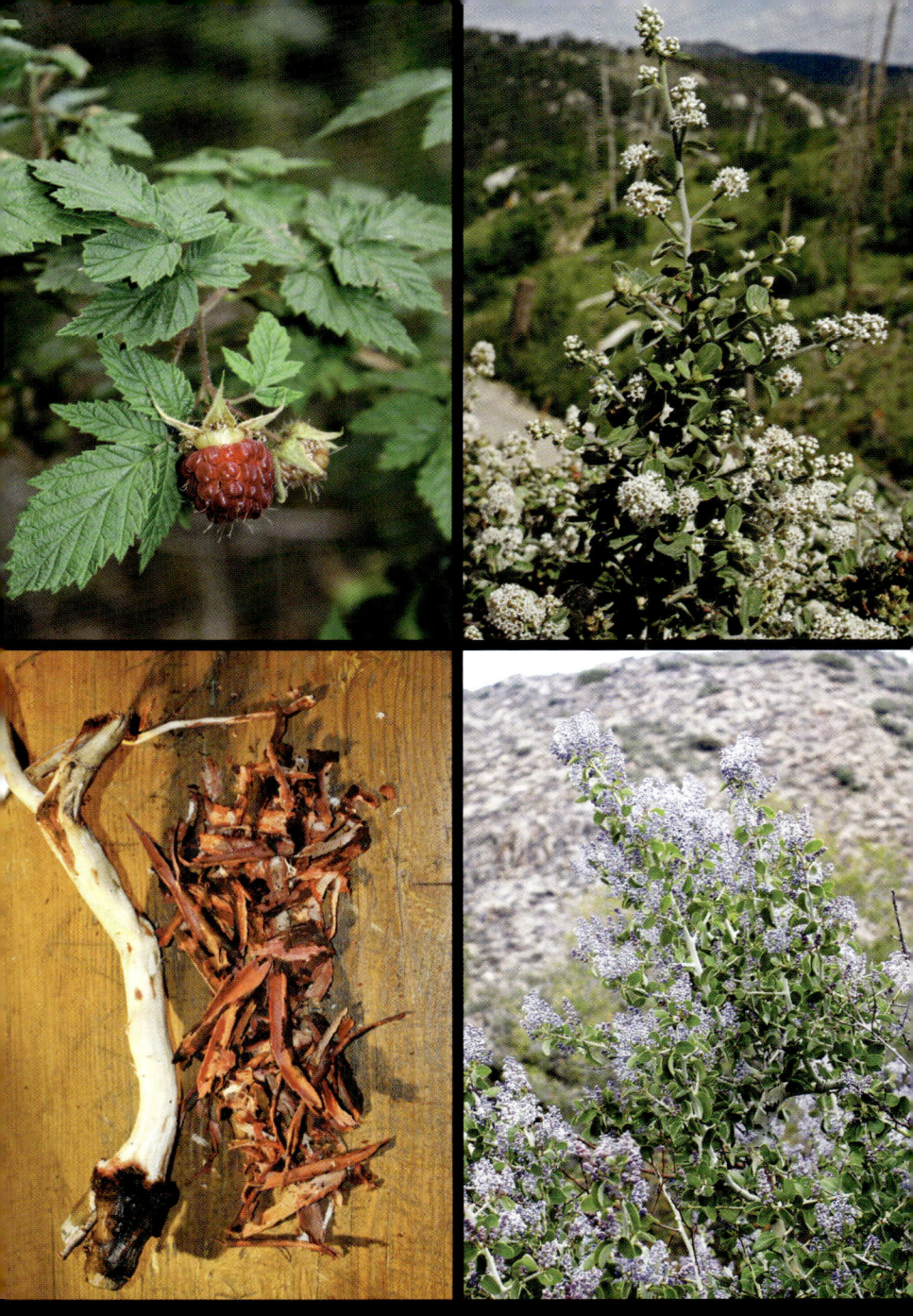

Clockwise from top left:
119. Red raspberry (*Rubus idaeus* var. *strigosus*); 120. Red root (*Ceanothus fendleri*); 121. Red root (*Ceanothus leucodermis*); 122. Red root (*Ceanothus greggii* var. *perplexans*)

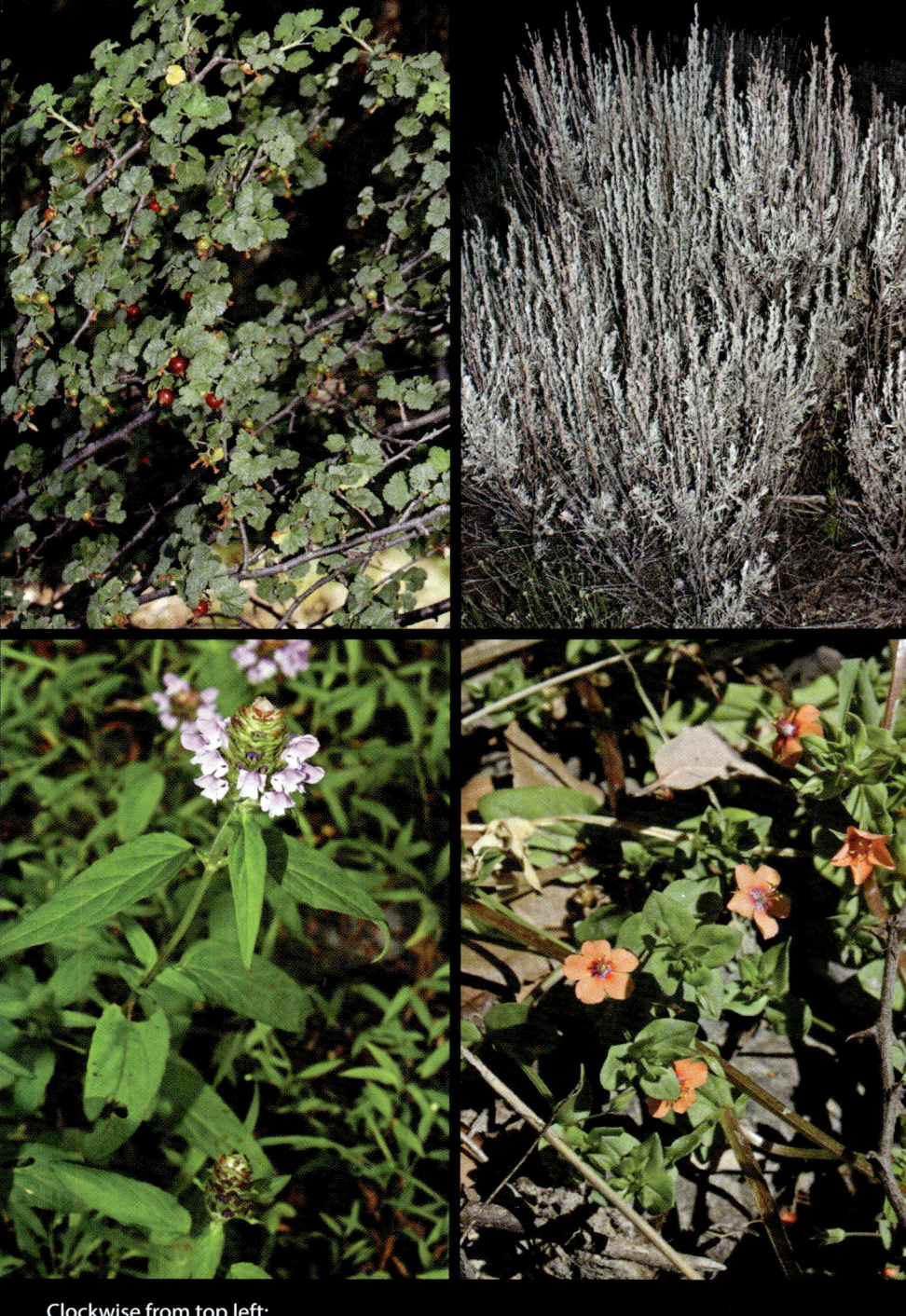

Clockwise from top left:
123. Ribes (*Ribes cereum*); 124. Sagebrush (*Artemisia tridentata*); 125. Scarlet pimpernel (*Anagallis arvensis*); 126. Self heal (*Prunella vulgaris var. lanceolata*).

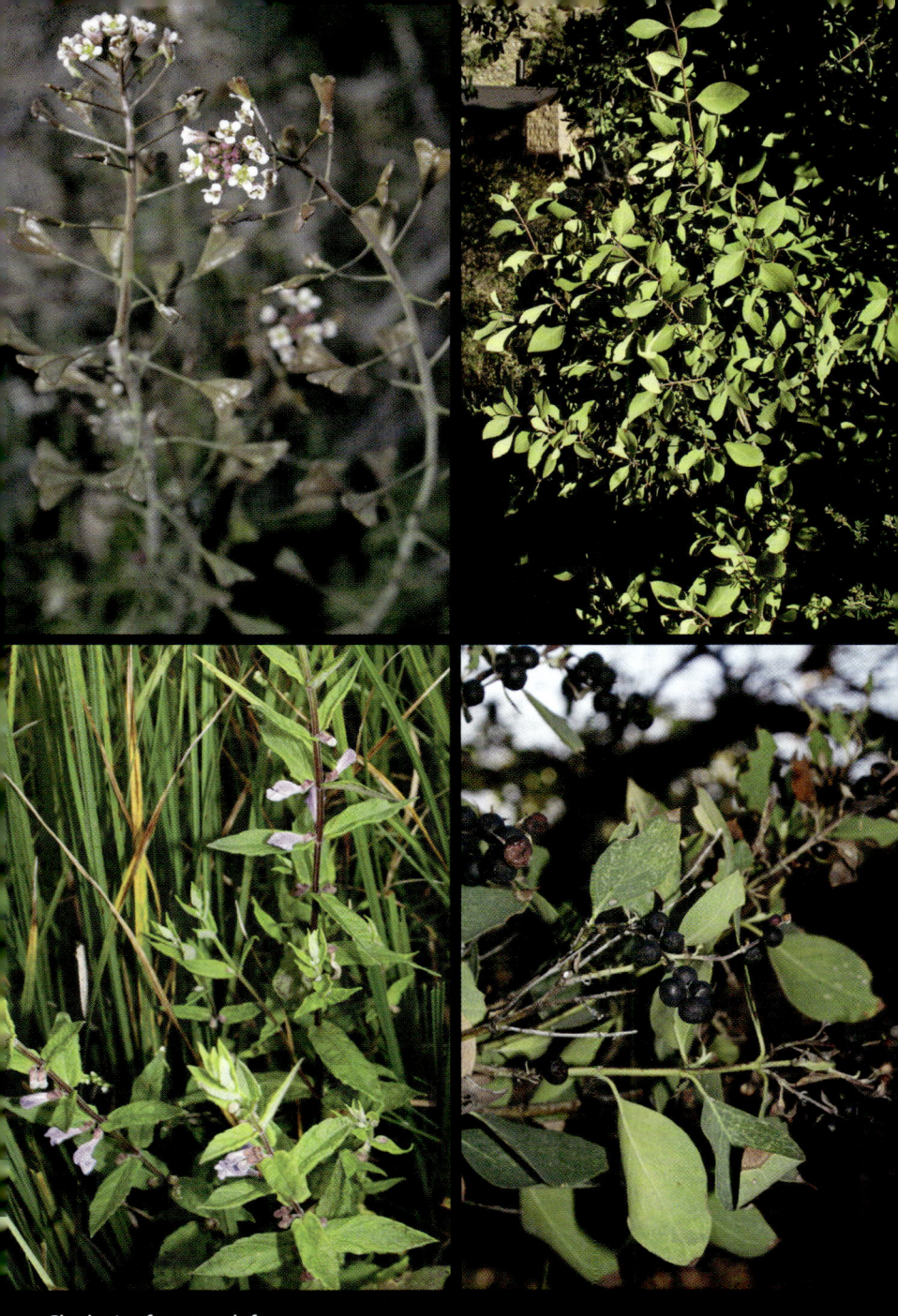

Clockwise from top left:
127. Shepard's purse (*Capsella bursa-pastoris*); 128. Silk tassel (*Garrya wrightii*); 129. Silk tassel (*Garrya wrightii*); 130. Skullcap (*Scutellaria galericulata*)

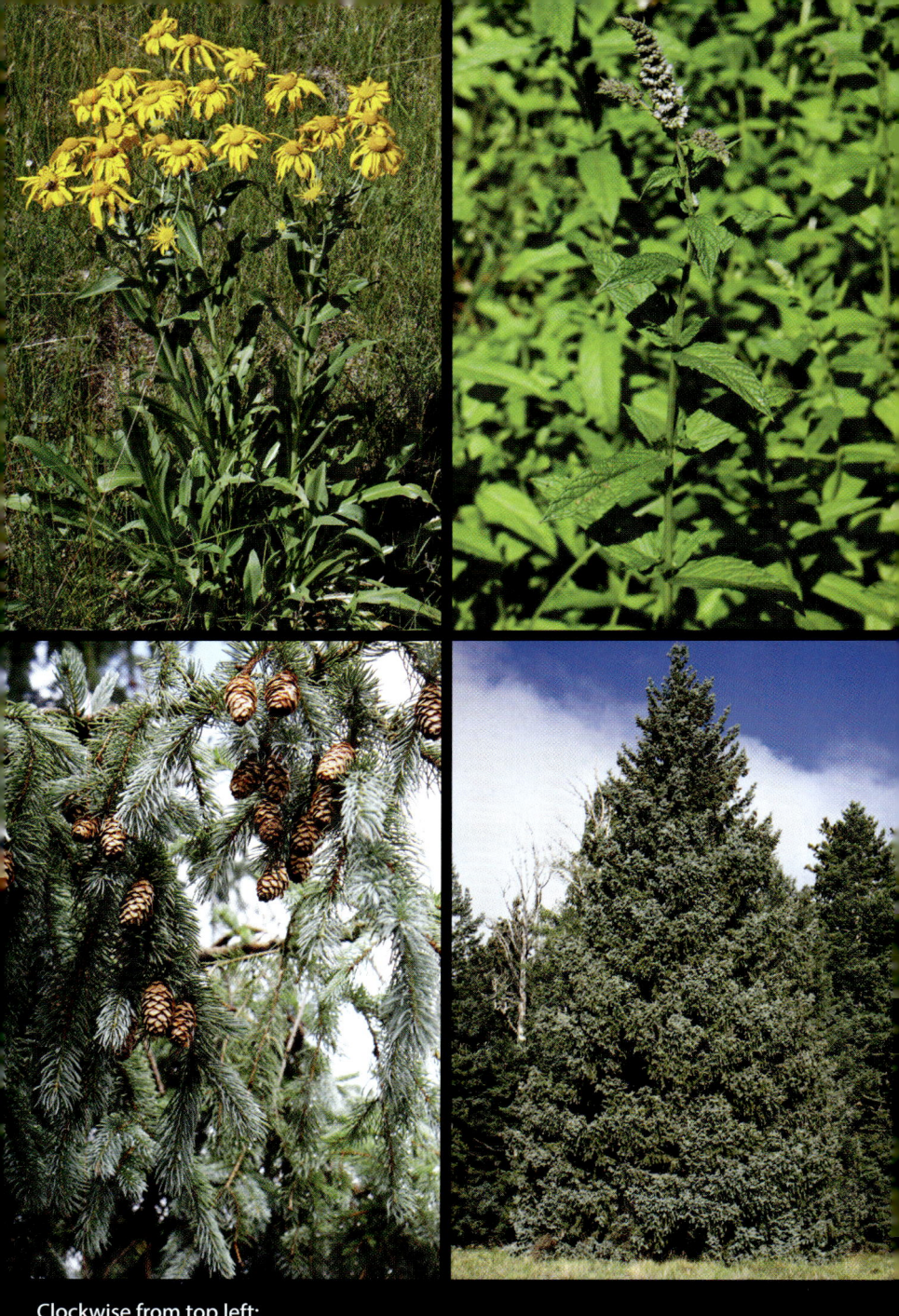

Clockwise from top left:
131. Sneezeweed (*Hymenoxys hoopesii*); 132. Spearmint (*Mentha spicata*); 133. Spruce

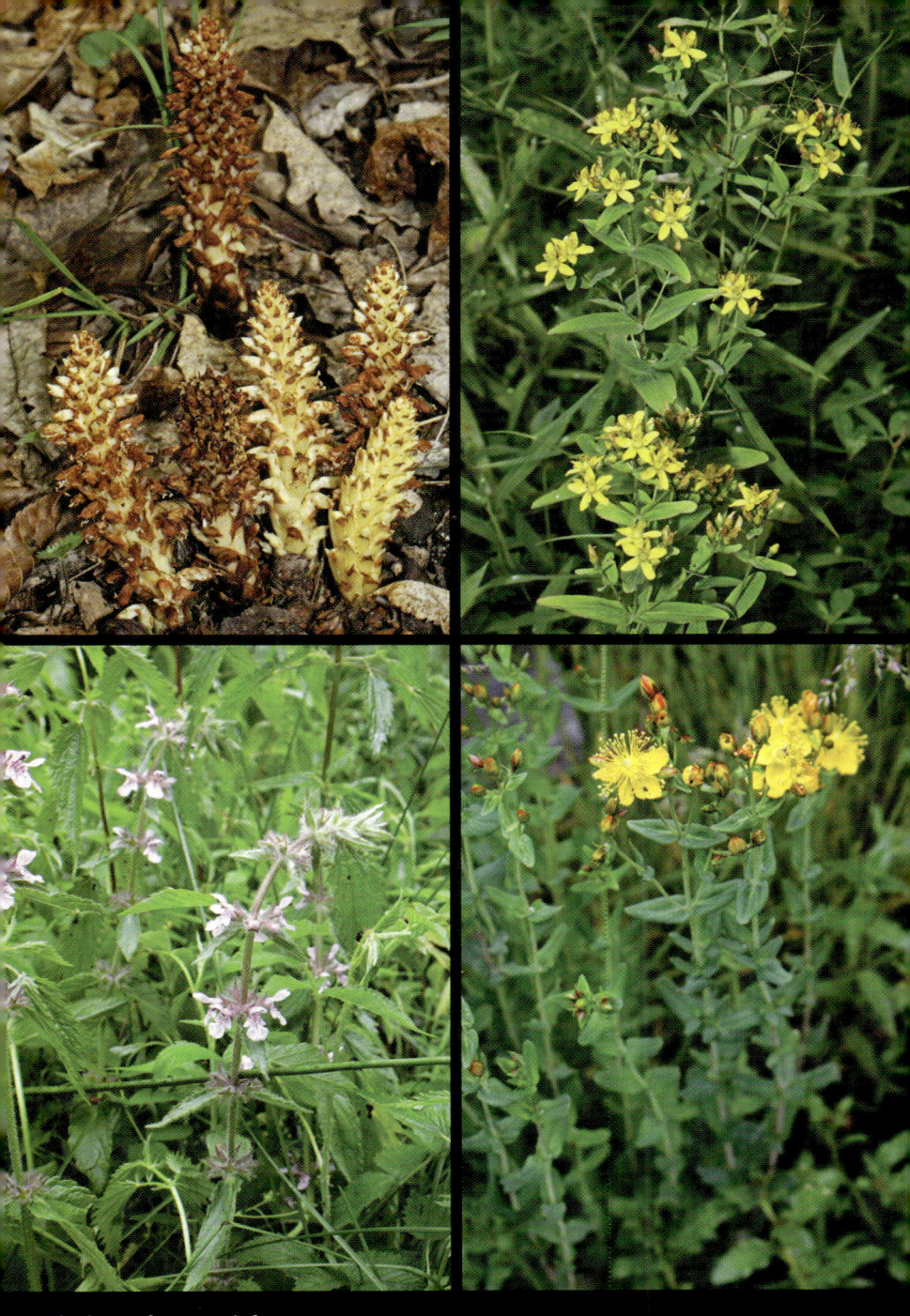

Clockwise from top left:
135. Squawroot (*Conopholis americana*); 136. St. John's wort (*Hypericum perforatum*); 137. St. John's wort (*Hypericum scouleri*); 138. Stachys (*Stachys pilosa*)

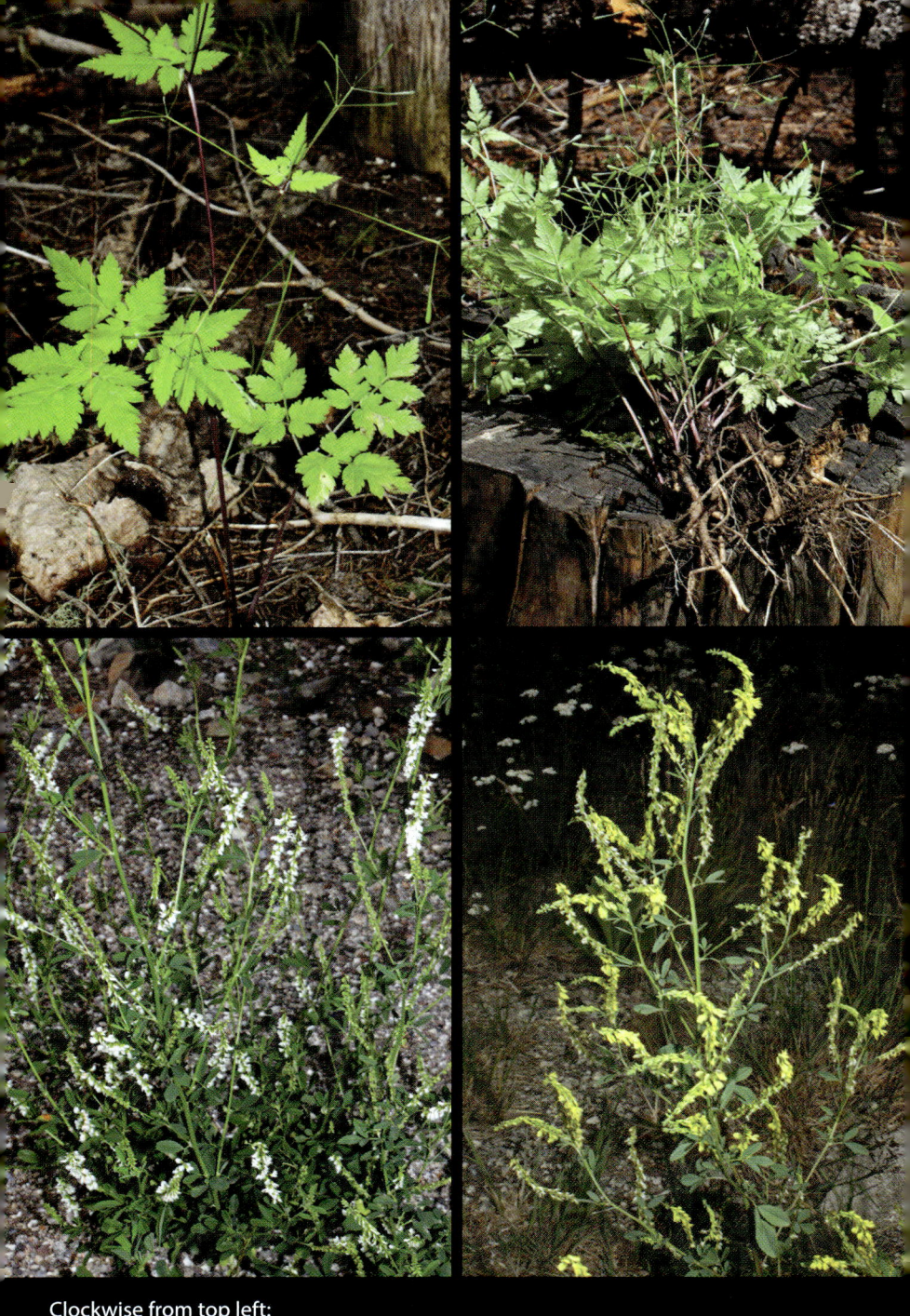

Clockwise from top left:
139. Sweet cicely (*Osmorhiza depauperata*); 140 Sweet cicely (*Osmorhiza depauperata*);
141. Sweet clover (*Melilotus officinalis*); 142. Sweet clover (*Melilotus albus*)

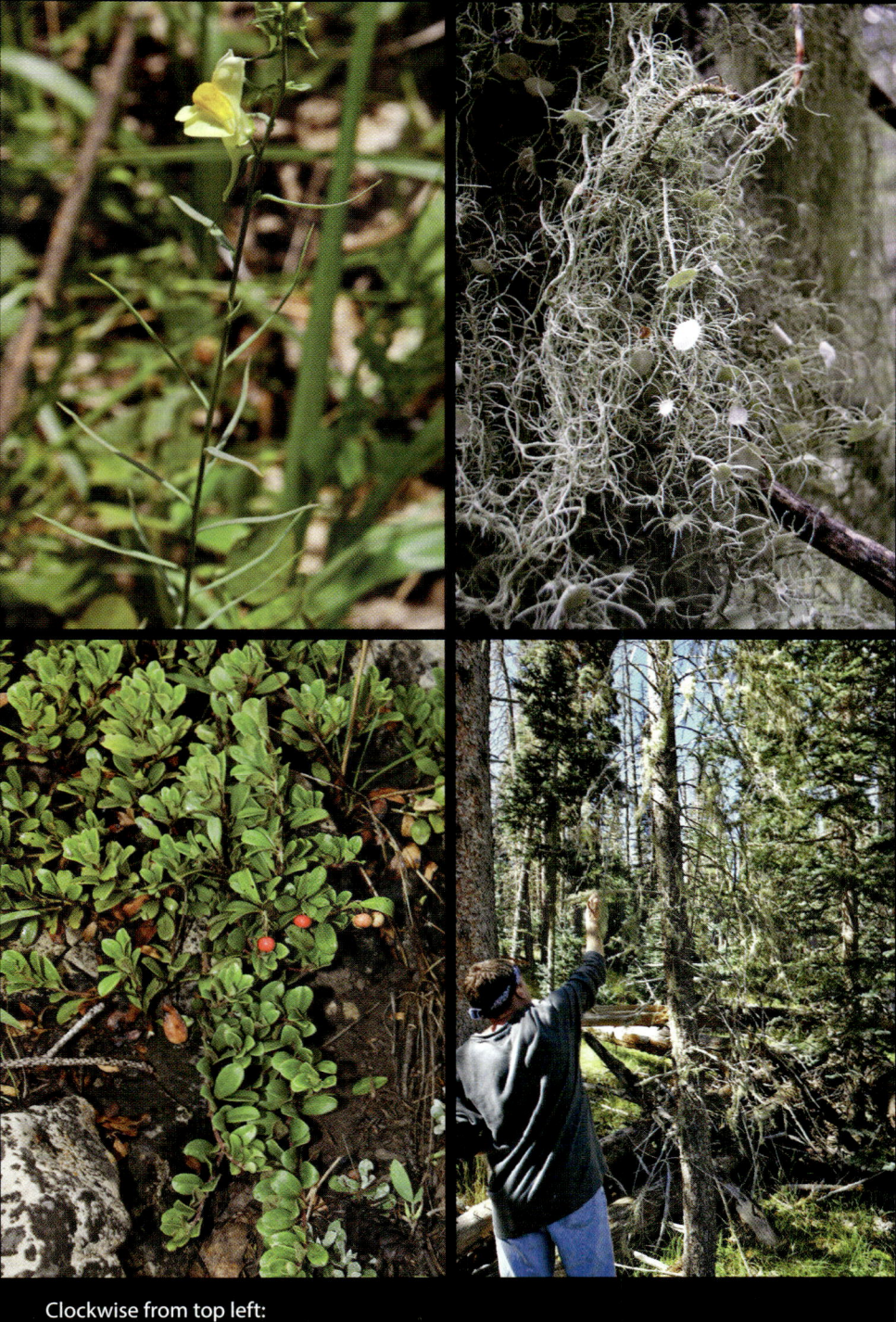

Clockwise from top left:
143. Toadflax (*Linaria vulgaris*); 144. Usnea (*Usnea spp.*); 145. Usnea (*Usnea spp.*); 146. Uva-ursi (*Arctostaphylos uva–ursi*).

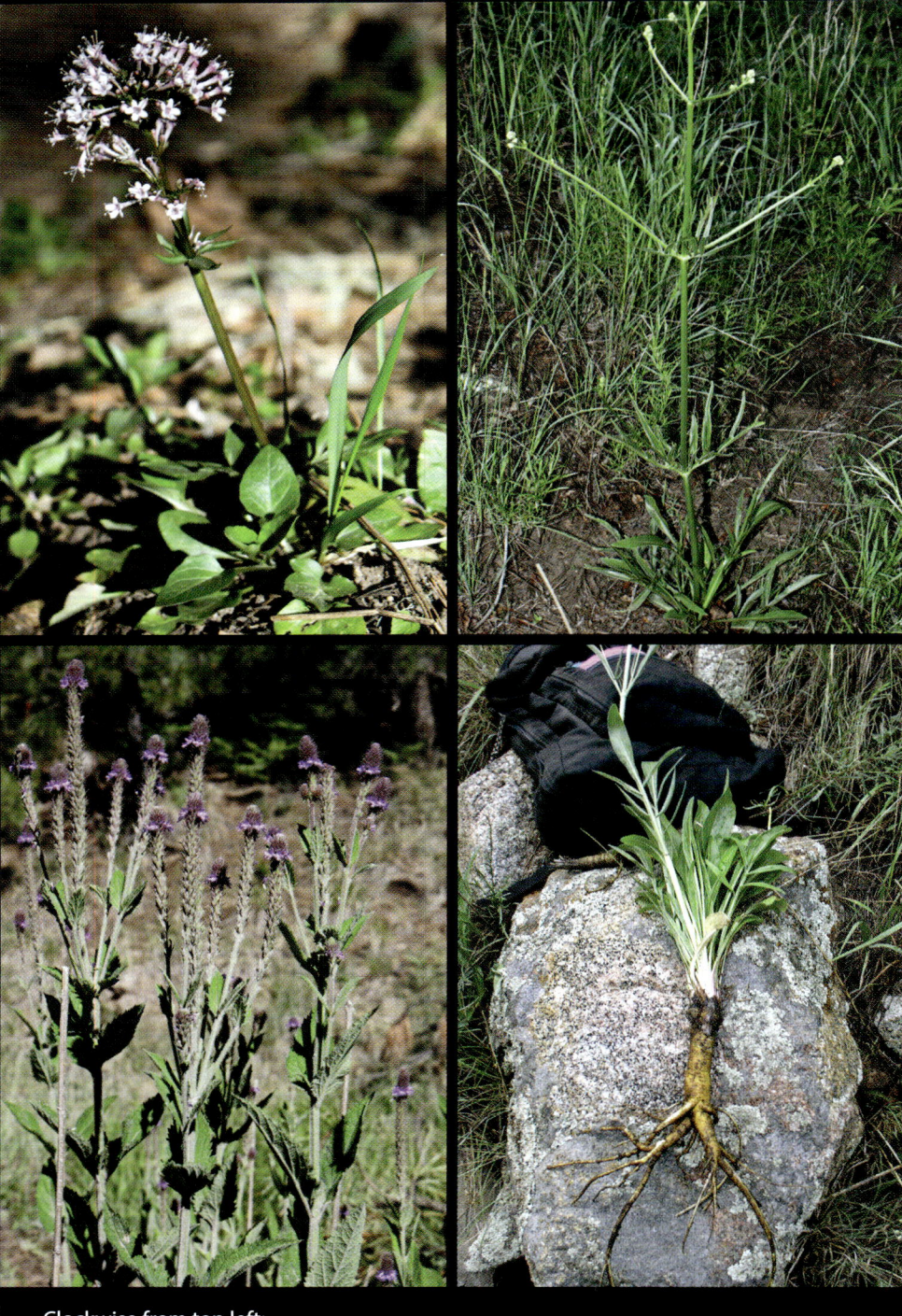

Clockwise from top left:
147. Valerian (*Valeriana arizonica*); 148. Valerian (*Valeriana edulis*); 149. Valerian (*Valeriana edulis*); 150. Verbena (*Verbena macdougalii*).

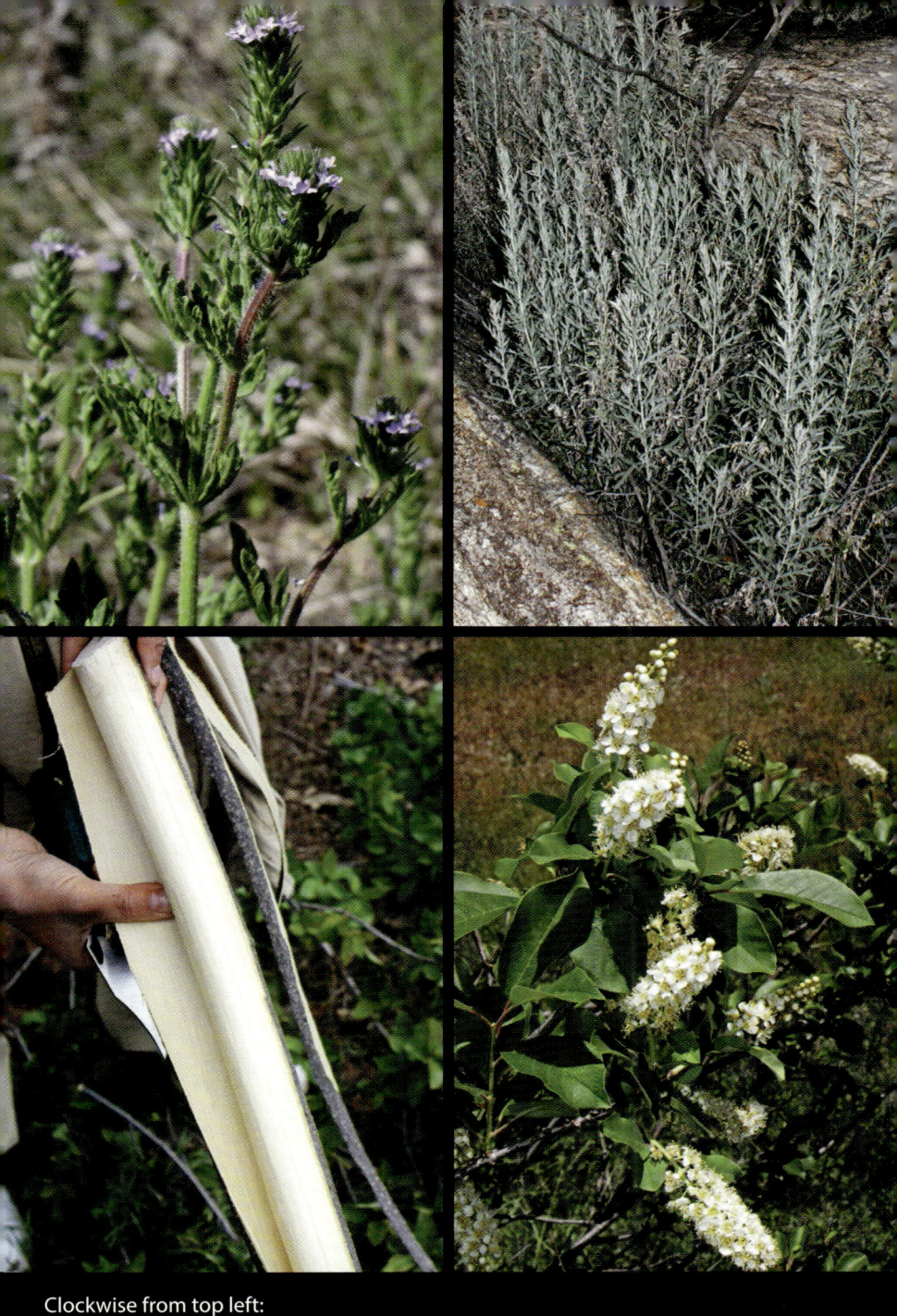

Clockwise from top left:
151. Verbena (*Verbena bracteata*); 152. Western mugwort (*Artemisia ludoviciana*); 153. Wild cherry (*Prunus virginiana var. demissa*); 154. Wild cherry (*Prunus virginiana var. demissa*)

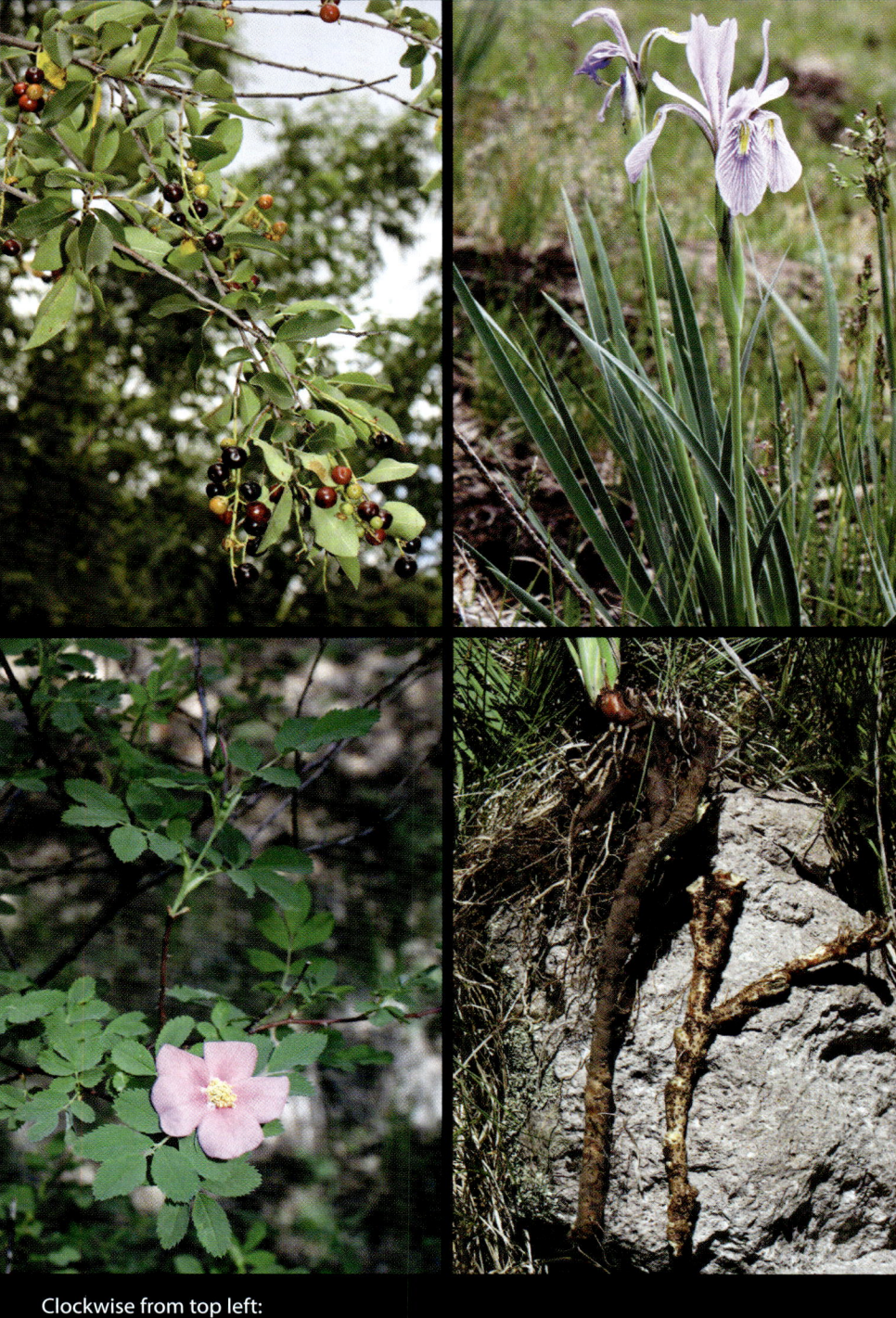

Clockwise from top left:
155. Wild cherry (*Prunus serotina* var. *rufula*); 156. Wild iris (*Iris missouriensis*); 157. Wild iris (*Iris missouriensis*); 158. Wild rose (*Rosa woodsii*).

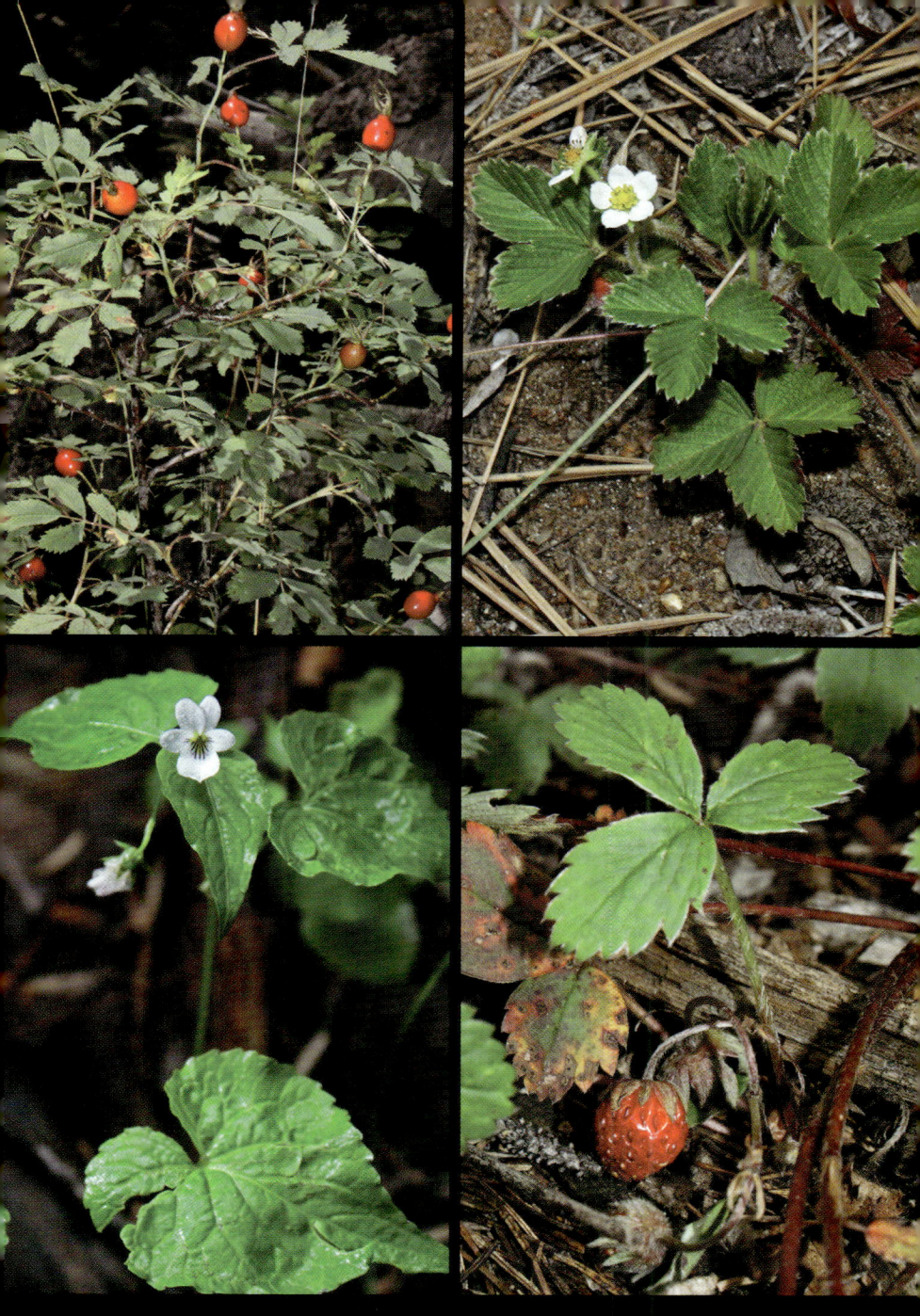

Clockwise from top left:
159. Wild rose (*Rosa woodsii*); 160. Wild strawberry (*Fragaria vesca*); 161. Wild strawberry

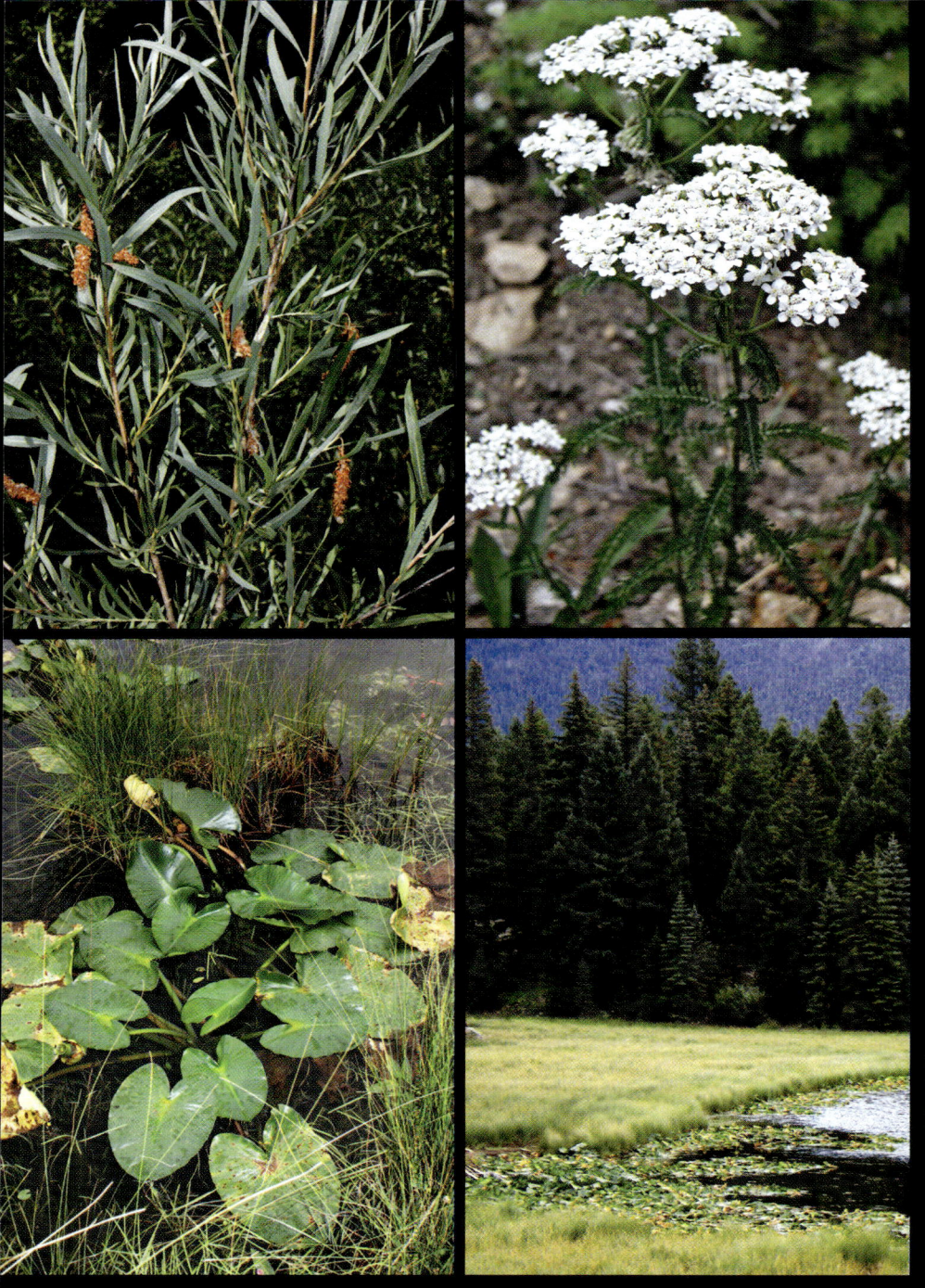

Clockwise from top left:
163. Willow (*Salix exigua*); 164. Yarrow (*Achillea millefolium*); 165. Yellow pond lily (*Nuphar polysepala*); 166. Yellow pond lily (*Nuphar polysepala*).

menstrual stimulant and is well used by women to relieve pelvic congestion if menses is suppressed.

Oil–based preparations, the dried and powdered root used as a dust, or the re–hydrated root powder used as a poultice are the choice modes for topical use. Distinctly antimicrobial, apply the root to infected cuts, scrapes, burns, sores, boils, and related issues. The room temperature tea as a sitz bath for bacterial or fungal vaginal infections has merit.

As for Lomatium's influencing of Epstein–Barr virus (Chronic fatigue syndrome), other herpesviruses, HIV[48] (as a co–therapy), and chronic Lyme's disease, or other related immunity/viral issues, I'm cautious to recommend the plant. That's entering panacea territory. Furthermore, there is some misapplied information in circulation: petri dish studies with a derivative rarely equate consistent success with the whole herb used with real people. I will say though, individuals with chronic systemic viral infections with few treatment options have little to lose – try it. If it makes you feel better than stay the course.

Indications
» Bronchitis, especially viral–related
» Bronchitis, thickened mucus
» Influenza, with lung involvement and fever
» As an expectorant
» Pharyngitis/Laryngitis
» Infection, skin (external)

Collection
Depending on the plant's age, root sizes will be small to very large. Most of the root's mass is centered around its crown and directly below. I recommend first digging down a couple of inches where the stem meets the ground. By doing so the collector will get a better idea of how much work is needed in removing the entire root. The wider the crown, the larger the root, and therefore the more labor intensive collection will be. Gathering a number of smaller to mid–sized roots in lieu of one large one, in most cases, is ideal. That way the gatherer can incrementally add to the collection as opposed to being stuck with excess material that may go to waste.

48 Most of the HIV studies (petri dish) are using suksdorfin, a constituent from Lomatium suksdorfii. It is total speculation whether Lomatium dissectum even contains this compound, let alone modifies HIV.

Lomatium is mostly a rocky hillside grower. And accordingly, the plant's forked roots often trace around subterranean rocks. Bring an array of tools – trowel, shovel, and pick axe.

Preparations/Dosage
» FPT/DPT (70% alcohol): 20–60 drops 2–3 times daily
» Standard/Cold infusion: 2–4 oz. 2–3 times daily
» Topical preparations: as needed

Cautions
5%–10% of people who take Lomatium develop the 'Lomatium rash'. Appearing like a hive outbreak, it's an inflammatory reaction to one or a number of the plant's compounds (furanocoumarins may be the culprit). If the rash occurs, stop taking the herb, or try using the tea or dry plant tincture instead of the fresh plant tincture. It's also not recommended during pregnancy, while nursing, or with babies. Dosed properly, Lomatium is fine with children.

Other Uses
Occasionally the roots are listed as having food uses. Like Cow parsnip, they are just too aromatic/balsamic/bitter to be eaten fresh. After much processing, maybe this species could be used as a survival food...but not as a staple. It's a medicine, not a food.

There do exist other Lomatium species that make fine root foods. These plants will have non–balsamic roots. For instance, Lomatium nevadense roots (and tops) are edible and need very little, if any, processing.

Madrone
Ericaceae/Heath Family

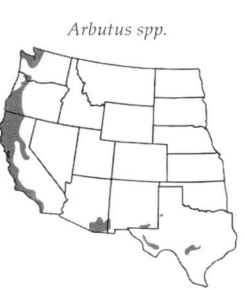

Arbutus spp.

Arbutus arizonica (A. Gray) Sarg. *(Arbutus xalapensis var. arizonica)*
Arizona madrone

Arbutus menziesii Pursh *(Arbutus procera)*
Pacific madrone, Madrono

Arbutus xalapensis Kunth *(Arbutus texana, A. xalapensis var. texana)*
Texas madrone

Description
Various species of Madrone are present in the both the New and Old World. Within America, three distinct species[49] are recorded. All sharing a majority of characteristics, Madrone's general growth pattern is that of a small to medium sized tree. Arbutus menziesii (Pacific madrone) is the largest of the three. It reaches stately heights of 60'–80', but usually maintains a lesser size. The smallest species, A. xalapensis (Texas madrone), grows to 12'–25' and is occasionally confused with Manzanita (another Heath family plant) due to its shrub–like growth when young.

    Madrone's exfoliating bark is its most unique feature. Arbutus arizonica's exfoliation is limited to young branches – here its thin red bark lifts and peels in flakes and strips. A. menziesii, easily having the greatest area of peeling dark red bark, exfoliates to leave new inner green bark, which then ages to dark red. A. xalapensis, also having dark to brick red thin bark, exfoliates in smooth flakes over most branch and limb areas. The older branch and lower trunk sections of all species are covered by non–peeling and roughened (squarish sections for A. arizonica) grayish bark.

    Generally evergreen, Madrone's leaves are ovate–lanceolate (Arbutus arizonica), elliptic (A. menziesii), or elliptic to ovate–elliptic (A. xalapensis). The hanging small flowers are urn–shaped and cream to tan (light green for

---

49   Arbutus arizonica is sometimes listed as a variety of A. xalapensis. The two species are also known to hybridize where their ranges overlap in the Animas Mountains of New Mexico.

A. arizonica). The reddish–orange to dark red fruit are semi–soft, globular, and range from pea to grape sized.

Distribution

The greatest numbers for both Arbutus arizonica and A. xalapensis occur in Mexico, with northern populations reaching into Arizona, New Mexico, and Texas. A. arizonica is limited to the mountains of southeastern Arizona and extends to the Animas Mountains of New Mexico. Almost always found on slopes and hillsides with intermittent drainages and/or streams not far below, look to 5500'–8000' with Oak, Juniper, and Pine.

Arbutus xalapensis has a significant elevation span (1000'–7000') due to the mountainous ascension[50] of isolated New Mexico and West Texas populations (Animas, Chisos, Davis, and Guadalupe Mountains). Throughout the Hill Country of the Edwards Plateau it is commonly encountered lower in elevation.

Arbutus menziesii has the greatest range of the three Madrones found within America. From isolated southern California pockets (San Diego County) it ranges north to coastal British Columbia. The densest populations occur in and around the Coastal Mountains of Northern California and Southern Oregon where coastal fog is a key meteorological influence. It grows as far west as the western foothills of the Sierras. Occasionally it is found in pure stands; however, it is mostly encountered periodically. From sea level to 4500', look to drainages, stream borders, and foothill slopes.

Chemistry

Arbutus general: phenols: arbutin, methylarbutin, hydroquinone; tannins: gallotannins, catechol tannins; flavonoids: quercetin; triterpenoids: betulinic acid, β–sitosterol, lupeol.

Medicinal Uses

Even though Uva–ursi (Arctostaphylos uva–ursi) and Manzanita (shrub–forming Arctostaphylos species) are the two best known Heath family medicinal plants of the group, Madrone is just as useful. Its activity as a urinary tract antimicrobial has much to do with two compounds – arbutin

50   Since the last Ice Age, many plant species have survived the earth's natural warming cycle by slowly transitioning to higher locales (as temperatures increase, greater precipitation levels are needed to meet hydration requirements, hence a plant's millennial upward movement).

and hydroquinone. Arbutin's conversion to hydroquinone, and then hydroquinone's local antimicrobial effect, is responsible for Madrone's influence. The process unfolds thusly: shortly after an arbutin–containing Heath family plant is ingested, the arbutin (remaining at least partly intact due to the presence of hydrolyzable tannin complexes) leaves the gut for the systemic system. Upon interaction with the kidneys, arbutin is cleaved to hydroquinone, which in turn is excreted in the urine (as hydroquinone glucuronide and possibly hydroquinone sulfate). In the presence of alkaline urine, conjugated hydroquinone is once again liberated to a free form, and only then exerts a strong antiseptic effect. Interestingly, if urine pH is normal, (slightly acidic) it stays largely inactive (as hydroquinone glucuronide/sulfate) and is of little infection–fighting value.[51]

Besides liberated hydroquinone's effect, another reason why Madrone works so well against the commonest UTI pathogen (Escherichia coli) is the low–level urinary acidification that occurs through its ingestion – in the presence of acidic urine, E. coli finds attachment (and budding) to urinary tract cells walls more difficult[52].

What all this means for the Madrone user is – take the tea daily for the treatment of non–complicated/non–organic UTIs, be them bladder or urethra oriented. Try 2–3 cups a day if in the throes of an active infection or 1 cup at the slightest urinary irritation. If Cranberry is found effective, Madrone should be as well.

If plagued by on– and off– again UTIs, and contributory factors have been eliminated (hygiene, dietary irritants, and/or more serious structural issues), basic dietary habits may need to be altered. High carbohydrate diets (vegan, vegetarian, and/or excessive consumption of refined sugars) tend to promote a more alkaline urinary environment and therefore a greater

51   This is just one example of how plant medicines, or their activities, can be misinterpreted by the well–meaning as having a kind of intelligence (descriptions common to the field such as 'modulator' or 'amphoteric' come to mind). That plants sometimes influence in difficult to understand ways is obvious; however, to suggest that there is a botanical–chemical intelligence within the plant that somehow 'knows best' is at best pseudo–science and at worst superstitious. There is always a rational answer to how plants affect the body, and if one is not apparent, it does the field a disservice to suggest otherwise.

52   Relatedly, some of the anthocyanins/anthocyanidins found in Cranberry, another Heath family member, have anti–adhesive effects. Even Corn silk (Zea mays), long touted for its positive urinary tract influence, has E. coli anti–attachment activity.

tendency for infection. For the fruitarian (dietary purity is not necessarily synonymous with health), the simple addition of animal protein several times a week will reduce infection prevalence.

Overtly, Madrone is a urinary tract astringent, though its tannin concentration is not quite as pronounced as Uva–ursi's or Manzanita's. Regardless, if the urinary tract tissues are lax and there is a combination of chronic irritation, dribbling of urine, and mucus discharge, then Madrone will be found useful.

Use Madrone leaf tea as a postpartum sitz bath. Soothing and tonifying to cervical and vaginal tissues it can be relied upon to reduce passive hemorrhaging, a not–uncommon occurrence from giving birth.

Indications
» Cystitis/Urethritis, alkaline urine
» As a postpartum sitz bath

Collection
New springtime or summer leaves are best. Clip them at their petioles and spread loosely on a cardboard flat or well–spaced in a paper bag.

Preparations
If decocting the leaf be sure to first soak them for 3–4 hours in a small amount of water. This will better facilitate arbutin's conversion to hydroquinone.

Dosage
» Leaf decoction: 4–6 oz. 2–3 times daily
» DPT (40% alcohol, 10% glycerin): 30–60 drops 2–3 times daily
» Sitz bath: as needed

Cautions
Arbutin, hydroquinone, and tannin compounds in large amounts are not completely benign substances, especially at organ–tissue target sites that see their medicinal effects. The areas of the body that experience a therapeutic gain from their proper use will also experience aberrations at greater quantities. Renal and gastrointestinal irritations are the most common side effects of large quantities or extended dosages. Due to its lower tannin content, Madrone can be taken a little longer than Uva–ursi or Manzanita, but still, everyday use should be kept to about two weeks. Due to the plant's

tannin–related uterine lining effects and the reproductive unknowns of arbutin and hydroquinone, Madrone should not be used consistently while pregnant.

Other Uses
Madrone fruit is a fair edible, and unlike Manzanita, is not as seed–filled and mealy. The berries are only mildly sweet, even at peak development, which supports their best use as a jam or preserve base. The fruit of North American Arbutus species are likely similar in nutritional content to the Mediterranean species, namely A. unedo, used locally for the previously mentioned items and as the base material for the alcohol beverage, known in Greece as Koumaro. Vitamins C and E, carotenoids, anthocyanins/anthocyanidins and other phenols, non–volatile acids (malic, citric, etc.) and sugars are reported for the fruit of Strawberry tree (A. unedo).

Marsh Marigold
Ranunculaceae/Buttercup Family

Caltha leptosepala

Caltha leptosepala DC. *(Caltha bicolor)*
White marsh marigold, Cowslip, Elkslip

Description
An herbaceous perennial, Marsh marigold's most notable characteristic is its rounded to elliptical thickened basal leaves. They are waxy to the touch, cordate–based, more–or–less toothed (leaf margins on some leaves can be crenate–wavy), and borne on sizable petioles (the large leaves may have petioles up to 8" in length). They are also distinctly net–veined. The white to cream flowers are solitary, 1"–1½" in diameter, and composed of 5–15 petal–like sepals. It's a tidy and symmetrically round flower.

Distribution
The Rocky Mountains, from Alaska to northern New Mexico, hold the largest concentrations of Marsh marigold. Occasional stands are also found in the higher reaches of the Sierra Nevada and the Pacific Northwest's Coastal Range and Cascades. Outliner groups are found in a number of Arizona's

high mountain ranges. Local habitats for the plant are fairly predictable: alpine/subalpine wet meadows, grassy bogs, and moist creek sides.

Chemistry

Caltha general: lactone: protoanemonin/anemonin; triterpene lactones: palustrolide, caltholide, epicatholide; aporphine alkaloids; pyrrolizidine alkaloid: senecionine[53] (C. leptosepala); oleanene glycosides, polysaccharides.

Medicinal Uses

Strongly stimulating (and potentially irritating) to mucus membranes[54], Marsh marigold's longest traditional application (Caltha palustris) is as an upper and lower respiratory tract stimulant – most often employed as part of a cough syrup formula. Loosening to thickened bronchial mucus, whether used alone or in combination (recommended), the tea or tincture will effectively increase lung secretions, helping to thin and expel ropey mucus. The sinuses may not be as obviously affected, but they too will benefit from Marsh marigold's secretory stimulation, especially if there has been a chronic infection and the local tissues are dry, sore, and plagued by re-infection.

Less documented, but still sensible, is Marsh marigold's usefulness when applied to gastrointestinal deficiencies – specifically secretory deficiencies. As with respiratory issues, the plant should be used in formula, ideally comprising no more than 25% of a well-crafted herbal combination. For example, Marsh marigold combined with bitters or chologogues could be considered in cases of poor gastric digestion or enteric assimilation. If secretory deficiency is part of the symptom picture, used as an accent, the plant will be found relevant.

The fresh plant (the dried plant is inert in this department) used topically as a field poultice (or the juice applied to a bandage) is diminishing to the pain and chronic inflammation of sores, swellings, bruises, contusions, and even arthritic complaints. Counter-irritant and rubefacient, its duration should be short-term, and the area should be monitored for a sense

---

53   Only one chemical workup (1976) found Caltha to contain senecionine. Additional studies should be performed to confirm its presence. The alkaloid set of veratrin and the glycoside helleborin (both poisonous compounds) were reported for C. palustris (1916); however, this observation, to my knowledge, has also never been duplicated by additional studies, yet many articles, books, and especially web sites, continue to list this likely flawed information.

54   This is most evident with the fresh plant. When chewed, it is acrid and biting.

of skin warmth. When the area begins to feel slightly stimulated, remove the application. If the preparation is left too long the area may blister. The protoanemonin in fresh Marsh marigold is usually more irritating to open wounds and cuts, so proceed with additional caution if the skin is broken.

In summation, use Marsh marigold (internally) in small combination-oriented doses. Used wisely it will stimulate and excite, and not irritate and inflame. This is definitely an herb where the 'more is better' approach does not apply.

Indications
» Secretory stimulant, respiratory, gastrointestinal
» Poorly healing and painful conditions (external)

Collection
If abundant, gather the whole plant – herbage and root. If the stand is isolated and/or not overly prolific, then just gather a leaf or two from random plants. Be sure to chew on a small piece of the fresh leaf. Why the term acrid is applied to Marsh marigold will become clear.

Preparations
The most energetic preparation for internal use is the fresh plant tincture (it has about $1/10$ of the protoanemonin of the whole fresh plant). It will maintain some minor acridity for 6–8 months, so for optimal potencies, Marsh marigold should be collected and prepared anew every year (like Anemone, Pulsatilla, and Clematis). This will be the preparation that is most apt to cause gastrointestinal irritation with overuse. The dried plant, as an infusion or dried plant tincture, is approximately half to quarter of the strength of the fresh plant tincture. More can be used per-dose, but its effects will be muted.

Dosage
» FPT: 10–15 drops 2–3 times daily
» DPT (60% alcohol): 20–30 drops 2–3 times daily
» Leaf infusion: 2–4 ounces 2–3 times daily
» Fresh plant poultice/Leaf juice: externally as needed

Cautions

Oral–esophageal–gastric–intestinal irritations are the most common complaints with internal Marsh marigold usage. Chances are if these symptoms are being experienced the dosage needs to be reduced (or the preparation changed from fresh to dried, or the herb stopped entirely). The difference between irritation (unwanted) and stimulation (wanted) is preparation and dosage. It is also wise to monitor for kidney and liver sensitivity. These symptoms too are unwanted. If they occur the herb should be stopped. Do not ingest the fresh juice. It potentially is the most acrid and should be left to counter–irritant external applications only.

At one least one pyrrolizidine alkaloid (senecionine) has been reported[55] for Caltha leptosepala (see previous footnote). The amounts are low (0.001%–0.005% of dry weight), but this is another reason why it's a good idea to keep Marsh marigold's internal use to reasonable amounts and short-term. The plant should not be used internally (a small topical area is fine), while pregnant or nursing.

Other Uses

This species (and Caltha palustris) is a well–known edible plant. The just-forming spring and early summer herbage (fleshy leaves and stems), as a cooked green, is surprisingly tasty. When cooked like spinach (boiled and rinsed), the plant's acridity dissipates (protoanemonin degrades rapidly in the presence of heat or through drying). The flower buds are also prepared the same way or even pickled and used like capers. Due to the (possible) presence of senecionine, I recommend eating Marsh marigold not as a seasonal staple, but as an occasional wild food addition.

---

55   Pyrrolizidine alkaloids in the Ranunculaceae are not the norm and should be considered extremely rare.

Monarda
Lamiaceae/Mint Family

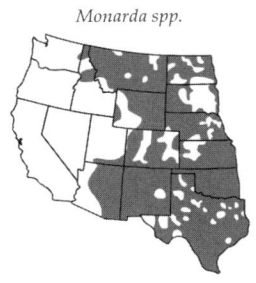

Monarda spp.

Monarda citriodora Cerv. ex Lag.
Lemon beebalm, Lemon horsemint, Lemon mint

Monarda fistulosa L. (*Monarda menthifolia*)
Horsemint, Wild bergamot, Wild oregano

Monarda pectinata Nutt.
Plains beebalm, Spotted beebalm, Spotted horsemint, Wild oregano

Description

Monarda citriodora is often divided into two subspecies: ssp. austromontana (M. austromontana) and ssp. citriodora. Although there are slight botanical differences, I'll treat the two plants here as one. Usually annual (occasionally biannual), it is a small, branched to single, square–stemmed herb. The leaf blades are 1"–2½" long and lanceolate to oblanceolate with serrate, subserrate, or entire margins. The flowers form in interrupted spikes. They are whitish to purple–tinged, often with purple dots on the lower lip. The flower bracts are densely canescent (fuzzy white) above or sometimes purplish and reflexed.

Monarda fistulosa, one of the easiest Monardas to identify, is a 2'–3' tall herbaceous perennial. Often growing in tidy mounds, it has ornamental appeal with its well–organized shape. Inversely, a just–developing stand can appear sparse due to its rhizomal–single stem growth. The upper portions are pubescent; the lower portions, lesser so. The leaf blades are ovate to lanceolate and 1"–3" (rarely 5") long. The lavender to purple flowers form in very distinctive solitary/terminal circular clusters at stem ends.

8"–16" in height, Monarda pectinata is typically an annual (but is also reported as an occasional biannual, or even a short–lived perennial). The branched stems are covered by a slight pubescence (as are most other parts). The ½"–2" long leaves are lanceolate or narrowly elliptic. The margins are serrate or subserrate. The flowers form in interrupted spikes and are white to pinkish with a dark–purple spotted lower lip. This Monarda is easily confused with M. citriodora. The flower bracts are the best identifier: M.

citriodora's bracts are fuzzy above and curl downward. M. pectinata's bracts are nearly erect and are smooth and hairless.

Distribution

The grassy plains of Texas hold the most Monarda species. In fact, only five of the (presently) seventeen species are found outside the state. As prairie plants, the majority of species exist in abundance throughout the southern Great Plains or micro–grassland pockets beyond this region.

From an isolated central California stand, Monarda citriodora ranges west through parts of Utah, Arizona, and New Mexico. Its greatest populations are found from Kansas and Oklahoma through to most of Texas. Its northern–most reach extends to Nebraska and Illinois. East of the Mississippi River it is encountered infrequently; from Kentucky and Tennessee to South Carolina and Florida. Look to pastures, rocky and sandy grasslands, and gravel–strewn hillsides.

Found in every state except Alaska, Hawaii, and Florida, Monarda fistulosa enjoys a wide distribution. Open woodlands, grasslands, roadsides, and the banks of intermittent streams are usual places for the plant. In the West, it is a plant of the mid–mountains, avoiding low deserts and alpine areas.

From western Missouri, Monarda pectinata is found from the Great Plains and Four Corner states (skipping Nevada), to California and Oregon. Sandy/gravely–soiled grassland regions as well as prairies and pastures are common environments for the plant.

Chemistry

Volatiles for Monarda punctata: α–thujene, α–pinene, β–pinene, α–phellandrene, α–terpinene, ϱ–cymene, carene, limonene, 4–terpineol, methyl carvacrol, thymol, carvacrol, β–caryophyllene.

Medicinal Uses

Spicy, aromatic, and stimulating, Monarda belongs to a class of plants within the Mint family best known for its strong/invigorating qualities. The majority of Monarda species, even beyond the profiled, have been used in near identical ways since people started using plants for medicine.

As a hot tea, Monarda is a stimulating diaphoretic. Take it to break a dry fever of mild to moderate temperature; readers may want to address higher temperature fevers with other herbs (Cottonwood/Willow) due to Monarda's potential of causing a slight spike, prior to diaphoresis[56].

As a fairly strong carminative, use Monarda for general states of indigestion and bloating. Pre- and post- vomiting nausea will be quieted with several ounces of tea or a strong dose of the tincture, though mothers-to-be should opt for other herbs for morning sickness (Spearmint for instance).

Though not as powerful as Silk tassel, intestinal cramp sufferers will find a strong cup of Monarda tea settling. It will also be of use if there is associated diarrhea with intestinal gas. For the day-after gastrointestinal upset of binge-drinking, some relief will be had with the plant's use, though for low-level systemic alcohol poisoning (hangover) Monarda will have little effect. Liver-oriented antioxidant herbs in combination with salicylate-type herbs, along with plenty of fluids, will help speed the recovery process in these situations.

The tincture or spirit ingested in small but frequent doses is a worthwhile therapy for the gastrointestinal effects of food poisoning, Candida overgrowths, and other microbial infections affecting the region. Having a trifecta of influences – anesthetizing, carminative, and antimicrobial – Monarda will be found specific and effective.

The tea or tincture is a traditional application for slow-to-start, painful menstruation. Its use will be found stimulating and soothing especially if there is a sense of poor circulation and congestion of the of pelvic region. If a hot water bottle helps when applied to the area, a strong cup of Monarda tea will likely do good.

The essential oil of Monarda, depending on species, contains typically between 50%–80% of thymol, a strongly antiseptic monoterpene also associated with the culinary herbs Thyme and Oregano. This high concentration of thymol makes the essential oil of Monarda of special note. Effective against a wide range of pathogens, topical application of the diluted essential oil (or essential oil-based preparation), is of value when applied to skin and nail fungi. In most cases continued daily application is needed

---

56   The body will resolve the majority of fevers caused by a viral or minor bacterial infection naturally, without much assistance. By allowing the body to do so, a greater capacity for immunological activity develops (especially for babies and children). Using Monarda in these cases does not halt an infection, but rather speeds the body's natural infection-fighting process. Pernicious infections, resulting in a continued elevated temperature, caused by more harmful organisms will likely need to be addresses with conventional antibiotics.

until complete eradication has been achieved (1 month or so for some stubborn infections). Poorly healing minor wounds, cuts, scrapes, and abrasions where local infection is visible (tissue redness) clears nicely with a 2–3 times daily application.

Thymol is one of several active ingredients that comprises part of the well-known mouthwash, Listerine. Along with eucalyptol (Eucalyptus) and menthol (Mint) the product is still used as an effective oral disinfectant. In lieu of Listerine, a daily mouthwash[57] composed of diluted Monarda essential oil (or even the diluted tincture or tea) is active against most harmful oral/periodontal microorganisms.

Indications
» Fever, dry, low to moderate temperature
» Dyspepsia, with gas and bloating
» Cramps, intestinal
» Infection, gastrointestinal
» Menstruation, slow to start/painful
» Infection, bacterial/fungal (external)
» As an oral disinfectant (mouthwash)

Collection
Like other Mint family plants, Monarda's leaves and flowers are covered by a dense concentration of volatile oil containing-glands. I recommend stripping the leaves and flowers from the plant while still fresh and using these parts only. The herbage can also be dried whole and the leaf and flower garbled from the stems and then stored.

Preparations/Dosage
» FPT/DPT (50% alcohol): 20–40 drops 2–3 times daily

[57] A simple mouthwash recipe is as follows: start with 1 pint of diluted alcohol (50% water/50% alcohol) as a base. Add 40 drops of essential oil to the water/alcohol solution. This mixture can be stored unrefrigerated. If tissue irritation or burning results, replace some of the Monarda essential oil with one, or a combination of, Mentha, Eucalyptus, Sage, or Cypress essential oil. Note: usually more than 40 drops of any essential oil in a 16 ounce base will be found too strong and will irritate sensitive oral tissues. Additionally, the base solution needs to be comprised of approximately 50% alcohol to fully dissolve the essential oil fraction – otherwise the essential oil part will remain floating.

- » Infusion: 2–6 oz. 2–3 times daily
- » Spirit: 10–20 drops 2–3 times daily
- » Steam inhalation: 2–3 times daily
- » Essential oil (diluted with a carrier oil): topically as needed
- » Ointment/Oil/Salve: as needed

Cautions
Monarda's effect as a reproductive tissue vasodilator makes it contraindicated during pregnancy. Excessive internal use of the essential oil may result in kidney and/or gastrointestinal irritation. Undiluted Monarda essential oil will blister the skin! It is especially irritating to more sensitive tissues and mucus membranes.

Monardella
Lamiaceae/Mint Family

Monardella spp.

Monardella Benth.
Western pennyroyal, Mountain pennyroyal, Coyote mint

Description
Monardella[58] is an aromatic Mint family herbaceous perennial (some species are annual). Most are low and bushy, with square stems and opposite leaves. The leaves are more–or–less gland dotted and entire to serrate. The majority have flowers clustered in dense terminal heads, subtended by surrounding leaf–like bracts that are often lavender to purple in color. Each flower corolla is white to light purple. Most Monardella species are easily distinguished by their large involucres.

Distribution
Of the thirty Monardella species throughout the West, most are found within California. Oregon hosts six species and Arizona has four. M. glauca, the widest ranging of the group, is found from Montana to New Mexico, then west to Oregon and California. M. odoratissima is found from British Columbia south through the Pacific Coast states, then east to Idaho

---
58 Meaning little or lesser Monarda.

and Nevada. The majority of species prefer dry and exposed soils of scrub, woodlands, and grasslands.

Chemistry

Volatiles for Monardella crispa (others are similar): α–pinene, β–pinene, camphene, myrcene, α–phellandrene, β–phellandrene, δ–3–carene, β–caryophyllene, trans–β–farnesene, linalool, citronellal, isoborneol, pipeitone, piperitenone, α–terpineol, pulegone.

Medicinal Uses

Belonging to a group of pulegone–rich[59], Pennyroyal–type plants, Monardella is medicinally equal to Poliomintha and slightly stronger than Hedeoma. Additionally, its historical use is similar to these related plants: Monardella is a stimulating emmenagogue, diaphoretic, and carminative.

Drink a strong cup of hot tea when menses is slow to start, particularly if the pelvic/lower back regions feel cold, crampy, and congested. As a good reproductive tissue vasodilator, area circulation is increased while smooth muscle/uterine cramping is decreased. These influences make the plant worthwhile in a whole set of self–limiting and very common menstrual situations. If curling up with a hot water bottle helps during this time of the month, it is likely that Monardella will too.

The tea is a minty–Pennyroyal tasting carminative. Use it or a dose of tincture in a little warm water if the gastric region is bloated, gaseous, and full after a heavy/rich meal. Most users find its settling effect a welcomed relief: trapped stomach gas will be expelled while the gastric lining becomes mildly anesthetized.

Like other Mints in its class, the hot tea is a moderate diaphoretic. Drink a stout cup or two if trying to break a dry, mild to moderate fever. A classic combination is its use in conjunction with a hot shower or bath before bed. This duo is nearly fool proof in promoting diaphoresis.

Monardella's pleasant scented aromatics are antibacterial. A whole array of external preparations can be employed to diminish infection–causing microbes. The essential oil will be the strongest preparation. Be sure to dilute it in equal parts of a carrier oil before its application to sensitive skin.

Indications

» Menstruation, slowed, with regional congestion

---

59   Most species contain 50%–70% pulegone per total essential oil volume.

- » Indigestion, with gas and bloating
- » Fever, dry, mild to moderate temperature
- » As a mild antiseptic (external)

Collection

Like other herbaceous plant medicines, gather the upper half of Monardella, preferably when in flower. If not in flower, the leaves alone are fine as long as they are strongly aromatic. If a particular species is not aromatic, forgo its collection. It will be an inferior medicine.

Preparations/Dosage

- » FPT/DPT (50% alcohol): 30–60 drops 2–3 times daily
- » Infusion: 2–4 oz. 2–3 times daily
- » Essential oil: 1–2 drops 2–3 times daily
- » Spirit: 10–20 drops 2–3 times daily
- » External preparations: as needed

Cautions

Monardella (and all pulegone–containing plants) has a controversial (and dangerous) history when used as an abortifacient. I sincerely caution against its use in this capacity. Monardella's moderate use as a tea while nursing (or small amounts with children) should cause no problem.

Mullein

Scrophulariaceae/Figwort Family

Verbascum thapsus L.
Common mullein, Woolly mullein, Gordolobo

Verbascum thapsus

Description

Like most biennials, Mullein's first year is spent producing basal leaves and a small anchoring tap root. Once mature its large woolly leaves are elliptic to oblanceolate. They radiate outward, with the lower leaves being the largest and most prominent. The upper, younger leaves are covered with a dense coating of fuzzy hair. Mullein's tall stalk begins to develop in the spring and matures with thick spikes of yellow 5–lobed flowers.

Distribution
Like many plants of Europe, Mullein is found in disturbed soils. Roadsides, field edges, and trailsides are common areas for the plant. Mullein seeds prolifically after forest fires. In some areas, it becomes nearly a ground cover during its first year of growth. These stands are typically transitory and disappear once soil stabilization occurs.

Chemistry
Iridoid glucosides: harpagoside, harpagide, aucubin; flavonoids: hesperidin, verbascoside; saponins.

Medicinal Uses
Mullein is a mild remedy that influences two main areas: the lungs and the urinary tract. The leaf tea/syrup is soothing to inflamed mucus membranes of the lungs, particularly those of the bronchi and trachea. Use it when there is a persistent dry cough that verges on being spasmodic. The plant is mildly inhibiting to Klebsiella pneumoniae and Staphylococcus aureus, both bacterial strains commonly involved in bronchial infections. Mullein combines well with expectorants like Lomatium and Ligusticum.

It has been proposed that Mullein root has a tonifying effect on the trigone muscle[60]. Although its mechanism of action is not clearly understood, the plant may prove useful if there is urinary incontinence from bladder weakness. The tincture or fluidextract for bed–wetting children is worth a try, but its effect is inconsistent due to potential psychosomatic factors that Mullein does not address. More consistently though, if there is irritation from chronic cystitis affecting the urinary situation, Mullein root will be found soothing.

Mullein flower oil is an age–old remedy for childhood earaches. 1–2 drops placed in the affected ear is quieting to pain and inflammation. Combined with Garlic oil, the duo is both soothing and antibacterial. The flower tincture can be used in the flower oil's place. It evaporates quickly, but its effect is still notable.

---

60 The trigone muscle controls much of the bladder's ability to store and release urine to the urethra. This muscle, which rests at the base of the bladder, is normally contracted. For urine to enter the urethra the trigone must relax. A lack of trigone tone is a factor in some cases of urinary incontinence.

Indications
- » Cough, dry and spasmodic
- » Bladder tone, poor
- » Cystitis, chronic
- » Earache, childhood (external)

Collection
Harvest the leaves during the plant's first year of growth or early into its second year, as these will be the most vital and healthy. Gather the slender tap root during the plant's first year. They will be fleshy and medically potent, as opposed to the second year's root which is woody and inert.

Preparations/Dosage
- » Leaf infusion/Root decoction: 4–6 oz. 2–3 times daily
- » FPT/DPT (50% alcohol): 30–60 drops 2–3 times daily
- » Flower oil/Tincture: 1–2 drops 3–4 times daily (ear drops)

Cautions
There are no cautions for Mullein.

Nettle
Urticaceae/Nettle Family

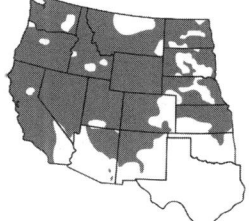

Urtica dioica

Urtica dioica subsp. *gracilis* (Aiton) Selander *(Urtica gracilis)*
American stinging nettle

Urtica dioica subsp. *holosericea* (Nutt.) Thorne *(Urtica holosericea)*
Giant creek nettle, Hoary nettle, Mountain nettle

Description
Nettle is a short-lived herbaceous perennial. Generally 2′–4′ tall with long, vertical, and angled stems, it has lanceolate to ovate, toothed, dark green leaves. Both the stem and leaf undersides have small stinging hairs (*Urtica dioica* subsp. *holosericea* more so). The plant's inflorescence is variable in shape, appearing spike, raceme, or panicle–like. The male clusters tend to

ascend; the female clusters droop. Nettle is monoecious – both male and female flowers form on the same plant.

Distribution

Urtica dioica subsp. gracilis is a wide-ranging Nettle found throughout most of America and Canada. However, it is largely absent from the Southeast and much of California, Nevada, Utah, and lower elevation Arizona. Throughout the mid and southern Rockies, it's a common streamside, moist meadow, and forest margin grower.

Though Urtica dioica subsp. holosericea is found in essentially the same habitats, its range is mainly limited to a few isolated stands in the mountains of Arizona and New Mexico to significant amounts in Utah, Nevada, California, Idaho, Oregon, and Washington. Essentially where subsp. gracilis leaves off, subsp. holosericea starts.

Chemistry

Polysaccharides, sterols: β–sitosterol, kaempferol; flavonoids: apigenin, quercetin, rutin; carotenoids: neoxanthin, violaxanthin, β–cryptoxanthin, lutein, zeaxanthin, lycopene, β–carotene; isolectins.

Medicinal Uses

Due to Nettle's organic mineral content, notably calcium and potassium, the tea serves as a reliable alkalizing and nutritive supplement. It is best used by individuals whom are plagued by acidosis (borderline) – a pH imbalance of the blood, caused by an overabundance of hydrogen ions and related acidic compounds. Although there are organic reasons for acidosis, Nettle will be most effective for low pH situations created by dietary indiscretions and constitutional tendency. If the diet contains large amounts of animal source protein (and little else) then Nettle tea will prove useful in its buffering activity. Consider the tea specific (alone or combined with Burdock, Dandelion, or Asparagus) for gout/uric acid conditions.

The tea tends to be mildly lowering to blood sugar levels. It is surmised that the plant affects both insulin secretion/sensitivity and dietary glucose absorption. There are stronger herbal medicines for such metabolic excesses, such as Prickly pear or Brickellia, but when dietary and exercise approaches are being utilized, and just 'a little' more is needed, the tea is often successful.

As an herb used to address constitutional issues, Nettle tea fits the middle-aged mesomorph. Anabolic, hyperglycemic, hyperlipidemic, and acidic are a number of functional tendencies that point to its successful application. It is not a tea to reverse an acute condition, but rather one to buffer metabolic excesses. These people should consider Nettle tea a tonic.

Nettle is one of the vegetable kingdom's most useful teas to offset the effects of nutrient malabsorption. Whether the reason is small intestinal inflammation, functional problems of gastric digestion, or a minor parathyroid imbalance affecting calcium levels, the tea will be found nourishing. Moreover, it should not to be over looked if in need of a rebuilding tea if recuperating from surgery or illness. In addition to food, the tea combines well with Alfalfa, vegetable juices, broths, and especially Yellowdock. Nettle–Yellowdock–Alfalfa is a suburb combination. For the anemic, the trio will do more good than any plant used alone.

Historically Nettle has been used for chronic bladder irritation with accompanying mucus discharge. Drink the tea when there is irritation and area sensitivity, particularly upon urination. Contributing to the plant's effect on the urinary tract, the leaf tea is a fair sodium leaching diuretic. As a simple approach to sodium related water retention and/or hypertension, 2–3 cups a day should produce an improvement.

The tea or tincture of the root is useful for age–related prostate enlargement (both aromatase and dihydrotestosterone dependent) and related irritation. Urine flow will be increased and urgency decreased with its use. For this application, it combines well with Saw palmetto and or Pygeum (see Wild cherry for a potential substitute). Although focus has been on Nettle root in regards to BPH (benign prostate hypertrophy), the leaf (most likely) has a corresponding effect, given its traditional urinary tract influence.

Nettle is also used during allergy season as a preventative for rhinitis, mainly in the form of the encapsulated dried or freeze–dried herb. My observation is that Nettle is hit–or–miss in this department. It is not unusual for any herb with a related tannin–flavonoid component to have an anti–allergy effect.

Similar to bee sting therapy, Nettle used topically over painful and arthritic joints is for some a surprisingly effective pain reliever. Rub the fresh leaves against the problem area until several stings are noticed. Done once or twice a day may seem like a sadomasochistic therapy; however, compared to regular Tylenol or Ibuprofen use, it's a whole lot better for the liver. Consider this a seasonal therapy for those whom live around the wild/fresh plant. The therapy's mechanism of action is probably several: placebo (some friendly encouragement from the mind never hurts), topical irritation (local vascular dynamics are shifted, which often is found relieving to deep seated pain), and lastly, a chemical effect from Nettle's compounds (the initial sting may give way to pain signal inhibition, or possibly trigger a cellular component that has a beneficial effect). It's anyone's guess really, but the application often works for rheumatoid and/or osteoarthritis.

Indications
» Acidosis, non–organic
» Hyperglycemia
» Malabsorption, nutrient
» Cystitis, with mucus discharge
» Benign prostatic hypertrophy/Prostatitis
» Rhinitis
» Arthritis, rheumatoid/osteo (external)

Collection
Gloves, a long–sleeved shirt, and pruners are essential when gathering Nettle. After clipping the upper half of the plant, band the stems together and hang them, or spread the cut herb out over an open flat and allow it to dry. Nettle root can be difficult to collect when growing directly in streambeds, not to mention these plants may be lesser in potency than those growing in drier soils. Often forming in colonies, one rhizome has many attached above–ground stems.

Preparations/Dosage
» Leaf infusion: 4–8 oz. 2–3 times daily
» Root decoction: 4–8 oz. 2–3 times daily
» FPT/DPT of root (50% alcohol): 30–60 drops 2–3 times daily
» Fluidextract of root: 10–20 drops 2–3 times daily

Cautions
The Nettle sting: in most cases the weal response subsides within an hour. Although rare, some people are sensitive to the tea and may develop a swollen tongue or irritated throat. If this is the case, discontinue the plant's use. Due to trichome pieces interacting with the skin, when garbling the dried herb (without gloves and sleeves) a mild form of the Nettle sting may

develop. It is of no concern. The plant is safe during pregnancy and while nursing. Like so many other plants, Nettle will absorb its share of heavy metals from contaminated soils, so care should be taken in choosing its collection site.

Other Uses

Use the fresh young leaves as a cooked green. Simmer them for 10–15 minutes and discard (or drink) the water. Boiling neutralizes Nettle's stinging ability. Sensitive individuals may want to re-simmer after a quick rinse.

Until the mid–1900s Nettle fiber, like Hemp fiber, held a substantial textile positioning due to its tensile strength and general abundance. The fiber's dominance peaked in Europe during the early 20th century when Germany outfitted her army with a majority of Nettle–based clothes, tents, and rucksacks. With Cotton's emerging dominance, Nettle textiles proved too costly to produce and soon fell into obscurity.

Oak

Fagaceae/Beech Family

Quercus gambelii

Quercus gambelii Nutt.
Gamble oak, Rocky mountain white oak

Description

Easily recognizable, Gamble oak is closely allied with eastern White oak. Growing to heights of 50' feet (though usually smaller) the leaves are its most characteristic feature. 5"–8" in length and deeply lobed, they are pubescent below and bright green above. The acorns are ½"–1" in length (and very astringent).

Distribution

Gamble oak is common throughout the interior mountains of several states: Colorado, Utah, Arizona, and New Mexico. A fast–growing and opportunistic Oak, this species is common to disturbed soils, either from fire, erosion, or road/trail maintenance. It's found at Ponderosa pine and Aspen elevations.

Chemistry

Oak general: phenolic compounds: condensed and hydrolyzable tannins, flavonoids.

Medicinal Uses

This is just one species of Oak that is medicinally useful. Whether it is a black, red, or white type, they are all active. Oak is a simple tannin–based astringent. Although it also contains an array of non–tannin phenolic glycosides, its crude tissue–tightening effect overshadows any medicinal direction that could otherwise be put to use towards issues that call for a bit of nuance. In other words: use Oak internally as a short–term strong astringent. Its use as a strict flavonoid source and/or low–level, longer–term intestinal or urinary 'tightener' is unwise due to the bark's high tannin[61] concentration.

A wash or fomentation is beneficial for cuts, scrapes, rashes, or any other skin condition that exhibits redness, swelling, and weeping from dermal trauma. Sun burn and mild heat burns are too soothed by a cool Oak bark soak or a cool tea–soaked towel. An oil, salve, or ointment made from Oak is well applied to poorly healing ulcerations and pressure–related bedsores.

As a short–term internal tea, the plant is appropriate for a number of conditions. Bleeding ulcers[62], be them esophageal, stomach, or intestinal centered are soothed and astringed. Diarrhea is symptomatically addressed with a strong brew of Oak tea. Best taken after most of the offending contents have been voided, it lessens hypersecretion which often leads to exhaustive emptying. If intestinal cramping is present, the addition of Yellow pond lily or Western peony will be found useful. For serious spastic activity, Silk tassel tincture (or Henbane...be careful) should be employed.

As a mouthwash, Oak tea astringes bleeding gums, though brushing with a little Myrrh powder or Goldenseal often better addresses gum–oriented poor circulation/healing issues. Additionally, the gargled tea is soothing to a sore throat. The tea also can be used as a nasal wash in order to shrink inflamed regional tissues. In either case, the tea is not strongly antibacterial, but simply antiinflammatory via its tannin content.

61 One exception: if the bark of a particular species or part is not overly astringent or has no characteristic pinkish–rust coloration denoting tannin concentration, it may pass as a more general tissue supportive flavonoid source.

62 Poor results will also be seen if the ulceration's cause is not addressed – alcohol, stress, etc.

Lastly, the insect galls that form on many species of Oak can be used as a concentrated tannic acid source. The older galls that are comprised of mainly an outer shell seem to be the choice article, as younger galls that still host insects are less potent. The crushed and powdered galls are extremely astringent. Use the powder as a dust for cuts, scrapes, and weepy rashes. I've seen it reliably clot deeper cuts (though not requiring stitches).

Indications
- Cuts/Scrapes/Abrasions/Burns (external)
- Bedsores and related ulcerations (external)
- Pharyngitis/Sinusitis (gargle)
- Diarrhea, acute
- Gums, spongy/bleeding

Collection
Gather the inner bark on larger branches where the outer bark is fissured or thickened. This is the traditional, yet labor intensive, part of Oak (the inner pinkish–rust colored cambium layer) that usually has the highest tannin concentration.

A less labor–intensive, but slightly inferior part of Oak is the immature secondary branch bark. Select a branch with no fissured bark that is less than wrist–size. Cut the branch away from the tree and then peel or cut the bark from the core wood.

Whatever branch size is selected, look for the pink to rust coloration of the inner bark. This is an indication of tannin content. When chewed, it should be astringent and drying.

Preparations
The bark dries easily. Even in humid climates there usually is no need to employ a dehydrator.

Dosage
- Bark decoction: 2–4 oz. 2–3 times daily
- External preparations: as needed

Cautions
There is little concern of toxicity with normal short–term use (several days to one week). Longer use may lead to gastrointestinal or renal irritation, which

is not uncommon for the extended use of most tannin–oriented plants. Relatedly, several days of Oak tea during pregnancy is not a concern, but several weeks of use may be.

Other Uses
Acorns, of course: depending on species and seasonal conditions, Oak's fruit is an important wild food source. To be made palatable, most species will need to be water leached. As a nutritious carbohydrate/protein–rich food source[63], the meal has grown in popularity due to a general resurgence in wild foods.

Oregongrape
Berberidaceae/Barberry Family

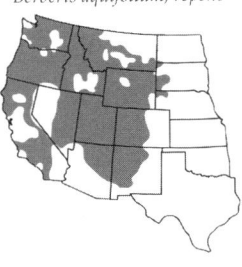

Berberis aquifolium, repens

Berberis aquifolium Pursh (*Berberis aquifolium var. aquifolium, Mahonia aquifolium*)
Holly grape

Berberis repens (Lindl) (*Berberis aquifolium var. repens, Mahonia repens*)
Creeping holly grape

Description
Mahonia aquifolium is a substantial and coarse evergreen bush. Usually between 3'–6' high, the plant's shiny leaves are comprised of 5–9 leathery, spinulose leaflets. The yellow, 6–petaled flowers develop in racemes. The purple–black fruit are grape–like in color and large seeded. They are tart–sweet in taste.

Berberis repens, B. aquifolium's smaller relative, also has Holly–like, stiff and shiny leaflets. They form in groups of 3–7. Typically no more than 1' in height, the plant is more apt to be walked on, as opposed to being waded through. The yellow flowers form in dense clusters. They are followed by a

---

63 'Acorn constipation' can occur from eating too much of the meal. It is easily remedied with a cup or two of Buckthorn bark tea. In fact, most California Indian tribes considered Cascara sagrada (a type of Buckthorn) an important medicine due to its laxative effect – an indigenous remedy for the side effect of an indigenous food.

clutch of blue–purplish berries. Both species discussed here often hybridize, making certain identification sometimes tedious.

Distribution

A plant of the Pacific Northwest, Berberis aquifolium is commonly found in Douglas–Fir forests as well as scrub areas. B. repens is found from the Pacific Northwest and Interior West, to higher elevation Arizona and New Mexico.

Chemistry

For Berberis repens (other species are similar): isoquinoline alkaloids: oxyacanthine, berberine, columbamine, corydine, isocorydine, glaucine, jatrorrhizine, magnoflorine, obaberine, obamegine, palmatine, thaliporphine, thalrugosine; lignan: syringaresinol.

Medicinal Uses

Berberis aquifolium makes up the bulk of commercial Oregongrape. B. repens (and B. nervosa) adds to the collective store – it's both collected as a separate Oregongrape and gathered and processed along with B. aquifolium, where it is technically an adulterant; however, one that causes no harm due to its identical activity.

Mainly due to Oregongrape's isoquinoline alkaloid content, it is inhibiting to a wide array of pathogens, be them bacterial or fungal. Topically, a wash, poultice, or fomentation is applied to infected cuts or wounds. These preparations are also effective for skin and nail fungi. Internally, use the root tea or tincture as a systemic support for the same issues. Its use is also indicated in bacterial or mold induced sinus infections and for sore/strep throat.

Oregongrape's berberine content (an isoquinoline alkaloid) is directly inhibiting to pathogenic gastrointestinal microbes and their harmful endotoxins. Take the plant if suffering from food poisoning, Giardia infection, amebiasis, and other GI tract parasitic/microbial infections. For these purposes, it should be combined with a carminative, which will lessen the griping often associated with these distresses.

As a bitter tonic, the tea or tincture is of use in relieving indigestion. Although not as direct in effect as Gentian or Bogbean, Oregongrape stimulates hydrochloric acid, pepsinogen, bile, and succus entericus secretion, facilitating food breakdown in the stomach and assimilation in the small intestine. Some even may experience a mild laxative effect through the plant's stimulation of these digestive secretions.

Like others in the family, the plant has an interesting effect on the skin and liver. Applied externally, Oregongrape slows excessive cellular proliferation, turnover, and lipid peroxidation, making it a valuable psoriasis treatment. Internally, the plant's effect on the liver is cooling and protective. It has been shown to normalize liver enzyme elevations, as well as other inflammatory markers associated with hepatitis, cirrhosis, and liver toxicity from environmental/dietary causes. It is hepatoprotective, possibly through its influence of the liver's cytochrome P450 pathway. Traditionally the plant was used for 'bad blood', and like Barberry, is considered a classic alterative, along with plants like Golden smoke, Stillingia, and Echinacea. It is especially indicated in conditions where the skin is dry, red, and heals poorly, or for what were once called scrofulous conditions.

Additionally, Oregongrape is broadly antiinflammatory and is well used internally in febrile states – it tends to clear systemic pyrogenic compounds. The plant also has use in auto–inflammatory conditions such as chronic allergies, psoriatic arthritis, and Lupus.

Indications
- Bacterial/Fungal infections (external and internal)
- Sinusitis/Strep throat (internal and gargle)
- Food poisoning/Giardiasis/Amebiasis
- Indigestion with insufficient protein/fat digestion
- Psoriasis (external and internal)
- Hepatic inflammation, sluggishness
- Fever/Autoimmune inflammation

Collection
The more yellow, flexible, and hydrated the roots are, the better. Compared to a number of desert–growing species (Berberis trifoliolata and B. fremontii) both Berberis' profiled here are easy to gather.

Preparations
Cut the roots into ¼"–½" sections. Tincture them fresh or dry the pieces for other preparations. The dried root is commercially available, as are various tincture/capsule preparations.

Dosage

- » Root decoction/Cold infusion: 4–6 oz. 2–3 times daily
- » FPT/DPT (40% alcohol): 30–60 drops 2–3 times daily
- » Capsule (00): 1–2, 2–3 times daily
- » Fluidextract: 10–20 drops 2–3 times daily
- » External preparations: as needed

Cautions

Berberine can cause hemolysis in babies with G6PD (glucose–6–phosphate–dehydrogenase) deficiency. Like other chologogues, do not use the plant if there is a gallbladder blockage.

Other Uses

Bitter–sour–sweet, the fruit of Oregongrape is an acquired taste; however, I would not call them unpleasant. They are fine eaten raw or used as a jam/jelly base.

Ox–Eye Daisy
Asteraceae/Sunflower Family

Leucanthemum vulgare Lam. *(Chrysanthemum leucanthemum)*
Great ox–eye, Field daisy, Maudlin daisy, Marguerite

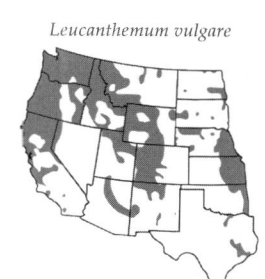

Leucanthemum vulgare

Description

An herbaceous perennial, Ox–eye daisy is clump–growing and rhizomatous. Its summertime flowers are well–composed and develop at branch ends. They are formed of white rays and yellow disks. The plant's leaves are variable: several inches long, longer than wide, with lobed or irregularly blunted–serrated margins. It's a handsome plant and is often sought after as an ornamental. The crushed foliage is mildly aromatic – it has a pleasant, fresh scent.

Distribution

Like many Eurasian plants, Ox–eye daisy does best in disturbed soils. Look to secondary roadsides, trailsides, and clearings. It's a full–sun grower and is also associated with grassy openings and meadows. Absent from most of the Southwest (low elevation), Ox–eye daisy is common to the middle Rockies and the Pacific Northwest states.

Chemistry
Sesquiterpenes: nerolidol, α–bisabolol, farnesol, farnesene; polyacetylenes; flavonoids.

Medicinal Uses
Little used today, Ox–eye daisy is a mild remedy, and can be thought of as an amalgam of Chamomile (Matricaria–Chamomilla), Garden Chrysanthemum (Chrysanthemum x morifolium), and Feverfew (Tanacetum parthenium). Its old–time use, as a waning fever tonic, has wide application, especially for children. Drink the tea when a fever's peak has past, yet perspiration is still excessive. The plant's consolidating non–tannin astringency is at work here and when used at the end of a feverish episode, leads to a more timely recovery. Most find Ox–eye daisy to be mildly sedative, like Chamomile, making it a nice fit for fever–related mental agitation.

The lungs are another area under Ox–eye daisy's influence. Inflamed bronchial tissue with excessive secretion, be it related to asthma or bronchitis, is quieted. It is also well used as a sitz bath (and internal tea) for vaginitis, characterized by discharge and inflammation, but if there is a bacterial/fungal/parasitic element, this simple approach will likely not be enough. A strong Berberis (antibacterial/antifungal) or Castela (trichomoniasis) sitz bath/douche will be a better application.

Topically, a general wash is cleansing, mildly antibacterial, and arresting to excessive secretion. Use it frequently on abscesses (after coming to a head/lanced), ulcers, bedsores, and other similar cutaneous problems.

Indications
» Fever, post–spike, excessive perspiration
» Bronchial inflammation, with excessive secretion
» Vaginitis, mild (external)
» Ulcerations and related cutaneous conditions (external)

Collection
A simple plant to collect, bunch the upper leaves, stems, and flowers together, and snip with pruners. Dry well–spaced in an open paper bag or on

a cardboard flat. Like Yarrow, the clipped flowering herb also dries well via bundling and hanging.

Preparations

Ox-eye daisy is a traditional tea plant. The infusion is best for overall use; however, its bronchial oriented influences are also communicated adequately through the dried plant tincture.

Dosage

» Infusion: 4–8 oz. 2–3 times daily
» DPT (50% alcohol): 60–90 drops 2–3 times daily

Cautions

A number of other Leucanthemum/Chrysanthemum species (i.e Chrysanthemum cinerariaefolium or Dalmatian daisy) contain pyrethrins, a group of naturally occurring compounds with well-documented insecticidal properties. These compounds also tend to be mildly to moderately toxic when ingested in sufficient quantities. There are no consistent reports of Ox-eye daisy containing these compounds, at least in greater than trace amounts.

Other Uses

The young springtime leaves, either fresh or cooked, are a fair edible. Mild and fresh-tasting, use them as a garnish or in larger amounts once boiled/rinsed.

Pedicularis
Orobanchaceae/Broomrape Family

Pedicularis groenlandica Retz.
Elephanthead lousewort, Pink elephants

Pedicularis procera Adams ex Steven A. Gray (*Pedicularis grayi*)
Giant lousewort, Towering lousewort

Pedicularis racemosa Douglas ex Hook.
Sickletop lousewort

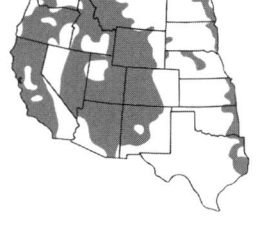

Pedicularis spp.

Description
Pedicularis groenlandica stands 1'–2' at maturity. The leaves are first to emerge in the spring. They are reddish due to a lack of chlorophyll. As the season progresses they mature to become deeply lobed, lanced–shaped, and fern–like. They are mostly basal, but also form alternately along the main stem's length. The magenta flowers develop in dense spikes; each appears as an elephant's head with galea appearing as an upturned tubular trunk.

Pedicularis procera, the tallest of the three species profiled, often grows to 4'–5' in height. Flowering stands command attention due to their striking appearance. The leaves are large and fern–like and mostly basal, though some also form along the flower stalk. The stalks are dark red and hollow when mature. The flowers are purplish–brown to greenish–yellow. The upper corolla lip is hood–like.

Pedicularis racemosa is a 1'–2' tall bunch–forming perennial. The toothed leaves are lance–shaped, undivided, and 2"–4" long. The white flowers develop in a leafy–bacted inflorescence. The galea forms into a long semi–circle beak.

Distribution
A circumpolar genus, China boasts the majority of Pedicularis species. Across North America these plants are common to temperate regions. In the West, most species are found in Aspen–conifer areas and surrounding meadows.

Chemistry

For Pedicularis procera: iridoids: aucubin, 6–deoxycatalpol, shanzhiside methyl ester, mussaenoside, 8–epiloganic acid, gardoside, proceroside; lignans; phenylpropanoids.

Medicinal Uses

A fascinating medicinal plant, Pedicularis[64] is effective for a number of central nervous system complaints. If plagued by restlessness use Pedicularis as a simple sedative before bed. Individuals whom exhibit more muscular tension than usual (this interfering with peaceful sleep) will respond well to the plant. As a bedtime sedative for hyperactive children it will be found more reliable than Valerian with its occasional circulatory stimulation. Although the plant always seems to fall behind other better known sedatives, its success often prompts repeat use and acknowledgment.

More so than many other sedatives, one Pedicularis specialty is its mild analgesic influence over muscular pain. Although not as powerful as a pharmaceutical, the plant will diminish soreness, inflammation, and related pain from muscular injury. Better for acute problems, Pedicularis can also be taken before bed if sleep is difficult due to pain sensitivity. Use it for sprains, contusions, muscle pulls, and a host of other sport–type injuries that are commonly encountered in these situations.

The herbaceous portions of Pedicularis, dried and smoked alone or in combination with other (non–drug) herbs, is reportedly relaxing. My experience is that internal (tincture or tea) preparations are more effective; however, the plant does have a small following as a smoking herb.

Indications

» Insomnia, with muscular tension
» Pain, muscular, as a sedative

Collection

Pedicularis is fairly straight–forward in its collection. If a large–growing species is being utilized, simply snip a leaf or two from each plant. If abundant and in flower, mix the upper flower spikes and leaves equally.

64   Because of related sedative effects, the name Betony or Wood betony is occasionally used for Pedicularis. This common name application for Pedicularis can be a source of confusion, as the Betonica/Stachys plants are really the true progenitors of the common name Betony.

Lower–growers may need to be more aggressively pruned in order to gather sufficient amounts. Regardless of species, the leaf and flower are the sought–after parts.

Preparations/Dosage
» FPT/DPT (50% alcohol): 60–90 drops 2–3 times daily
» Infusion: 4–8 oz. 2–3 times daily

Cautions
Pedicularis is known to be parasitic in varying degrees to other plants in its proximity. Be cautious about its collection if found growing intermingled with Senecio, Helenium/Hymenoxys, Thermopsis (Lupinus too), or other toxic plants.

Pine
Pinaceae/Pine Family

Pinus spp.

Pinus L.
Ponderosa pine, Limber pine, Lodgepole pine, Pinyon pine, etc.

Description
All pine trees have several characteristics that make them easily identifiable. They are evergreen. The bark is either furrowed or scaled. The leaves are needle–like, more or less aromatic when crushed, and found in groups of 1–6 (usually 2, 3, or 5). They form from small branch nubbins and are sheathed at the base as a group.

The small cylindric/ovoid pollen–bearing cones form in clusters mostly below the larger seed bearing cones or 'pine cone'. The female cones mature at the end of the second or third season.

Distribution
With over seventy species represented country–wide, nearly thirty species of Pinus exist throughout the West. Most species flourish at temperate latitudes/elevations, with some existing in expansive stands (P. ponderosa or Ponderosa pine). In the Southwest, P. edulis or Pinyon pine is a significant tree of grassland and upper desert areas.

Chemistry

For Pinus ponderosa: volatiles (needles): α–pinene, β–pinene, δ–3–carene, β–myrcene, limonene, β–phellandrene, methyl chavicol; diterpene resin acids (needles/oleoresin similar): abietic acid, dehydroabietic acid, neoabietic acid, imbricataloic acid, isocupressic acid, acetylisocupressic acid, succinylisocupressic acid, palustric acid, pimaric acid, isopimaric acid; piperidine alkaloids; arabinogalactan–proteins; procyanidins.

Medicinal Uses

Currently, various species of Pine and their products are recognized (or have been recognized) as source materials for medicine, the arts, and industry. Forgoing the obvious (lumber), medicinal/edible Pine parts can be separated into a number of categories.

1. Oleoresin: this is often referred to as Pine resin, Pine gum, Pine sap, Pine pitch, or turpentine[65]. Pine oleoresin naturally seeps from mechanically or insect damaged bark and is initially sticky and pliable but later crystallizes with exposure to the air and sun. Chemically it is a combination of a volatile fraction (approximately 20%–35%) and a non–volatile fraction or 'rosin'[66] (approximately 65%–80%). The volatile fraction (in most species pinene is the predominant monoterpene), basically the essential oil part of Pine oleoresin, is the most medicinally active element.

2. Inner Pine bark: the official Pine species utilized for its bark, of longest traditional medicinal use (North America), is Pinus strobus (White pine). Even today, the bark of White pine can still be found as an ingredient in some cough syrups. It is probable that other Pine barks that have piney–aromatic scents are good substitutes for White pine bark. Another potential for Pine bark that deserves more research is its arabinogalactan content (immune stimulating starches). Although Larch (Larix) bark, another conifer, is

---

65 Technically, turpentine is the accurate definition for Pine's viscous oleoresin. Today though, 'turpentine' usually refers to various distillates of Pine. For instance, 'Gum turpentine', mainly used by artists to thin oil–based paints, is the distillate of Pine's oleoresin. 'Wood turpentine' is a distillate of Pine parts left over from paper–lumber processing.

66 Although it is the essential oil fraction of Pine's oleoresin that is most well documented as having medicinal influence, new research suggests that the non–volatile portion of oleoresin (resin acids or what is known as 'rosin' after separation) is also worth attention. Anticarcinogenic and antiinflammatory effects are only two attributes recorded for this part in recent studies.

well known in the alternative health field as an immune stimulant, the bark of other Pine species may be of similar value. Ascorbate complexes (vitamin C) and phenolic compounds (similar to pycnogenol) found within the bark also make most species of Pine interesting. Furthermore, Pine bark, of whatever species, will contain fair quantities of volatiles, making it a good base material for essential oil distillation.

3. Pine cones: the females cones of most species are covered at some point (usually spring or summer) by oleoresin. When coated and sticky, they can be used as another base distillation item, if the essential oil is desired.

4. Pine seeds or 'Pine nuts': found within the successfully pollinated and mature female cone, the seeds of a number of species (Pinyon pine in the West) are a fine food source. Nutrient rich, they contain fair amounts of protein and essential fatty acids.

5. Pine needles: actually modified leaves, green Pine needles contain sizable amounts of aromatics and chlorophyll, and smaller amounts of ascorbate. Use them as another base material for essential oil distillation or a tea of the needles for medicinal/nutritional applications.

It is the secreted oleoresin from nearly all Pines that most concerns us here, as this portion can be easily prepared without expensive equipment for both internal and topical use. Ponderosa pine (Pinus ponderosa) and Limber pine (Pinus flexilis) are two common mountain–growing western Pines that usually yield large–to–moderate oleoresin quantities, though any other oleoresin–producing species will generally work as well.

A tincture made with the oleoresin is the best preparation for internal use. It is also well mixed with other tinctures in a formula, as alone the oleoresin tincture added to water will separate into its respective parts and form a gummy top layer. If this water and floating–oleoresin mixture is imbibed, some of the oleoresin will stick to the teeth and gums, and if allowed to linger, will cause redness and burning.

As part of a formula, oleoresin tincture imparts a stimulating–antimicrobial influence. After ingestion, the oleoresin's aromatic terpenes are secreted/excreted into the bronchial environment. Here they serve to loosen thickened bronchial mucus and inoculate the surrounding airspace/lung tissues with antimicrobial volatiles. Coughing become more productive and any potential bacterial (and likely viral) growth is inhibited. Formulated as a syrup ingredient (10%–25%), the oleoresin tincture complements cough suppressants like Wild cherry or Pleurisy root very well.

Of influence to the gastrointestinal region, the tincture can be combined with a bulking mucilage for a time–released coating effect. The essential oils found within the oleoresin are powerfully antimicrobial, making its use in bacterial diarrhea, dysentery, and most other intestinal infections worth noting. In fact, before the advent of modern antibiotics, Pine essential oil ('turpentine spirits') was often a successful treatment for cholera infections.

The oleoresin tincture should also be tried as a urinary tract antimicrobial. It is best suited for lower urinary tract infections that have been slow to resolve or are on–again–off–again in nature. Like bronchial formulations, use it as part of a tincture formula. Adding an oleoresin urinary formula to a 2–3 times–a–day tea of Corn silk or Hollyhock is fine way to proceed.

Although the internal use of oleoresin certainly has application, it is its external use that is most documented in older medical texts. Rarely used alone, but almost always as a formula ingredient, Pine oleoresin adds a stimulating–anesthetizing–antimicrobial element to topical combinations. Keeping the oleoresin content of the formula to about 10% is a good rule–of–thumb. At these levels, it makes a worthy ingredient as a topical chronic muscle/sport's injury formula. Both stimulating and reducing to sensitivity, it especially combines well with other aromatics such as Mint or Eucalyptus essential oils or Camphor. Relatedly, in similar ratios it's also well–used for chronic arthritic pain.

The needles, seeds, and even the inner bark of Pine (most conifers) contain small amounts of ascorbate (vitamin C) complexes. A simple Pine needle infusion makes a fine wintertime cold and flu tea. Its trace vitamin C content will be accented nicely by the needle's antimicrobial volatiles, evidenced by the piney aroma the steeping infusion produces. The tea can also be applied as a gargle for sore throats or as a nasal wash.

Indications
» Bronchitis, non–productive cough
» Infection, urinary tract, chronic
» Infection, intestinal
» As a stimulating/anesthetizing/antimicrobial medicant (external)
» As a cold and flu tea

Collection
In former times Pine oleoresin was manually collected in large quantities using the 'boxing' and 'cup and gutter' techniques. Although the boxing

technique was much more destructive to the tree, both relied upon making large cuts or incisions into the sap–producing bark and collecting the oleoresin that resulted from the injury over a span months (as with any tree, sap production is highest in spring and summer, tapering off when temperatures start to drop in the fall).

For our purposes, low–impact collection is all that is needed. Throughout various times of the year most Pine species will have semi–liquid new drippings (spring–summer) and/or semi–hardened and crystallized nodules (fall–winter) of oleoresin adhering to injured areas (insect holes, animal–initiated damage, and wind–damage are the most likely causes). The less pliable the nodule, the longer it has been on the outside of the tree and exposed to the elements. These nodules have a reduced essential oil content. Oleoresin that is viscous and molasses–like is newly secreted. Oleoresin in an in–between state (semi–soft and nodule–formed, yet not fully crystallized) has likely been exposed to the elements for only several months. Both the molasses–like and the semi–hardened oleoresin will be fine for tincture and salve use. But if a sizable quantity needs to be gathered, you may not have the luxury of being choosy – collecting an array of different oleoresin types in various states of crystallization is equally fine.

After finding a Pine stand, begin to examine the trees for bark damage, insect holes, etc. At this point, it should not be difficult to locate secretions of various quantity and quality. Some trees will have barely a spot of oleoresin, then others will have entire sides dripping, like crystallized waterfalls. Although hardened and semi–hardened nodule collecting is easy enough, fresh oleoresin collecting is a sticky business. The use of a putty knife or similar implement and a mason jar will make collection less difficult. After removing the oleoresin from the tree, scrape the lump off on the lip of the jar. If tincturing directly, know the weight of the jar before adding oleoresin and alcohol. Then, by weighing the oleoresin and the jar together, the weight of just the oleoresin can be easily determined and tincturing can proceed with one less step. Use a high–proof alcohol to wash hands and tools afterwards.

Pine needles need to be green, still on the tree, and preferably collected during the spring or summer (old Pine needles on the ground are good for two things: they make a comfy area to take a nap and if dry they are a good tinder). Containing volatile oils, make sure to dry Pine needles away from the sun and without artificial heat.

Preparations

Technically not a tincture, but a solution used like a tincture, place 1 part (weight) of oleoresin in 5 parts (volume) of alcohol (95%). If using crystallized oleoresin chunks first use a mortar and pestle or wrap the chunks in a cloth and pound them between two bricks to break the nodules into smaller pieces. Fresh oleoresin that is malleable needs no preparation, just add the correct amount of alcohol. Shake daily for 7–10 days. Strain from the solution what has not dissolved; bottle the oleoresin solution. Last step: decant the oleoresin solution after it stands for several days. There is often a layer of dirt and oleoresin precipitants at the bottom of the solution. Discard this layer.

Using oleoresin for topical applications is straight forward. Keep concentrations to around 10% of the total oil or salve weight/volume. Greater concentrations may be fine for unbroken skin but the chance of irritation increases with the amount of oleoresin in a formula. Simply apply low heat to an appropriate herbal oil (9 parts). Add the oleoresin (1 part) and slowly heat/stir until it is totally dissolved. Beeswax can be added at this point if a salve is desired (often less beeswax is needed due to the thickening effect of oleoresin).

Infuse the dried Pine needles for tea like any other aromatic–containing herb: be sure to cover the tea while it steeps.

Pine essential oil[67] is commonly available at health food stores. I recommend purchasing a pure aromatherapy grade for both internal and external use. Add the essential oil to herbal oils and salves at a 1%–2% concentration. 1–2 drops of the essential oil can be dropped in a capsule and swallowed or a spirit can be made enabling its mixture with other tinctures. Another noted internal preparation is the addition of the essential oil to a mucilage (bran, psyllium, Aloe gel, etc.) for a 'time–released' gastrointestinal effect. Pine essential oil's therapeutic effects are basically the same as oleoresin preparations – only without the occasional gastrointestinal upset that occurs with oleoresin consumption (due to the resin acid portion of oleoresin).

67 Pine essential oil, 'gum turpentine', and 'wood turpentine' are all very close in composition – their main monoterpene is pinene, either alpha or beta. For these distilled oils, I stress the use of pure Pine essential oil for both internal and external use. The reason being, industrial solvents (or solvent residues) may or may not have been used in the distillation/extraction process for 'gum turpentine' (a distillate of the oleoresin) and 'wood turpentine' (a distillate of various parts of the tree as a by–product of the paper and lumber industries).

Dosage

- » DPT of oleoresin (95% alcohol): 10–20 drops 2–3 times daily
- » Essential oil (needles, cones, inner bark, or oleoresin): 1–2 drops 2–3 times daily
- » Spirit: 10–20 drops 2–3 times daily
- » Oil/Salve: as needed
- » Needle infusion: 4–6 oz. 2–3 times daily

Cautions

Stomach upset is the most common complaint with the internal use of oleoresin–based medicines. The rosin fraction of oleoresin is somewhat difficult to digest. Lessening the dose or amount of oleoresin tincture in the formula should remedy this problem. I also advise against swallowing a pea or grape–sized oleoresin piece as an internal preparation, for whatever medicinal reason, due to the same stomach–upset issue; also, most of the oleoresin in this concentrated pill–like form will be non–assimilable.

As with any internal essential oil–based herbal medicine, liver and kidney inflammation is a possibility with over use. Central nervous system symptoms have also been reported with heavy dosing. The internal use of Pine oleoresin or Pine essential oil should be considered only for short–term durations: 1–2 weeks at a time, and only at sensible levels. Fatalities have been reported for excessive Pine essential oil consumption. Sadly, the majority of cases involve babies and children drinking large amounts (several ounces at a time) while unsupervised. This is no different than what has occurred with the improper/unsupervised use of Tea tree, Pennyroyal, Thuja and other essential oils. Don't be frightened of oleoresin and essential oil based medicines, just be prudent. Do not use them internally while pregnant or when nursing (or with children), though its external use is fine. Pine needle tea is safe during pregnancy/nursing and with children.

Pine oleoresin (and essential oil) is flammable – proceed with the necessary caution around an open fame.

Other Uses

As a primitive patching agent, joint–filler, or fixative, melt hardened oleoresin nodules using a low heat. Once softened, apply it as needed and then allow the oleoresin to dry. Its use as a sealant to water–going vessels is ancient.

Using an incense burner, small nodules of oleoresin can be burned like any other resin–type nugget or copal. Even 5–10 drops of the oleoresin tincture can be dropped on a hot plate. The resulting smoke is piney and aromatic.

A number of species of Pine in the West are known as Pinyon pines: Pinus edulis and P. monophylla are fairly common, though there are other species that are just as useful. Aside from the oleoresin and needle uses already mentioned, Pinyon pines' seeds (or 'nuts') are larger than other Pine species making collection (and eating) worthwhile. Gather the cones when still green, just before opening (after the cones begin to open the birds and other animals greedily eat the seeds). Throw the green cones in a campfire (or use a barbecue grill or large wok over a fire), watching closely for them to begin to open. Once they start to expand take the cones out of the fire. Let them cool a little and remove the seeds. Crack the shells between your teeth (if the shells are not yet too formed fingers alone should be adequate) like a large Sunflower seed. Discard the shell; eat the inner seed. Very close in relation to store–bought European Pine nuts, these are the wild American version of a pricey item found in gourmet markets.

The inner bark of young Scotch pine (Pinus sylvestris) has a long tradition of being used as a emergency food throughout parts of northern Europe. After roasting/baking/boiling the bark to remove as much of the oleoresin as possible, it was then ground into a meal/flour. It was best added to other grain flours in bread making as a supplement (10%–20%). Used alone as an emergency staple, toxic reactions were not uncommon (though still better than starving to death).

Pipsissewa
Ericaceae/Heath Family

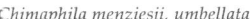

Chimaphila menziesii, umbellata

Chimaphila menziesii (R. Br.) Spreng.
Little prince's pine

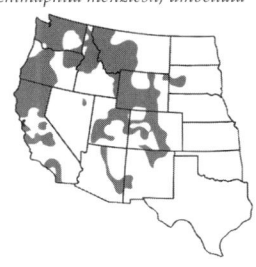

Chimaphila umbellata (L.) W.P.C. Barton
Prince's pine, Ground holly

Description
Pipsissewa is a small evergreen perennial. Forming in colonies from below–ground creeping rhizomes, the plant's leaf growth is thickened and somewhat leather–like. The singular leaves are linear to linear–ovate and more or

less serrated. Chimaphila menziesii's leaves are dull–green and occasionally have a mottled midvein area. C. umbellata's leaves are glossy–green with no lighter middle.

The nodding dish–shaped flowers develop on long stems and are neatly composed of 5 whitish–pinkish petals and 10 stamens. The seed capsule is approximately ¼" in diameter.

Distribution

Chimaphila menziesii's core territory is the Pacific Northwest. It's also found in western parts of Idaho, Montana, Nevada, southern California, and a number of isolated stands in Utah. A sporadic grower, look to mountainous coniferous forests. More abundant than C. menziesii, C. umbellata is found from the Pacific Coast ranges, then east to New Mexico and Montana. Skipping most of Great Plains region, this species is also common from the north–central states to northeast and mid–Atlantic states. The plant is found in mountainous forests, often in thick Pine needle litter.

Chemistry

Phenolic acid: homogentisic acid; phenolic glycosides: arbutin, isohomoarbutin; flavonoids: avicularin, hyperoside, kaempferol; triterpenoid: β–amyrin; sterols: β–sitosterol, taraxasterol, ursolic acid; quinones: chimaphilin, renifolin; flavanol: epicatechin gallate; waxes: hentriacontane, nonacosane; methyl salicylate.

Medicinal Uses

Sharing many of its medicinal attributes with related Heath family plants, Pipsissewa is primarily a urinary tract medicine. Slightly astringent and curiously spicy–stimulating in taste and action, the herb tea (or tincture in water) is best applied to chronic irritations and mild/moderate infections of the urinary area. It most reliably remedies lower urinary tract infections: urethritis and cystitis are its best applications, especially if the infection is chronic or subacute. Cloudy and mucus–containing urine and pain upon urination indicate Pipsissewa's use. Additionally, it will be found specific for chronic lower urinary tract infections dependent upon alkaline urine (i.e. Escherichia coli proliferation). Use Uva–ursi or Madrone if the infection is acute, but if a maintenance herb is needed try Pipsissewa instead.

Men whom suffer from urinary complaints from prostate enlargement and related prostatitis, should see symptomatic relief with Pipsissewa. Not really prostate shrinking but rather antiseptic and inflammation reducing to the surrounding urinary tissues, it is best used when scanty urination and chronic infection from incomplete voiding are the main symptoms.

More advanced upwardly moving infections such as ureteritis and pyelitis are treated less reliably by Pipsissewa, especially if the plant was used with no success when the lower regions were affected. But if Pipsissewa has just been discovered, and the renal pelvis (pyelitis) and/or the ducts leading from the kidney to the bladder (urethritis) are affected, try it for two or three days. If the symptoms of scanty and/or cloudy urine and dull pelvic ache begin to diminish, stay the course until the infection has resolved; if no betterment is sensed within two to three days, resort to conventional medicine. Note though – the plant will have an optimal effect on these mid to upper urinary infections when they are in their beginning stages (unlike the plant's indication for chronic lower infections).

Pipsissewa's application to an established kidney infection (nephritis) and even matured pyelitis are its least reliable usages. Remember: the longer an unchecked kidney infection is allowed to fester, the greater chance of permanent kidney damage and systemic infection. Use the herb initially, but if more severe symptoms develop (lower back pain, fever, and blood in the urine), it would be prudent to seek the greater potencies of pharmaceutical antibiotics.

Pipsissewa's best tonic use is for low–level autoimmune non–bacterial kidney inflammation. Many will find the plant diminishing to the general lower–back ache, extremity edema, and joint–tissue pain that often accompanies flare–ups. Often protein (albumin) tainted urine will clear with the plant's consistent usage.

Indications
» Urethritis/Cystitis, chronic/subacute
» Urethritis/Cystitis, with alkaline urine
» Urethritis/Cystitis, with prostate involvement
» Ureteritis/Pyelitis, mild/beginning stages
» Inflammation, renal, autoimmune causes
» Albuminuria, autoimmune causes

Collection
Simply snip the top half of Pipsissewa from its base. The leaves will yield the greatest bulk for the tea and tincture, but if some of the flowers and even stems are collected this is also fine.

Preparations/Dosage
» Infusion: 4–8 oz. 2–3 times daily
» FPT/DPT (50% alcohol): 30–60 drops 2–3 times daily

Cautions
Pipsissewa is a relatively safe medicinal plant. Due to its astringency, some stomach upset and/or bladder/kidney irritation may result from excessive amounts. Limited quantities are acceptable during pregnancy and are also not a problem while nursing or with children.

Plantain
Plantaginaceae/Plantain Family

Plantago major

Plantago major L. *(Plantago borysthenica, P. dregeana, P. latifolia)*
Broadleaf plantain, Ribwort

Description
Plantain is a small herbaceous short–lived perennial. Originating from the plant's stalkless center, the leaves are ovoid, dark green, hairless, pleated, and have wavy margins with or without serrations. The flowers are inconspicuous and small. They are clustered in elongated spikes, rising upward from the plant's center. The seedpods contain numerous, small, reddish–brown seeds.

Distribution
Plantain is a European native. It has extensively naturalized throughout America and Canada. Look for it in moist and disturbed soils. Lawns, gardens, and roadsides are usual spots for the plant.

Chemistry
Mucilage composed of polysaccharides; tannins; iridoid glycosides: aucubin, catalpol; silicic acid; protocatechuic acid; flavonoids: apigenin, luteolin.

Medicinal Uses
The fresh plant chewed or crushed and then placed on insect bites or stings is soothing and antiinflammatory. Like Chickweed, it is also quieting to heat rashes and burns and will assist in wound healing.

Internally, the tea or fresh juice diminishes mucus membrane heat. Use it for intestinal inflammation with corresponding diarrhea. It's also a soothing diuretic that lessens urinary tract irritation and burning urination. Additionally, the plant reduces bronchial irritation particularly when the lungs feel hot and dry.

Indications
» Inflammation/Injury, skin
» Bites/Stings/Rashes (external)
» Inflammation, intestinal, with diarrhea
» Urination, painful
» Irritation, bronchial

Collection
Gather the plant's herbage. Use it fresh or dry.

Preparations/Dosage
» Poultice/Oil/Ointment/Salve: as needed
» Infusion (cold or standard): 4–8 oz. 2–3 times daily
» Fresh juice: ½–1 oz. 2–3 times daily or topically as needed

Cautions
There are no cautions for Plantain.

Other Uses
Plantago ovata and P. psyllium are two species of Plantain that are widely used for their mucilage/fiber–containing seed coats (or husks). 'Metamucil' is a popular psyllium seed husk supplement.

Pulsatilla
Ranunculaceae/Buttercup Family

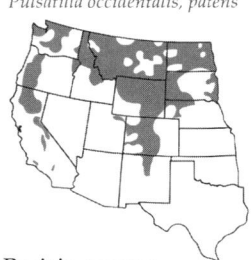

Pulsatilla occidentalis, patens

Pulsatilla occidentalis S. Watson *(Anemone occidentalis, A. occidentalis var. subpilosa)*
Western pasqueflower, White pasqueflower

Pulsatilla patens (L.) Mill. *(Pulsatilla hirsutissima, P. ludoviciana, Anemone patens)*
Pasqueflower, American pasqueflower, Wild crocus, Prairie crocus

Description
Due to the shifting winds of botanical classification, Pulsatilla is also found labeled as Anemone. And that is fine, botanists do have their reasons after all. However, I believe (as did historical classifiers) these two groups are morphologically different enough to warrant separation. What distinguishes these two plants from their Anemone brethren? Much longer styles and shaggy seed heads.

Both Pulsatilla species profiled here are known to emerge and bloom early in the season. With little concern for conditions that keep most other plants suspended, they occasionally even push up through lingering patches of snow.

Nearly all parts of both plants are covered by long hairs. The smaller of the two, Pulsatilla patens, grows to be 10" in height, but usually it is less with its divided leaves being mostly basal (and a whorl at mid–stem). Its striking blue to whitish flowers are composed of 5–7 petal–like sepals. The flowers are borne singly on each stem. At maturity, the styles can reach lengths of 1½" and appear in mass as a spreading head of silvery fluff.

P. occidentalis' leaves are also basal (with a mid–stem whorl) and divided into 2–3 short and narrow triangular segments. Its flowers are one per stem and composed of 5–7 showy white sepals. The fluffy styles are 1½" long, and unlike P. patens', are flexed downward, appearing like an upturned mop.

Distribution
Pulsatilla occidentalis is found in California, Oregon, Washington, Idaho, and Montana. It's a high mountain plant, associated with open coniferous

forests and meadows, generally from 8000' and above. Good winter snow cover is a habitat prerequisite.

A circumboreal plant, in North America Pulsatilla patens is found from New Mexico, north to Montana (and Canada), west to Washington, and then east to Michigan. High elevation grasslands/meadows and open prairie where the soil is rocky and winters hard, are prime locales for P. patens.

Chemistry

Lactones: protoanemonin, anemonin; triterpene glycosides; anthocyanins/anthocyanidins (flowers).

Medicinal Uses

The medicinal use of American Pulsatilla is patterned after the once official European plants: Pulsatilla vulgaris (alternately, Anemone pulsatilla or European pasqueflower) and Pulsatilla pratensis (alternately, Anemone pratensis or Small pasqueflower). Due to quality problems, American homeopaths and Eclectics began to use native species of Pulsatilla (mainly the more easterly grower, P. patens) as replacements for the European plants during the mid–1800s. Not only did the European sources produce a poor medicine due to shipping/age deteriorations from the transatlantic journey, Pulsatilla, whatever species, poorly maintains its potency once dried (the vast majority of herbal imports at the time were dried and shipped in bulk).

Pulsatilla affects both somatic and psychosomatic parameters. Its physical influences are related to its protoanemonin content. Although its effect on the mood and emotional outlook likely has to do with a related group of acrid volatiles, the specific constituents responsible for its subtler uses are not precisely known.

Small doses of the fresh plant tincture (5–10 drops per dose dropped directly in the mouth) are useful in relieving episodes of depression, gloominess, and fear, particularly if these symptoms exist alongside mental agitation, hysteria, and insomnia. Individuals whom struggle with issues of physical deficiency and poor circulation will respond better to Pulsatilla than those of robust yet excessive temperaments, i.e. ectomorph versus mesomorph. For this type of individual, it will be of use in calming the mind from overwork, extended periods of intense focus (late night driving for instance), and other issues that take on a fatigued yet 'too tired to sleep' quality.

For women of atonic temperament, premenstrual mood fluctuations or 'hysteria' associated with this time of the month tends to be calmed with Pulsatilla. Stimulating to core vascular, its positive influence will be noticed if slowed menses, pelvic congestion, and first–second day period cramps are the norm. Even ovarian pain during ovulation or otherwise will be sedated by the plant.

Men suffering from chronic forms of epididymitis, orchitis, seminal vesicle and cowper's gland inflammations often see betterment with Pulsatilla. It's not that the herb is strongly antibacterial (these inflammations are often bacterial/STD–related and should be addressed accordingly); however, its influence is nonetheless symptomatically sedating to these regional problems. Even the progression of beginning–stage varicoceles, caused by weak venous circulation, will at least be slowed with the herb.

For both men and women, if there is decreased libido and lack of sexual interest from stress, overwork, and nervousness, try small doses throughout the day. Similar to the herb's other indications, it will be more effective for individuals whom are atonic and easily influenced emotionally/physically. Relatedly, use Pulsatilla as a supportive formula ingredient if plagued by chronic urinary inflammations, particularly if genetic urinary weakness seems to be at the problem's core.

As a headache remedy Pulsatilla often excels, particularly if there is a stress factor. Sinus and menstrual headaches too are relieved by the herb. Even if used in the early stages of a migraine, particularly during the aura phase, it's not uncommon for it to halt its development. It's thought that Pulsatilla's cerebral vasodilator properties are at least partly responsible for its activity: 5–10 drops directly on the tongue is an approximate dosage for these problems. If Pulsatilla worsens the headache, it usually means cerebral vasoconstrictors are a better choice, i.e. Coffee, Kola nut, or Periwinkle (Vinca major).

Pulsatilla is a gastric stimulant: through a dilatory effect it provides more blood to the stomach walls. For indigestion and digestive atony combine the plant with bitters and take the combo before meals, particularly if the constitutional picture fits as previously described.

An eyewash made with the fresh plant tincture (see Preparations) is of use in chronic conjunctivitis, ocular irritation (hayfever reaction for instance), and styes. Like Marsh marigold, topically Pulsatilla is rubefacient. It causes vasodilation, quickly bringing more blood to surface tissues. A fresh plant poultice is well–applied to chronic arthritic conditions; however, be sure to remove the plant at the first sign of redness, or else blistering may result.

Indications
- Depression, with mental agitation/insomnia
- Dysmenorrhea/Amenorrhea
- Debility, genital/urinary system
- Libido, decreased
- Headache/Migraine, beginning stages
- Indigestion, due to vascular weakness
- Conjunctivitis/Styes (eyewash)
- Arthritis, as a counter–irritant (external)

Collection
Gather the foliage (leaves, flowers, and stems) in early spring. Chew a leaf to better understand the plant's medicinal effect. It should be acrid...if not, an incorrect plant may have been selected.

Preparations
Pulsatilla's potency degrades through drying (and storage) so it is best to tincture a fresh batch every year or two. For the eyewash mix 10 drops of fresh plant tincture in 2 ounces of isotonic water; make fresh daily.

Dosage
- FPT: 5–15 drops 2–3 times daily
- Fresh poultice: apply as needed (remove at first feelings of warmth)
- Eyewash: 3–4 times daily

Cautions
Pulsatilla can be mentally unsettling for some people (mesomorph body type). Too much of the plant will cause gastric irritation and diarrhea. Do not use it in acute vascular conditions that are inflammatory in nature. Like most Buttercup family plants do not use it during pregnancy due to its dilatory effect on the uterine environment.

Pussytoes
Asteraceae/Sunflower Family

Antennaria Gaertn.
Catspaw, Catstoes, Everlasting

Antennaria spp.

Description
Carpeting and patch–like in growth, Pussytoes is mainly composed of small woolly leaves growing in basal formations. Individually they are linear to spoon–shaped, often densely hair–covered and sessile (reminiscent of a cat's paw or toe). Usually in the range of 6"–1', the plant's small flower stalk is topped by small, unisexual, papery, bract–composed inflorescences.

Distribution
A Northern Hemisphere genus, North America hosts the greatest number of species. Common to forest clearings and meadows, Pussytoes is almost always found in semi–moist soils with good sun exposure.

Chemistry
Very little information exists on Pussytoes' chemical makeup, but most Antennaria[68] species are closely affiliated with Anaphalis, Gnaphalium, and Pseudognaphalium.

Medicinal Uses
Nearly all traditional information on Pussytoes indicates its use as a lung–oriented tea. Bronchial inflammation with related pectoral soreness, particularly if there is a painful cough, is its main indication. Its medicinal use will fit most lung conditions at some level, as it's not particularly stimulating, unlike Lomatium or Ligusticum, nor potentially nauseating (via vagus nerve affinity) like most Asclepias species. Also, because it is mild, there will be little harm done if used at random with not much thought. It combines well with herbs that are more directed (stronger expectorants, antitussives, etc.) due to its underlying antiinflammatory and diffuse nature (Pussytoes

---

[68] Plant geneticists surmise that Antennaria likely arose (during the Oligocene or Miocene) from Mexican Gnaphalium. The genus then migrated into more distal parts of the Northern Hemisphere (and South America).

shares many lung similarities with Mullein). One last note regarding the plant's bronchial effects: a number of species are agreeably aromatic and more or less glandular. If this is the case with any species of interest, then it will have a stronger expectorating effect on the lungs.

The plant is also a soothing and mildly astringing remedy for irritative diarrhea and loose stools. If there is any spastic activity, 30–60 drops of Silk tassel tincture can be added to the tea for a stronger effect. A number of species were once utilized by North American Indians as a postpartum medicine. Use both a sitz bath and the internal tea if in need of its reproductive tissue soothing qualities.

Indications
» Bronchitis with lung soreness and cough
» Diarrhea, with intestinal irritation
» Reproductive injury, postpartum (internal and external)

Collection
Find a good–sized blanket–like stand of Pussytoes and up–root the outlying plants. This process will be easier than using pruners on the short leaves. Knock off any attaching dirt and debris and dry the whole plant normally for tea preparations.

Preparations/Dosage
» Herbal infusion: 4–8 oz. 2–3 times daily

Cautions
I am unaware of any specific cautions for Pussytoes. It is a mild herbal medicine.

Other Uses
A number of Antennaria species were mixed with Tobacco and other herbs as an ingredient of Kinnikinnick, a highly customized and varied smoking mixture employed at one time or another by most American Indian tribes. For instance, Antennaria rosea (Rosy pussytoes) was used by the Blackfoot for this purpose. The fluffier the leaf of any species, the more likely it will be a good smoking candidate.

Pyrola
Ericaceae/Heath Family

Pyrola spp.

Pyrola L.
Shinleaf, Canker lettuce, False wintergreen

Description
Pyrola is a small perennial herb. Including the flowering stem, it grows to about 1' in height. The leaves are basal, generally ovate to elliptic, and depending on species, either entire or slightly toothed. Most species have thickened leathery leaves; several species' leaves are shiny. The greenish–white to pinkish flowers are complete and 5–parted.

Distribution
With the southern Great Plains states and Southeast as exceptions, Pyrola is found country–wide. Conifer–covered mountains throughout the West is its core area. Usually found in deep forests, often next to springs or around moistened and rich soils, look for the plant underfoot. Coral root is a common associate.

Chemistry
Phenolic glycosides: arbutin, catechin, epicatechin gallate, procyanidin, hyperin; flavonoids: quercetin, rhamnetin, kaempferol.

Medicinal Uses
In use and potency consider Pyrola to be a diminutive Pipsissewa. Sharing most of the latter's therapeutic qualities (stimulating antimicrobial astringent), yet to a lesser degree, Pyrola is mainly indicated in chronic lower urinary tract irritations. It's particularly indicated in cloudy and mucus tinged urine with accompanying irritation and pain upon urination.

Like other Heath family plants, due to Pyrola's arbutin content, it is found useful if an infection is commingled with alkaline urine (which is common). Although Uva–ursi will be more acidifying to the urine and therefore more inhibiting to Escherichia coli, Pyrola (and also Pipsissewa) will too have a positive impact.

Men should try Pyrola (or Pipsissewa) if troubled by urinary complaints stemming from an enlarged prostate. For the peripheral symptoms of urine backlog, scanty urination, and chronic bladder infection/irritation, it often provides some relief. Although it likely has no direct shrinking effect on the prostate, the surrounding urinary tissues that are secondarily affected by prostatic hypertrophy are well influenced by the plant.

For the initial stages of mid and upper urinary tract infections (ureteritis and pyelitis) Pyrola should be tried. Though it does little good in advanced bacterial infections, especially if the kidneys are affected, Pyrola often gives relief, especially if urine production is scanty (from duct–tissue inflammation). Use the herb initially, but if pelvic/lower back pain, nausea, and fever develop (or become more advanced), seek the greater potencies of pharmaceutical antibiotics.

Also like Pipsissewa, Pyrola is used as an antiinflammatory for the kidneys, especially if chronically affectedly by autoimmune disturbances. On–and–off again autoimmune related nephritis is a specific for the herb. Although it is only a mild to moderate antiseptic, if used daily, urine levels of albumin, occult red blood cells, and white blood cells should lower.

Use the herb tea as a mouth rinse/gargle for oral ulcerations (canker sores) and sore throat. The warm tea used every couple of hours will be found most effective.

Indications
» Urethritis/Cystitis, chronic/subacute
» Urethritis/Cystitis, with alkaline urine
» Urethritis/Cystitis, with prostate involvement
» Ureteritis/Pyelitis, mild/beginning stages
» Inflammation, renal with autoimmune causes
» Albuminuria, autoimmune causes

Collection
Snip a few leaves from one plant, then move on to the next. Dry the herbal portions normally for tea (or the dried plant tincture) or tincture these parts fresh.

Preparations/Dosage
» Infusion: 4–8 oz. 2–3 times daily
» FPT/DPT (50% alcohol): 30–60 drops 2–3 times daily

Cautions
As with any tannin oriented plant, overuse may result in gastric upset and/or bladder–renal irritation. Simply reduce the dosage or discontinue Pyrola if these unwanted effects arise. Reduced dosages/amounts are fine during pregnancy and will pose no problem while nursing or with children.

Rattlesnake Plantain
Orchidaceae/Orchid Family

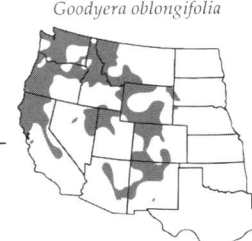

Goodyera oblongifolia

Goodyera oblongifolia Raf.
Giant rattlesnake plantain, Green–leaved rattlesnake plantain, Western rattlesnake plantain, Rattlesnake orchid

Description
At first emergence Rattlesnake plantain is composed of a funnel–like rosette of basal leaves. When mature the ovate to elliptic leaves are pointed, flat, and have whitish central molting. From each rosette, a central flower stalk (1'–2' high) develops bearing an inconspicuous spike of whitish–green to pinkish flowers. Colony–type stands form from underground rhizomes.

Distribution
Significant in distribution, Rattlesnake plantain is found throughout the western mountains, Canada, and the Northeast. Densely shaded and moist coniferous forests is its usual habitat. Coral root is a common companion plant.

Chemistry
Orchids general: alkaloids, flavonoids, sterols, carotenoids, anthocyanins/anthocyanidins.

Medicinal Uses
As a simple topical soother, use a field poultice (freshly bruised/crushed) on burns, scrapes, stings, and insect bites. It also can be dried and made into an oil/ointment/salve and applied for similar things.

Gargle the warm tea (or diluted juice) to soothe oral ulcerations, sore throats, and hoarseness due to voice–overuse. Swallowed, the tea or juice becomes a gastrointestinal soother. Use it for stomach and intestinal inflammations. It will not correct any major problem, but as a low–level counter to irritation, Rattlesnake plantain is worthwhile.

Indications
» Burns/Scrapes/Stings/Bites (external)
» Irritation, oral (gargle)
» Irritation, gastrointestinal

Collection
As long as soils are non–compacted and comprised of forest litter, Rattlesnake plantain is an enjoyable and easy plant to collect. I recommend simply working your hands under the plant's shallow roots. Gently pull up the plant, root and all. Some of the smaller tendrils may break off but the majority of roots should remain connected. More compacted soils will necessitate a shovel.

Preparations/Dosage
» Infusion: 4–8 oz. 2–3 times daily
» Fresh juice: ½–1 oz. 2–3 times daily
» Fresh plant poultice/Oil/Ointment/Salve: as needed

Cautions
There are no known cautions for Rattlesnake plantain.

Red Osier Dogwood
Cornaceae/Dogwood Family

Cornus sericea

Cornus sericea L. *(Cornus stolonifera)*
American dogwood, Creek dogwood, Red dogwood, Red twig dogwood

Description
A large shrub, Red osier reaches heights (and widths) of nearly 10′–12′. One notable characteristic is its red–purple stems, which are especially apparent in the winter when the leaves are absent. Lanceolate to ovate, they are about twice as long as wide (2″–3½″ long is average),

prominent–veined, point–tipped, green above, and lighter (appressed hairs) beneath. The white–cream, small, 4–petaled flowers develop in flat–topped cymes at branch ends. The fruit are also whitish. They are one–seeded, pea–sized, and form in clusters. Red osier is particularly adept at stem–rooting. Large and dense stands of the plant are mostly comprised of clones.

Distribution

The northern latitudes of the United States (from Washington to Maine) and Canada contain the greatest populations of Red osier. It's very common in the western mountain states (especially in the Rocky Mountains) and is known also to the higher mountains of the Southwest. Absent from grasslands, basins, and drier mid–mountains, it's mainly found in montane habitats and almost always next to streams in moist soils.

Chemistry

Cornus general: iridoid glycosides: dihydrocornin, cornin, phlorin; triterpenoids; flavonoids; tannins

Medicinal Uses

The use of Red osier is more old fashioned than that of most better–known herbs. Even by the mid to late 1800s its use had become infrequent at best, as most physicians preferred Cornus florida[69] (Flowering dogwood) for its similar yet more vigorous effects.

There is not much modern–day research on Red osier (let alone Flowering dogwood) in regards to its medicinal activity. Even the Asian species of Cornus, which gets slightly more scientific attention, are mostly researched for their antioxidant and glucose regulating properties. For Red osier, I rely upon my own observations, a few mentions by the Eclectics, and sensible hypothesis.

Malarial infections and most other 'intermittent' feverous states thought to be caused by 'bad air', were the plant's main historical indications. For us this means Red osier should be taken when sick and feverish; however, not at the high–temperature peaks but rather at the lulls (during a multi–day fever temperatures are often lower earlier in the day, then spike in the evening). In other words, Red osier should be used at sub–feverish

[69] Distribution had much to do with the preference of Cornus florida. It simply was more available: Cornus florida is common to most of the eastern part of the county, as opposed to Red osier's domain of the less populated western mountains.

times during a multi-day sickness (headache and general weakness during this time also point to its use). This nuance in dosing is somewhat important due Red osier's low-level pulse/circulatory stimulation. I do not believe Red osier strongly counters any systemic infectious principle (virus, microbe, or other), at least no more than similar tannin-containing plants, but rather it potentially augments some immunological parameter, and therefore helps the body to rally against an infection.

Red osier is astringent and bitter (though not as bitter as Flowering dogwood). Standard doses will lessen diarrhea and loose stools (not uncommon symptoms in feverish infections); however, too much of the tea often has a nauseating effect[70].

The bark used topically does have some antibacterial influence. Festering cuts, ulcerations, and other similar conditions in need of healing will show improvement with the wash or fomentation.

Indications
» Fever, low-temperature with weakness and circulatory deficiency
» Cuts/Ulcerations, poorly healing (external)

Collection
Dig the root/rooting stem. Remove the outer layer from the roots (referred to as the rootbark) and lower stems. The smaller flexible roots can be gathered and processed without stripping. Dry the rootbark/lower stem bark/smaller roots for tea or tincture preparations.

Preparations
At least one important glycoside (cornin) in Red osier (and in other Cornus species) has been shown to diminish significantly in the presence of heat. This means the cold infusion is a choice preparation for the plant; however, a regular infusion of the rootbark will also be found adequate. The decoction, due to its continued application of heat, will be of some use, just not optimal. If in need of a condensed preparation (nausea being an issue with the poor-tasting tea), the dried plant tincture of the rootbark should be considered. Red osier rootbark should always be first dried due to the fresh material's more pronounced nauseating effect.

---

70   A number of American Indian tribes (Navajo for instance) used bark preparations as a ceremonial emetic.

Dosage
» Rootbark infusion (cold or standard): 2–4 oz. 2–3 times daily
» DPT (50% alcohol) of rootbark: 20–30 drops 2–3 times daily

Cautions
Red osier is probably not the best herb to be used while pregnant, at least not in larger quantities. I say probably because there is little written information on the subject. The plant while nursing should be fine.

Nausea is the most consistent complaint with Red osier; however, this can be mitigated by keeping dosages to the recommended amounts, or add 60 drops of Field mint or Monarda tincture as an offset.

Other Uses
Red osier's ripe white fruit are marginal tasting at best. They can be eaten (sparingly) alone; however, they were almost always mixed with better tasting wild berries (usually Serviceberry or Chokecherry). The young flexible stems are a good basket–making item. Used by many western mountain tribes, the inner stem bark was a common smoking ingredient in Kinnikinnick.

Red Raspberry
Rosaceae/Rose Family

Rubus idaeus

Rubus idaeus L.
American red raspberry, European red raspberry

Description
Red raspberry is an herbaceous, bristly sub–shrub. The leaves are odd–pinnate and formed of 3–5 serrate leaflets. They are dark–green above and gray–white, pubescent–tomentose below. The flowers form in axillary or terminal racemes. Each cluster contains 4–7 flowers. Like most Rose family plants, Red raspberry's white flowers are perfect and have 5 petals and 5 sepals. The red fruit is hemispherical and ⅖"–½" in diameter.

Most classifiers consider American and European red raspberry one species. Morphological differences for independent groups (often influenced by locale) are currently reflected by numerous subspecies and varieties.

Distribution
With much of the Southeast and Texas as an exception, Red raspberry is found throughout most of North America. It is common to coniferous forests, usually along streams, and on rocky slopes and hillsides. The plant is also found throughout similar temperate regions of Eurasia.

Chemistry
Flavonoids: rutin, isoquercitrin, quercitrin; caffeic acid derivatives; phenolic acids; anthocyanins/anthocyanidins (fruit).

Medicinal Uses
Of all the Rose family astringents, Red raspberry is the best known. A time-tested and kindly remedy, its heralded reputation is not without founding. 1–2 cups daily (no more), started at the beginning of the last trimester of pregnancy, has a tonifying effect, lessening the possibility of miscarriage. Through its influence of area vascularity, it also makes the birthing process better defined and efficient.

Used as sitz bath and internal tea, Red raspberry is additionally a mild postpartum tonic. It too reduces the inflammation and discharge of vaginitis and cervicitis. For heavy menstruation, if there is red blood when menses should be at its end, the internal tea is useful. Even mid-cycle spotting will be curbed with the tea. For urinary irregularities, such as mild cystitis or urethritis, it will also prove soothing.

Besides Red raspberry's active tissue influence, the tea contains a fair amount of calcium. Although the mineral's quantity is not large (compared to supplementation), due to its absorbable form most of it is bioavailable. For the plant's nutrient uses it combines well with Horsetail or Nettle.

Indications
- As a prepartum tonic
- As a postpartum tonic (external and internal)
- Vaginitis/Cervicitis (external and internal)
- Menstruation, heavy
- Cystitis/Urethritis
- As a nutritive tea

Collection

When in their prime, snip the leaves from the plant. Once dried, garble the leaves (and flowers) from the stems. Discard the stems. Red raspberry leaf is commercially available, though wildcrafted material will usually be of better quality.

Preparations/Dosage

» Herb infusion: 4–8 oz. 1–3 times daily
» Sitz bath: 1–2 times daily

Cautions

There are no cautions for Red raspberry.

Other Uses

The fruit is a well-known edible. The fresh berries from wild plants are usually better tasting than store bought and also make a fine base for preserves, syrups, etc.

Red Root

Rhamnaceae/Buckthorn Family

Ceanothus L.
Buckbrush, Deerbrush, Wild lilac

Ceanothus spp.

Description

Western species of Red root can be generally divided into 3 separate camps. Group A: like Ceanothus fendleri, these are low growing shrubs, more–or–less spiny, and have alternating elliptic to oblong leaves. The flowers are white and form in umbel–like clusters on branch ends. Group B is comprised of stiff–branched large shrubs, like Ceanothus greggii (this particular species has opposite leaves, grayish bark, and whitish flowers). Members of Group C are semi-flexible large shrubs with branches that are covered by a thin green bark. Their elliptic to ovate leaves are larger than the leaves of the other two types. The densely–clustered flowers, depending on species, are either bluish–lilac or white to cream in color. Certainly, there are exceptions to these three main types: Red root is notorious for hybridizing, which often makes species identification troublesome.

Distribution

Sixty–plus species of Red root are found throughout the West, particularly in California, where dozens of species exist side–by–side. Look to the mid–mountains with chaparral vegetation and Yellow pine.

Chemistry

Triterpenes: ceanothic, ceanothetric, and betulinic acids; flavonoids: kaempferol, delphinidin, cyanidin, quercetin, rhamnetin, chrysoeriol, malvidin, petunidin, luteolin, velutin; tannins; peptide alkaloids: americine, ceanthamine, ceanthine, adouetine nonacosane; 1–hexacosanol, cinnamic acid.

Medicinal Uses

The medicinal use of western Red root is patterned after Ceanothus americanus (New Jersey tea or simply Red root), a ubiquitous shrub found from the edge of the Great Plains, then east to the coast. This plant saw traditional American Indian use prior to the Colonists arriving in America; however, its recorded beginnings started around the country's formative years. In those times, it was best known as a medicine for splenitis, then referred to as 'ague cake', a term most often used to describe an enlarged spleen, a common symptom of malaria. I'm not suggesting Red root, whatever species, as an herbal remedy for malaria (a rather serious mosquito–borne protozoal infection); however, its early history does help to shed light on its sensible application.

I believe most, if not all, western Ceanothus species can be used like Ceanothus americanus, just as long as the root or root bark is non–woody and reddish–tannin pigmented. My personal favorites, due to their flexible reddish roots, are the young shrubs of 'Group C', often called Lilac bush (blue flowers), but if those types are not in your local area: unearth, investigate, and utilize what's nearby.

Considering no other group in the Buckthorn family has Red root's unique effect on the lymphatic system[71], the plant is sort of an anomaly. At the core of Red root's therapeutic influence is its effect on lymphatic tissue, immunologic cells, and blood–lymph lipids. The plant is not necessarily a

---

71 It's interesting to note that a number of Ziziphus species (also Buckthorn family) have recently been reported to contain several triterpenes also found in Ceanothus.

strong white blood cell stimulant, like Echinacea or Stillingia, but rather an organizer/stabilizer of these cells and tissues. The low–level immunological stimulation (mainly due to the triterpenes) that does occur is most pronounced in the viscera – particularly the spleen and liver.

It has been postulated that Red root is additionally therapeutic due to its influence on surrounding cellular charge[72]. This stabilizing effect is evidenced by its activity on swollen adenoids, or in the extreme, tonsillitis. Alone or more effectively with Echinacea, Red root's application here has a successful history of use. General pharyngitis, with or without swollen lymph nodes, also responds well to a gargle of the diluted tincture. Where Ocotillo is indicated for trunk/pelvic lymphatic swelling due to less than ideal lipid/lymph interactions, Red root is better for throat centered swollen lymphatic tissue when there is a clear immunological issue.

The plant's (Ceanothus americanus) main application throughout the Revolutionary War period was for splenitis, or 'ague cake' as it was once called. Due to modern–day constituent research and analysis, we can postulate how Red root most likely works for this and other visceral inflammations (hepatitis for instance). It reduces organ swelling due to a mild regional leukocyte stimulation (or organization). Applications for Red root in this area include: visceral swelling from minor physical injury, infection (bacterial, viral, or parasitic), and autoimmune disturbances (such as Lupus erythematosus) that affect the organs.

Defining Red root's amplitude is important. Consider it a long–term low–level approach for these conditions. The plant occasionally gets touted as an 'anti–viral' herb. I believe that is over stating Red root's influence, as its most pronounced effect is not against a particular virus, but rather its reduction of the disorganization that a virus may cause.

For mastitis, internal use of Red root in concert with external Poke root oil (and/or Sweet clover) will prove an effective combination. Poke root, being the stronger of the two herbs, may even cause the area to 'sweat'; this

---

72 Insults that affect systemic and lymphatic cellular charges are myriad: bacteria/viruses and the inflammatory response they trigger, waste materials, and unorganized lipids are just several factors that have a disruptive effect. Incidentally, the late Michael Moore was the first to suggest that Red root had an influence on cellular charge and congestion. By viewing his own blood sample (after ingesting Red root) with a dark field microscope, he observed micelles having less attraction to cell walls and other blood constituents compared to samples without Red root.

being the result of Poke root's powerful lymphatic stimulation. Fresh Poke root applied as a poultice will be the strongest preparation.

Like other alteratives, women may experience benefit through using Red root for fibrocystic breast disease and uterine fibroids[73]. Exact mechanisms are unknown, but the plant most likely exerts a positive effect through its organizational/clarifying influence over lymph and blood. Additionally, hepatic stimulants like Oregongrape or Barberry are also indicated in these situations due to their augmentation of detoxification pathways.

Indications
» Pharyngitis/Tonsillitis
» Splenitis/Hepatitis, chronic
» Mastitis

Collection
A general rule is: the roots will be as stout and robust (i.e. difficult to collect) as the top portion is large. Unearthing a 6'x6' plant will necessitate a backhoe. Select smaller (and younger) plants. Not only will the roots be easier to gather but they will be less woody, and therefore more medically vital.

I have also encountered a number of species (Ceanothus integerrimus and C. greggii var. perplexans for instance) with a distinctly two-parted root: an outer red root bark and an inner woody core. With these types, strip the root bark from the core and utilize this outer layer; discard the woody inert core. Lastly, Red root is more difficult to collect if found in dry, rocky, and compacted soils – the drier the environment, the woodier the root. In any case, if any part is pink to reddish and flexible, use it.

Preparations
If possible tincture the roots fresh. Once dried, they become difficult to powder, plus preparations from dried material tend to be less potent – good for the tannins, but lesser so for Red root's lymphatic qualities. If making the dry plant tincture be sure to include 10% glycerin in the menstruum. This will inhibit the tannins from forming unwanted complexes.

---

73   Breast/uterine fibroids are often hormone metabolite dependent. It is interesting to note that fibroids usually diminish or disappear upon starting perimenopause (innate reduction of estrogen/progesterone). Relatedly, chronic stress/caffeine increases fibroid occurrence.

Dosage
» FPT/DPT (50% alcohol, 10% glycerin): 30–60 drops 2–3 times daily
» Root decoction: 4–6 oz. 2–3 times daily

Cautions
Although remote, there may be blood coagulation issues with excessive usage.

Ribes
Grossulariaceae/Currant Family

Ribes spp.

Ribes L.
Currant, Gooseberry

Description
Over sixty shrub–forming species comprises Ribes. Perennial and shrubby, its leaves are alternating, palmately lobed, and veined. Depending on the species, the stems are non–armed and smooth or have nodule or inter–nodule spines or bristles. The flowers are small and inconspicuous. They vary widely in shape, with some plants having tubular flowers and others having squat flowers with a flared opening. The mature fruit is a several–seeded, bristled or smooth, orange, red, or purple–black berry (several species even remain green when ripe).

Distribution
The Pacific Coast states host the greatest number of plants. With the exception of Mississippi, various types are found country wide. Woodland margins and open woods are typical habitats. Yellow pine and Aspen are common companion trees for Ribes.

Chemistry
Leaves: phenolic acids, flavonoids: quercitin, kaempferol. Fruit: ascorbic acid, flavonoids, anthocyanins/anthocyanidins.

Medicinal Uses
The general use for any species of Ribes is as a mild astringent. Gargle the herb tea for mouth sores, bleeding and inflamed gums, and to soothe a sore

throat. The same tea preparation is ingested to remedy mild gastric irritation and as a similar astringent for diarrhea. Moreover, most will find the plant soothing to inflamed urinary tract tissues. The crushed leaves are applied as a quick field poultice or the tea as a wash for scrapes, cuts, and sun burn.

The leaves of European Ribes species have long been used for various complaints, especially as a pain–relieving tea for arthritic conditions. Given the plant's abundance of phenolics, it's reasonable to hypothesize that North American species have corresponding effects on inflammation. If the choice is available, use the leaves of black–fruited species. They have higher amounts of antiinflammatory compounds.

Indications
» As a mild astringent
» Mouth sores/Bleeding and inflamed gums (gargle)
» Sore throat (gargle)
» Irritations, gastrointestinal
» Diarrhea
» Scrapes/Cuts/Sun burn (external)

Collection
Snip 1'–2' from the leafing branch ends and place these in an open paper bag or well–spaced on a cardboard flat. Once dry garble the leaves from the branches. Keep the now dried leaves for tea material (discard the branches).

Preparations/Dosage
» Herb infusion: 4–8 ounces 2–3 times daily

Cautions
There are no cautions for Ribes.

Other Uses
Ribes is well known for its vitamin C containing edible fruit. Most species have good to fair tasting berries that can be eaten directly from the plant, prepared as a jam/jelly, or dried for future use. The bristly–fruited species need some extra care when eaten fresh – just be sure to crush the bristles (they are not thorns) first with teeth before chewing. American Indians considered most local species an important supplemental fruit.

Compared to the red, orange, and green species, black–purple berry plants have the highest amounts of flavonoids and anthocyanins/anthocyanidins (in the fruit, and leaves too). These plants will be best as providers of an antioxidant–berry 'superfood'. Black currant seed oil is pressed/extracted from the seeds of European species, Ribes nigrum. It's used as an essential fatty acid supplement.

Sagebrush
Asteraceae/Sunflower Family

Artemisia tridentata Nutt. *(Seriphidium tridentatum)*
Big sagebrush, Mountain sagebrush

Artemisia tridentata

Description
Generally evergreen and size–variable, in ideal circumstances Sagebrush reaches 6'–8' in height, but 3'–4' is more common with average soil, rainfall, and warmer temperatures. The trunk is woody and thickened. On older plants, it's covered by grayish–brown stringy bark. The leaves are wedge–shaped and typically have 3 blunt teeth; however, they sometimes have 4–9 teeth, and occasionally are completely lacking teeth and are entire. The leaves' silvery–blue appearance results from the plant's dense coating of leaf hair. When crushed, they smell distinctly Sage–like. In the fall the small yellow flowers form in panicles at branch ends. Sagebrush is a prolific seeder, demonstrated by various removal programs designed to clear it from western grazing lands.

Distribution
Extremely common in the western United States, look for Sagebrush on flats, basins, and exposed hillsides. It is found from British Columbia and South Dakota south to the Rocky Mountains, New Mexico, central Arizona, and California.

Chemistry
Artemeseole, camphor, carvacrol, 1–8–cineol, α–pinene, β–pinene, thujol, and thujone, among other essential oils.

Medicinal Uses

Sagebrush is a strong and multi-faceted plant medicine, capable of affecting several organ systems more profoundly than the best Mugwort, a closely related herb. As a remedy for asecretory indigestion, Sagebrush excels. Stimulating to hydrochloric acid, pepsinogen, and other gut secretions, as well as being quieting to fullness and bloating, the room temperature tea before meals is efficacious. Like other Artemisias, it tends to stimulate hepatic and biliary secretions, making its (occasional) use in area sluggishness prudent.

The cold tea is diuretic. The hot tea is strongly diaphoretic, particularly if the skin is hot and dry, the pulse is strong, and there is a general feeling of contained body heat. The plant can break the most stubborn of fevers.

Broadly antimicrobial and anti-parasitic, Sagebrush has long been hailed as a treatment for food and water borne illnesses, be them from Salmonella spp., Escherichia coli, or other pathogenic organisms responsible for food poisoning. Modern and traditional findings support the plant being used in amebic infections (i.e. montezuma's revenge/traveler's diarrhea) and as a broad spectrum vermifuge. Pinworms and roundworms are the surest parasites Sagebrush will eliminate.

The plant is stimulating to menses mainly through its essential oil content. The hot tea (or tincture placed in hot water) is particularly useful in dilating uterine capillary beds, thus delivering more blood and activity to the area.

When applied topically, the herb is significantly antimicrobial and antifungal. External preparations are useful in inhibiting numerous Staphylococcus, Streptococcus, and fungal species. From ringworm and athlete's foot to wounds and ulcers that need some infection fighting help, the plant is powerful. Compounding this influence is Sagebrush's mild analgesic effect. Acute pain from contusions, sprains, and blows along with chronic pain from rheumatoid arthritis or bothersome old sport injuries, are all quieted.

A warm poultice or fomentation is decidedly sedative to menstrual, intestinal, and stomach cramps. Moreover, the plant makes a strong antimicrobial respiratory tract medicine. Inhaling the volatile oil filled steam of the tea is useful for bronchitis, especially when lung mucus is thickened and difficult to expectorate. The inhaled steam rivals White sage and Eucalyptus in treating strep throat and sinusitis.

Indications

» Indigestion, asecretory

- » Cramps/Flatulence, gastrointestinal
- » Congestion, liver/gallbladder
- » Fever, dry skin
- » Food poisoning
- » Diarrhea, amebic
- » Pinworm/Roundworm infestation
- » Amenorrhea with water retention and feelings of coldness
- » Infection, fungal/bacterial (external)
- » Contusions/Sprains (external)
- » Cramps, menstrual (external)
- » Cramps, gastrointestinal (external)
- » Bronchitis (inhaled steam)

Collection/Preparations
In the spring, before flowering, snip the last 8"–10" of new growth from the branch ends. These clippings can either be wrapped in small bundles or chopped into smaller manageable pieces for drying.

Dosage
- » Leaf infusion (cold or standard): 2–4 ounces 1–2 times daily
- » FPT/DPT (60% alcohol): 10–30 drops 1–2 times daily
- » Inhaled steam: 2–3 times daily
- » External preparations: as needed

Cautions
Due to Sagebrush's thujone and related essential oil content, do not use it during pregnancy or while nursing. Additionally, its use should be discontinued if dizziness, nausea, or headache occurs. Consider Sagebrush for short–term use only (1–2 weeks concurrently).

Other Uses
Although the smoke is harsh on the eyes and respiratory tissues, Sagebrush smudge has a rich ceremonial history. It is known as the 'other' Sage.

Scarlet Pimpernel
Primulaceae/Primrose Family

Anagallis arvensis L.
Red chickweed, Weatherglass

Anagallis arvensis

Description
Scarlet pimpernel is a low-growing herbaceous annual. Spreading in habit, it tends to be many-branched and mat-forming. Its opposite leaves are entire, ovate, and about an inch long. They tend to clasp (or are sessile) the ridged stems and have spreading-parallel veins. Each 5-parted flower develops solely on its own axil-originating pedicel. For the most common form (var. arvensis) they are salmon colored. The other type is blue (var. caerulea). The flower is followed by a small many-seeded globe-like capsule.

Distribution
Native to Eurasia, Scarlet pimpernel is now naturalized extensively throughout North America. Most abundant in eastern parts of the United States, it is also found in several western states. Look to coastal regions of California and Oregon for the largest populations. It's locally available throughout parts of Arizona and Texas too. Next to springs and seeps, and damp and disturbed soils will potentially host the plant.

Chemistry
Oleanane glycosides: anagallosaponins VI–IX; triterpene saponins: cucurbitacins; flavones.

Medicinal Uses
In ancient times, when the arcane was mixed with the practical, Pliny, Dioscorides, Gerard, and Culpepper all agreed, Scarlet pimpernel affected the liver. More energetic than Dandelion, but not as active as Wild iris, the tincture/tea is a moderate hepatic stimulant. Its benefit will be seen when applied to simple cases of poor bile production and release, particularly if symptoms include constipation and achy joints. Like other chologogues/choleretics, a key indication for its use is poor fat digestion – distension and fullness after a rich/fatty meal. Try the tincture in a cup of Field mint or Monarda tea prior

to an especially fatty meal. Also, if prone to skin eruptions and outbreaks in conjunction with a poorly preforming liver, its internal influence will help to clear the skin.

An area that has seen some scientific inquiry lately involves Scarlet pimpernel's microbial/viral effects. Apparently, it inhibits HSV–1 replication and Bacillus subtilis, Escherichia coli, and (especially) Candida albicans growth. These finding give merit to the plant's (topical) use in poorly defined skin afflictions, as a wound healer, and as a general 'cleanser'[74].

Indications
- Hepatic congestion, non–organic/non–viral
- Biliary insufficiency, without gall stones
- Constipation, liver/gallbladder related
- Indigestion, especially lipids
- Infection, bacterial and fungal (external)
- Infection, Candida albicans (external)

Collection
A simple herb to collect, clip the flowering–leafing upper portions. Tincture these parts fresh or dry them loosely for other preparations.

Preparations/Dosage
- FPT/DPT (50% alcohol): 10–30 drops 2–3 times daily
- Herb infusion: 2–4 ounces 2–3 times daily
- External preparations: as needed

Cautions
Scarlet pimpernel is not a completely benign herb. It does contain a number of triterpene saponins, some of which are hemolytic (damaging to red blood cells) at higher concentrations. Consider its use at the above internal doses safe for a week or two at a time; side effects may be seen if the plant is taken for extended periods. It's also not recommended during pregnancy or while nursing.

---

[74] In the 1800s Scarlet pimpernel had a significant following as a cosmetic herb.

Self Heal
Lamiaceae/Mint Family

Prunella vulgaris L.
Heal all, Carpenter weed

Prunella vulgaris

Description
Easily overlooked and diminutive in statue, Self heal forms from creeping rhizomes. Its opposite leaves are lance–ovate to lance shaped and 2"–4" in length. They are somewhat hairy and entire (or shallowly dentate). The flowers form in stubby terminal clusters and are intermingled with purplish bracts. Each flower is 2–lipped and purple. The lower lip is 3–lobed; the upper lip is hooded.

The two main plants in the region are of the same species, yet separate variants. Prunella vulgaris var. lanceolata is our native variety. P. vulgaris var. vulgaris is introduced. Variety lanceolate has a leaf much longer than wide. Variety vulgaris's leaf is more broad and is lance–ovate in shape.

Distribution
Variety lanceolata enjoys a wide range throughout America and Canada. It is common to temperate/high elevations in the West. Moistened and semi–shaded soils next to streams and springs are its common places. Variety vulgaris has a more limited disbursement. Semi–common throughout California (northern), Oregon, and Washington, the plant often overlaps var. lanceolata's territory.

Chemistry
Flavonoids, monoterpenes, polysaccharides, sterols, tannins, triterpenoids.

Medicinal Uses
Self heal, like so many western North American herbs with Old World affiliations, is steeped in ancient application, which if properly interpreted gives insight into how to better utilize the plant in today's health/disease environment.

Drink (and/or gargle) the tea, or a tablespoon of the freshly pressed juice in a little water, for oral, esophageal, and gastrointestinal inflammations. Best used in the pre–ulcerative stages of epithelial irritations/inflammations, the plant's traditional application of reducing intestinal sensitivity during and after a bout of diarrhea or dysentery is practical and effective.

Due to a number of studies showing several isolated constituents having inhibitory power over HSV –1/–2 viruses, Self heal has been touted as a treatment for these infections. I find this doubtful. Here's why: the difference between an isolated, single plant chemical affecting petri–dish parameters versus a whole, crude plant (or preparations thereof) affecting an in–vivo situation is massive.

The best that can be hoped for with the use of Self heal on this issue is the more speedy resolution of an active outbreak when applied topically. Simply, it quickens healing of tissue injury, whether virally induced, or otherwise. And though there may be some small viral inhibition occurring (via its polysaccharide fraction), crude herbal forms of Self heal only have miniscule effects on the stand–alone virus (in situ). If HSV benefit is perceived it is due to the plant's general influence of inflammation and tissue healing.

Self heal's common external uses are sound: as a healer of ulcers, wounds, cuts, scrapes, and abrasions. A towel or cloth soaked in the fresh juice or the freshly pureed herb applied to burns and insect bites has merit, though the ointment, oil, or salve for topical injuries will have better penetration and/or coating ability.

Indications
» Irritations/Inflammations, oral, gastric, intestinal
» Diarrhea/Dysentery
» As a mild systemic antiinflammatory
» As a vulnerary for stings, scrapes, cuts, etc. (external)

Collection
Due to Self heal's diminutive size it can be a tedious plant to gather. If possible, gather equal leaf and flower portions – stems in moderation are fine.

Be aware of look–alike plants – Plantago and Senecio are two of note. Without a flower, leaf characteristics of these plants can be similar. Mixing an occasional Plantago leaf with Self heal is not a problem, but mistakes with toxic Senecio may be.

Preparations/Dosage
» Infusion: 4–8 oz. 2–3 times daily
» Fresh juice: ½–1 oz. 2–3 times daily or topically as needed

- » FPT/DPT (50% alcohol): 30–60 drops 2–3 times daily
- » Fresh plant poultice/Oil/Ointment/Salve: as needed

Cautions
Self heal is a safe (very mild) plant medicine. Even at higher doses there are no cautions for its use.

Shepherd's Purse
Brassicaceae/Mustard Family

Capsella bursa–pastoris (L.) Medik.
Shepherd's heart, Pickpocket

Capsella bursa-pastoris

Description
Shepherd's purse is a small herbaceous annual. Its leaves are mainly basal and form in clustered rosettes. They are varied in shape, entire to pinnately lobed, and usually clasp the stem. The very small white flowers form in elongated racemes. The plant's most characteristic feature is its wedge–shaped seed capsules. They appear as inverted hearts. Each is borne on a small pedicel.

Distribution
Ubiquitous and practically universal, a little soil and water are all that Shepherd's purse needs to thrive. It is common to lawns, garden plots, and grassy areas. Although originally native to Eurasia, it is now a worldly plant, seeking out disturbed soils, only avoiding the hot and humid tropics.

Chemistry
Fatty acids; flavonoids; tyramine and fumaric acids, diosmin.

Medicinal Uses
Truly a unique medicinal mustard, Shepherd's purse is a special hemostatic, not acting through any tannin source, but rather through yet another unexplained constituent group. Influencing tissue capillary beds, its astringency is penetrating, yet not gross like Geranium or Oak.

For the urinary tract, use the plant when there is passive hemorrhaging or blood in the urine, particularly if there is accompanying sediment. It curbs chronic irritation of the bladder and urethra, and is especially indicated if the urine is dark or contains mucus. Shepherd's purse is not particularly antibacterial, so in these situations, if there is an active infection, the herb is best mixed with a urinary disinfectant.

As a lithotropic agent, use Shepherd's purse if there is irritation, hematuria, and general stone formation. If suffering from a tendency towards elevated uric acid levels or phosphaturia, the plant is doubly indicated. It is also soothing if there exists urogenital pain from sexual activity, and for men, seminal vesicle irritation.

For women, the fresh plant tincture will be of benefit during the first days of menses if bleeding is heavy. During pregnancy if there is threatened miscarriage, and spotting is the main symptom, Shepherd's purse is specific. For minor postpartum hemorrhaging, the plant seldom fails to stop bleeding.

A property of Shepherd's purse that is common to most other pungent mustards, is its menses stimulating potential. Although in opposition to the plant's previously mentioned uses, if taken in large doses it is often stimulating in amenorrhea (a quality of most Mustard family plants).

As an astringent, the plant also lessens gastrointestinal tract bleeding from gastric or duodenal ulcers, as well as from other intestinal injuries. Taken internally (with Collinsonia root), the combination shrinks and is hemostatic to hemorrhoids.

Indications
- Hemorrhage, passive, urinary tract
- Deposits/Sediment, urinary
- Irritation, seminal vesicle
- Menstruation, heavy
- Miscarriage, potential, with spotting
- Hemorrhage, passive, postpartum
- Hemorrhage, GI tract
- Hemorrhoids, bleeding

Collection
Gather the entire plant, small tap root and all.

Preparation
The fresh plant tincture is Shepherd's purse primary preparation. The recently dried herb prepared as a tea is second best.

Dosage
» FPT: 30–60 drops 2–3 times daily

Cautions
There are no cautions for Shepherd's purse.

Silk Tassel
Garryaceae/Silk Tassel Family

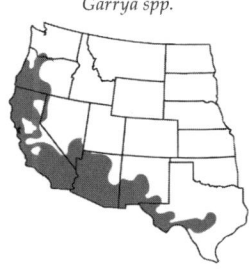

Garrya spp.

Garrya flavescens S. Watson
Ashy silk tassel

Garrya fremontii Torr.
Bearbush

Garrya wrightii Torr.
Wight's silk tassel

Description
Silk tassel is an evergreen or semi–evergreen large bush/small tree. Its leaves are opposite, leathery, and elliptic, ovate, or oval. Male and female flowers from in catkins on separate plants. Male catkins develop in clusters of three; females are solitary, and mostly appear tassel–like. The fruit are ovoid, purple–black, and ¼" in diameter.

Distribution
Garrya flavescens ranges from southern New Mexico and Arizona to southern Utah, southern Nevada, finally to California. It is abundant on desert slopes, throughout chaparral areas, and scrub woodlands.

Garrya fremontii is common from California to southern Washington. In Oregon it is abundant west of the Cascades. G. wrightii is found throughout Arizona, southern–central New Mexico, and western Texas. Another chaparral grower, look to dry slopes and hillsides.

Chemistry
Garrya general: polyisoprene (trans–1,4–polyisoprene); iridoid glycosides: aucubin, geniposide, geniposidic acid; diterpenoid alkaloids: veatchine, garryine, garryfoline, isogarryfoline, cuauchichioine, isocuauchichicine.

Medicinal Uses
Silk tassel's alkaloid content affects an array of smooth muscle groups throughout the body. One of its most reliable uses is to quiet spastic intestinal episodes from amebiasis or giardiasis. For these purposes, it is best used in conjunction with antimicrobial herbs such as Tree of heaven or Crucifixion thorn. In many cases this herbal combination is able to replace the use of conventional drug therapies (Flagyl).

Sufferers of spastic diarrhea (unrelated to infestation), borborygmus, or the dull ache of lower intestinal spasm, will find the tea or tincture relieving. If anxiety is a contributing factor, it combines well with a nervous system sedative such as Pedicularis or Skullcap, or if ulcerative colitis is the principle concern, then Canadian fleabane. Moreover, the plant's tannin content adds to its therapeutic influence when diarrhea exists as a symptom.

Used alone or in tandem with Yellow pond lily, Silk tassel is superb at limiting the pain of menstrual cramps. For women whom are sensitive to the twinges of ovulation, it is also well applied.

Although there are more specific herbs (Chelidonium), try a strong dose of Silk tassel if troubled by gallbladder spasms – most find its influence symptomatically relaxing to the smooth muscle contractions that accompany a gallbladder attack and stone passage. However, it will do little towards gall stone development or to encourage their dissolution.

Silk tassel is best thought of as a 'drug plant': a medicinal plant that has little nutritional or constitutional value, but rather like a low–level pharmaceutical, is used for symptom suppression.

Indications
» Spasm, intestinal
» Spasm, uterine/ovulatory
» Spasm, biliary

Collection
Gather the recent leaves in the spring or summer. If the leaves are too environmentally stressed, the rootbark can be thought of as a more potent substitute.

Preparations/Dosage
» DPT (50% alcohol) of leaf: 30–60 drops 2–3 times daily
» DPT (50% alcohol) of root bark: 15–30 drops 2–3 times daily

Cautions
Do not use Silk tassel during pregnancy or while nursing. Due to its potency and unknown interactions, it is best not to mix it with most other pharmaceuticals.

Skullcap
Lamiaceae/Mint Family

Scutellaria angustifolia Pursh
Narrowleaf skullcap

Scutellaria galericulata L.
Marsh skullcap

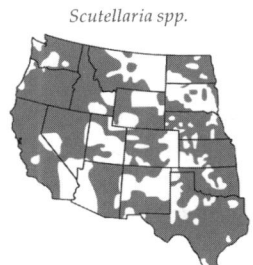

Scutellaria spp.

Description
Scutellaria angustifolia is a small herbaceous perennial. Reaching sizes of 1' or so, the slender stems are simple or branched and arise from creeping rhizomes (as do most Skullcaps). The leaves are narrow to ovate–lance shaped and reach lengths of 2"–3". The flowers are solitary and form from axils of the upper stem's reduced leaves. They are deep blue–violet.

Branched or simple, Scutellaria galericulata stands 1'–2' high. Herbaceous, pubescent, and perennial, the plant often forms in colonies from creeping rhizomes. Its square stems and opposite leaves are notable: individual leaves are 1½"–3" long and lance–shaped with toothed margins. The leaf bases vary from truncate to subcordate. The flowers are intermingled with the upper leaves. Tubular and 2–lipped (upper lip hood–like), they are blue–violet.

Distribution

Scutellaria angustifolia is found from British Columbia, eastern Washington, and Oregon to western Idaho, Nevada, and northern Utah. Unlike a number of the moisture–loving Skullcaps, this species prefers more rocky and dry environs.

Widespread throughout temperate regions of the Northern Hemisphere, Scutellaria galericulata is common in the West. It is a wetland indicator and usually found in low–lying meadow areas, along grassy streamsides, and mountain fens. St. John's wort, Stachys, and Field mint are usual companion medicines.

Chemistry

For Scutellaria latifolia (other species similar): flavones: baicalein, baicalin, chrysin, wogonin, oroxylin a, genkwanin; flavonols: quercetin, rutin; flavanones: hesperetin, hesperidin, naringenin; isoflavone: daidzein; neo–clerodane diterpenoids.

Medicinal Uses

Skullcap's activity is due to its mild inhibition of the central nervous system. Although research points to several potential mechanisms, it is widely acknowledged that Skullcap's most significant effect is on GABA (γ–aminobutyric acid) oriented synapses (either as a mimic that stimulates GABA receptor sites or that which allows native GABA to linger).

As a sleep facilitator, take a full dose before bed. Use it if the mind is restless (emotional/mental stress) and the body (following the mind's lead) is unable to relax. Its effectiveness will be reduced if insomnia is the result of a physical malady and associated pain.

Use lesser amounts during waking hours as an anti–anxiety calmer. The tincture is fairly effective when taken ten minutes prior to performances in order to curb stage fright. Consider using it before any social situation that causes stress and unease. For these purposes, it mixes well with an equal part of Kava. Feelings of work or family related anxiety will too lessen with Skullcap.

Where smaller doses gently relax, larger doses diminish mild seizure activity, tics, and stress–emotion related tremors. Best case scenario for Skullcap is its ability to defuse heightened neuronal activity from developing into a full tonic/clonic seizure. In these situations, it is important to use it before the seizure's manifestation while in the 'aura' phase. One tablespoon of tincture is a strong but effective dose for an average-sized adult. Reduce the dose accordingly for smaller adults and children. I've seen fair to good results when Skullcap is used as a 3–4 times a day medicine in epilepsy or epilepsy-like conditions. If used diligently the reduction or even the discontinuation of gabapentin or related pharmaceuticals is sometimes possible.

Most species of Skullcap are bitter (don't be afraid to experiment with a species not profiled here – in fact the more bitter a particular species is, the more likely it will be an effective medicine). Aside from poor tasting species often being stronger sedatives, Skullcap's bitterness usually simulates appetite and stomach activity (and for some, heartburn if taken on an empty stomach).

The more resinous a species is, the more apt it is to be a mild diaphoretic. These plants will make fine sedative-sweating agents (sudorifics) particularly when stress and lack of sleep are factors in prolonging a dry feverish condition (wintertime cold/flu, etc.).

Indications
» Insomnia
» Stress/Anxiety
» Seizure activity/Tics/Tremors
» Fever, dry

Collection
Ideally when in flower, clip the upper herb. Clump growing, drier climate Skullcaps are usually less time consuming to gather. Wetland growing Skullcaps are more tedious to collect – snip a sprig here, snip a sprig there, and continue.

Preparations
Although most Mint family plants should have their stems discarded due to this part's lower potency, in Skullcaps's case, the stems are so slender and light, it really isn't necessary. The fresh plant tincture is the strongest preparation, particularly in reference to the plant's sedative-seizure reducing qualities. The tea from the recently dried material is a fair second.

Dosage
» FPT/DPT (50% alcohol): 30–60 drops 1–3 times daily
» Herb infusion: 4–8 oz. 1–3 times daily

Cautions
Skullcap has a very safe usage history. It's generally thought of as being side effect free. It is theoretically possible that heavy use may potentiate the benzodiazepine class of drugs (i.e. Valium/Diazepam) so caution should be applied if using these drugs and the herb in tandem.

Sneezeweed
Asteraceae/Sunflower Family

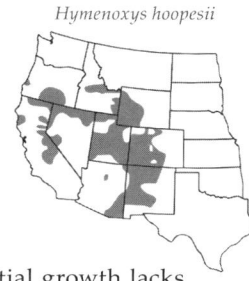

Hymenoxys hoopesii

Hymenoxys hoopesii (A. Gray) Bierner (*Helenium hoopesii, Dugaldia hoopesii*)
Owl's claws, Orange Sneezeweed, Raíz del lobo, Yerba del lobo

Description
A 2′–3′ tall herbaceous perennial, Sneezeweed's initial growth lacks any significant center stalk. The basal leaves are oblanceolate and reach lengths of about 1′. The stalk leaves are sessile, smaller, and lanceolate to ovate. The leaves/stems have varying degrees of hair – usually greater when young.

The flowers are orange to yellow and composed of both disk and ray florets. The rays are ½″–1″ in length and usually notched. The achenes (seeds) are attached to a fibrous tuft (pappus) making air disbursement likely.

Distribution
Common throughout the Rocky Mountains, Sneezeweed is mostly encountered in the moist soil of mountain meadows, surrounded by mixed conifers and Aspen. Often growing in abundance, it paints meadows and grassy expanses in yellow–orange during the summer.

Chemistry
Sesquiterpene lactones: guaianolides, pseudoguaianolides, secohelenanolides: hymenovin; flavonoids; dugaldin.

Medicinal Uses
As a liniment or short–term soak, Sneezeweed's external use is medicinal due to an array of aromatic lactones and volatiles. It's diminishing to the

acute pain of contusions, blows, and falls – essentially injuries that have left the skin unbroken, but are likely to bruise and swell. Relatedly, it makes a useful after–practice liniment for any contact sport participant.

Indications
» Injuries, acute, unbroken skin (external)

Collection
From Sneezeweed's root crown, the underground rhizome bends at a near right angle and is usually just beneath the soil's surface. It's anchored by many fine rootlets.

Begin digging 1' from the plant's central leaf area. If the soil is non–compacted the job sometimes can be done with hands alone. Often the roots of multiple plants will be found intermingled. Discard the leaves/stems/flowers.

Preparations/Dosage
» FPT/DPT (60% alcohol) as a liniment: apply as needed
» Decoction (as a wash/soak): apply as needed

Cautions
There are several cautions for Sneezeweed's use. First, it should not be used internally. This plant and other Hymenoxys species are known to cause livestock poisonings ('spewing sickness') due to several of its sesquiterpene lactones. There are traditional accounts of its internal use, but these uses are somewhat nebulous (and could easily be matched with different herbs that are non–toxic).

Its topical use should be avoided during pregnancy and with babies and children (there exist risk–free herbs that are just as effective – see Therapeutic Index). Otherwise, keep Sneezeweed's use to short–term: several times a day a for a week or so, then rotate to another herb. Discontinue its use if nausea occurs at any point during its application.

Spearmint
Lamiaceae/Mint Family

Mentha spicata L.
Mint, Bush mint, Yerba buena

Mentha spicata

Description
Spearmint is a small herbaceous perennial and reaches heights of 2′–3′. The plant's leaves are lanceolate–ovate, glabrous above, and gland–dotted below. They have serrated margins, rounded bases, and short petioles. The spiked flower clusters form near stem tips. Each flower has a 5–lobed toothed calyx. The corollas are white to lavender. It reproduces through both seeds and clones.

Distribution
Due to Spearmint's lengthy cultivation its exact Eurasian point of origin remains a mystery. Now found world–wide as an escapee, in the West look to streamsides, ditches, or really any wet area, especially if a homestead or an old ranch was in the area. The best stands are made up of feral plants from a by–gone herb garden.

Chemistry
Main volatile compounds: myrcene, limonene, cis–carveol, carvone, β–bourbonene, β–caryophyllene, β–farnesene, γ–muurolene, n–octacosane, n–tricosane.

Medicinal Uses
Prosaic in application, Spearmint should first be thought of as a gentle carminative, soothing to indigestion, gas pain, and nausea. The tea can be used liberally in these cases. Even for colicy babies a tablespoon or two of the tea will be found relieving.

The hot tea is specifically used in childhood fevers. Not as vigorous as Peppermint, Spearmint will stimulate perspiration, making it indicated in mild to moderate fevers if the skin is hot and dry. The internally used essential oil or spirit may be too strong for little ones, but for adults it is a more active preparation.

Indications
- » Indigestion/Gas/Nausea/Colic
- » Fever

Collection
Gather the upper herbal portion, with or without the flower. Once dry, garble and discard the plant's stems. Store the herb in a sealed jar, which helps to maintain its potency.

Preparations/Dosage
- » Herb infusion: 4–8 oz. as needed
- » Essential oil: 1–2 drops in a capsule 2–3 times daily
- » Spirit: 10–20 drops 2–3 times daily

Cautions
Excessive internal amounts of the essential oil may stimulate menses, so it should not be used during pregnancy. The tea is fine during this time and also there is no problem when given to babies/children.

Spruce
Pinaceae/Pine Family

Picea spp.

Picea Link.
Blue spruce, Engelmann spruce, White spruce, etc.

Description
Spruce is a conical, evergreen tree with thin–scaly bark and whorled branches. The linear leaves are four–sided (as opposed to Fir's flattened leaves), short–stemmed, and spirally arranged, where they spread equally on all sides (younger twigs). Roughened leaf scars remain after the leaves fall from their bases (smooth scars for Fir). The small male cones form in clusters. The larger female cones are pendulous and mature in one season.

Distribution
A common conifer throughout the mountainous West (and East), Spruce is often found with Douglas fir, Fir, and Aspen. Montane valleys and slopes are its usual habitats.

Chemistry
Picea spp. (needles): monoterpenoids: myrcene, limonene, β–phellandrene, α–pinene, β–pinene, 3–carene; piperidine alkaloids; resin acids (general conifer): abietic acid, neoabietic acid, palustric acid, pimaric acid, isopimaric acid.

Medicinal Uses
Spruce belongs to a group of trees (Pine, Spruce, and Fir) that share nearly all uses and preparations. Here I cover the medicinal basics for this tree (and related parts), but let me refer readers to the Pine profile for the most complete account of how to use this and any other terpene–rich conifer oleoresin, needle, or related essential oil.

Like Pine and Fir, medicinal applications for Spruce are historically well recorded. Both New and Old World utilizations were common and often interlinked with other conifers – it was not unusual for an array of related genera/species to be gathered and utilized collectively.

The oleoresin (sap) portion of Spruce and its essential oil content most concerns us here, as this is its strongest medicinal part. Although the non-volatile 'rosin' segment is also being consumed (and used topically) with oleoresin usage, its greater therapeutic influence (aside from being viscous and sticky) has yet to be discovered[75].

A simple 1:5 oleoresin tincture (technically a solution) is the most convenient preparation for internal use. It is also best mixed with other tinctures as part of a formula, as used alone it will quickly separate when added to water or tea. Furthermore, if the oleoresin tincture is dropped in the mouth directly the resin part tends to adhere to teeth and gums, and will cause some irritation if allowed to linger.

Oleoresin tincture has a three–parted influence. It is equally stimulating, antimicrobial, and anesthetizing. One of several regions that reacts predictably to its ingestion is the respiratory area. The oleoresin's volatile

---

[75] Research suggests that this non–volatile portion of oleoresin (resin acids or what is known as 'rosin' after separation) is also worth attention. Anticarcinogenic and antiinflammatory effects are only two attributes recorded for this part in recent studies.

aromatics enter the bronchial environment as a route of elimination. Their effects are as follows: bronchial mucus becomes thinned and more easily dislodged via coughing and lung tissues are exposed to antimicrobial/antiviral aromatics. These influences will especially help sufferers of non–productive bronchitis and lung–centered influenza get well in a more timely manner. The oleoresin tincture can be successfully formulated with other tinctures as a cough syrup ingredient. It also combines well with cough suppressants such as Wild cherry or Pleurisy root.

As a gastrointestinal remedy, the oleoresin tincture or essential oil is strongly disinfectant to a number of common pathogens that are responsible for bacterial diarrhea, dysentery, and related enteric fever (in older times Pine essential oil [Spruce is nearly identical] was considered a successful medicine for cholera infections). As a lower urinary tract disinfectant the oleoresin tincture or essential oil is used to resolve on–and–off–again infections. It is best used in combination with regional soothers such as Checker mallow or Hollyhock.

External applications of oleoresin are multi–faceted. Like internal usages, its influence falls into three categories: stimulating to tissues, reducing to sensitivity, and antibacterial. As a formula ingredient, keep oleoresin levels at about 10% (or less) – anymore and tissue redness and irritation may develop. Add it to combinations designed to heal long standing ulcers and bedsores, particularly if they become infected easily. Additionally, topical oleoresin formulations are well–applied to arthritic joints, general rheumatic pains, and even chronic sport's injuries.

A Spruce needle infusion makes a fine wintertime cold and flu tea. Containing small amounts of vitamin C complexes and antimicrobial volatile oils, the tea will bring about a speedier resolution to these episodes. Equally, use it as a gargle for sore throats and as a nasal wash for sinusitis. Even children find the piney aroma and taste of the needle tea tolerable, if not enjoyable.

Indications
» Bronchitis, non–productive cough
» Infection, urinary tract, chronic
» Infection, intestinal
» As a stimulating/anesthetizing/antimicrobial medicant (external)
» As a cold and flu tea

Collection

Spruce oleoresin is collectable most times of the year, though new spring-summer oleoresin which is viscous and semi-liquid is the best for medicinal uses. Later in the year this same oleoresin hardens due to exposure. These hardened nodules are generally less potent due to a reduced essential oil content, but are still of some value if fresh secretions are not available.

Begin by locating a healthy Spruce stand. Examine the trees for oleoresin deposits, most often the result of bark damage from boring insects or other mechanical damage. Once a collectable quantity of viscous oleoresin is located remove it by using a putty knife. Scrape the lump onto the lip of a mason jar. If the oleoresin tincture is desired (know the weight of the jar before gathering; weigh the jar and oleoresin together; then subtract the pre-calculated jar weight) add the appropriate amount of alcohol. Afterwards use a high-proof alcohol to wash hands and tools.

Spruce needles, like Pine and Fir, should be gathered when green (and on the tree), preferably during the spring or summer. Crush a few – they should be aromatic. When drying them for tea, be sure to set the needles away from direct sunlight, yet in a dry place.

Preparations

The oleoresin tincture (actually a solution) is very easy to make. If the oleoresin is soft and malleable the next step is not necessary. If crystallized, the nodules first need to be crushed. Use a mortar and pestle or place the nodules in a bag and lightly pound them with a heavy object or hammer. Once crushed/powdered, simply combine 1 part (weight) of oleoresin with 5 parts (volume) of alcohol. Shake the mixture for a minute or two daily for 7–10 days. Strain from the tincture what has not dissolved, then bottle the liquid. Last step: decant the oleoresin tincture after letting it stand for several days (there is often a precipitant layer of dirt and undissolved oleoresin that settles to the bottom – discard this layer).

When using oleoresin topically, keep concentrations to 10% or less – at least initially. Some people are fine with stronger concentrations; however, if experimenting with higher oleoresin amounts, be sure to increase the percentage incrementally. Greater oleoresin concentrations are almost always found irritating to exposed cuts and wounds.

To prepare: apply low heat to a pre-selected herbal oil (9 parts). Add the oleoresin (1 part) and slowly heat/stir until it is completely dissolved.

Beeswax can be added at this point if a salve is desired (often less beeswax is needed due to the thickening effect of oleoresin).

Infuse dried Spruce needles for tea. Like other aromatic-containing herbs: be sure to cover the tea while steeping. Spruce essential oil is not as readily available (commercially) as Pine essential oil; however, regardless of whether Spruce, Fir, or Pine essential oil is decided upon, I recommend purchasing a pure aromatherapy grade for both internal and external use. Add the essential oil to herbal oils and salves at 1%–2% concentrations. 1–2 drops of the essential oil can be dropped in a capsule and swallowed or a spirit can be made enabling its mixture with other tinctures. Another noted preparation is the addition of the essential oil (1–2 drops) to a mucilage (bran, psyllium, Aloe gel, etc.) for a 'time-released' effect on the gastrointestinal walls. Spruce (and other conifers) essential oil's therapeutic effect is basically the same as an oleoresin preparation – only without the occasional gastrointestinal upset that occurs with oleoresin consumption (due to the resin acid portion of oleoresin).

Dosage

» DPT of oleoresin (95% alcohol): 10–20 drops 2–3 times daily
» Essential oil (needles, cones, inner bark, or oleoresin): 1–2 drops 2–3 times daily
» Spirit: 10–20 drops 2–3 times daily
» Oil/Salve: as needed
» Needle infusion: 4–6 oz. 2–3 times daily

Cautions

The most common complaint with oleoresin use is stomach upset, likely caused by the rosin fraction (swallowing a pea-to-grape sized hardened nodule plucked directly from the tree is a stomachache waiting to happen). Lessening the dose in most cases will solve the problem.

Toxicities[76] from Spruce (also Pine and Fir) can occur with the ingestion of excessive amounts of the essential oil. Liver, kidney, and central nervous system irregularities have been reported. Historical accounts do also list baby and child fatalities – almost always due to the accidental ingestion of very large amounts (ounces not drops).

76 Toxicity from oleoresin is somewhat self-limiting due to the digestive upset that occurs with excessive ingestion; also, the essential oil amount of oleoresin is at best 25%.

No different than other medically active substances: emphasis should be placed on proper dosage. Small internal drop doses (of the essential oil) are therapeutic. Larger doses are often dangerous. Even dosed properly both oleoresin and essential oil preparations should be treated as short–term use items. A sensible regiment is their use for one or two weeks at a time. Do not use the oleoresin or essential oil internally while pregnant, nursing, or with children, though their external use is fine. There is no problem with the needle tea. Lastly, oleoresin (and essential oil) is flammable.

Other Uses

Use a low heat to soften crystallized oleoresin nodules. Apply the now–softened oleoresin to cracks, gaps, and seams in wooden constructions and other creations as a sealant. Its use as a water–repellent/patching agent is ancient. Nuggets of oleoresin are also burned on a hot plate or incense burner for their piney–aromatic smoke.

Squawroot
Orobanchaceae/Broomrape Family

Conopholis alpina

Conopholis alpina Liebm. (*Conopholis alpina var. mexicana, C. mexicana, C. panamensis, C sylvatica*)
Mexican squawroot, Cancer root, Groundcone

Description
Squawroot[77] belongs to a family of plants that lacks chlorophyll and are root parasites. There are two Squawroots in the United Sates – Conopholis alpina, the one being profiled here, and C. americana, the eastern species. Both are nearly identical in appearance, and likewise can be used the same way.

This parasitic perennial appears like a small, elongated, cream–yellowish Pine cone. The flowering 'cone' part rests on a small above–ground

[77] The name Squawroot for Conopholis is the longest in use. The common name Cancer root is confusingly applied to any number of Broomrape family plants, as is Groundcone, which can refer to any related plant appearing like a Pine cone. The following common/scientific names are the most consistently used: Broomrape for Orobanche spp., Beechdrops for Epifagus spp., Groundcone for Boschniakia spp., and Squawroot for Conopholis spp.

stalk, which is often partially hidden by surrounding leaf litter. It is usually no more than 6"–8" tall (up to 10" with stem) and is composed of Pine cone–like scales, with the upper ones serving as bracts for the tubular, pale, and 2–lipped corollas. The fruit develops into a small many–seed containing capsule. Squawroot's roots are shallow, bulbous, and nodular masses, not appearing unlike a lesion or cancerous growth[78].

Distribution
Squawroot does not have an extensive range. However, locally it is abundant and stable. Core stands of the plant are found further south in Mexico. In America, look to southeastern Arizona, south/central New Mexico, and West Texas. Isolated mountain ranges, between 5000'–6000', under Oak (Oak roots are its most common host), Cypress, Madrone, or transition zone Pine, where leaf litter accumulates, are usual habitats.

Chemistry
Unknown, but I suspect Oak–oriented tannins and flavonoids are common to the plant.

Medicinal Uses
This species and the more easterly grower, Conopholis americana, were once used topically for cancerous growths and poorly–healing ulcerations. Likely more effective in the applicant's mind due to the root's nodular and cancerous appearance than truly arresting to cancer, Squawroot's most sensible use is as a topical astringent.

Both above–ground stems and sub–surface roots are drying and astringent, though the roots are more so. Crushed and applied as a fresh poultice, Squawroot is reducing to skin redness and inflammation. Use it for sunburn, rashes, and minor cuts and scrapes. More involved ulcerations and poorly healing wounds that usually have a bacterial or diminished circulatory element will be bettered with Squawroot (plus the addition of Echinacea or Wild indigo).

Additionally, the tea or tincture in a little water makes a soothing gargle for sore throats, and if swallowed will help to diminish idiosyncratic diarrhea. The name Squawroot harkens back to the day when American Indian women used the tea (and likely a topical wash) of the stem/root to arrest

78 The name Cancer root may also have a Doctrine of Signatures connection: what appears like a particular disease, treats (or was thought to) that disease.

passive hemorrhaging of traumatized tissues after childbirth – much like other tannin/flavonoid plants such as Potentilla or Wild rose.

Indications
- Sunburn/Rashes/Scrapes (external)
- Sore throat (gargle)
- Diarrhea
- As a postpartum astringent (external and internal)

Collection
Squawroot typically grows in sizable colonies. I recommend gathering from a stand's edge (above ground spikes and roots or just spikes if the stand is not that large).

Preparations
The plant is well hydrated and may develop mold growth if not sliced thinly and spaced well before drying. The use of a dehydrator in most cases is optimal. The plant can always be crushed when fresh and used topically or made into a fresh plant tincture.

Dosage
- FPT/DPT (50% alcohol): 30–60 drops 2–3 times daily
- Infusion: 4–6 oz. 2–3 times daily
- Poultice: as needed

Cautions
Like any other astringent–oriented plant: gastrointestinal and/or kidney irritations may develop with extended use.

Other Uses
Occasionally Squawroot is listed as an edible plant (bears do seem to relish it, at least Conopholis americana, also known as Bear corn). Maybe after multiple boiling rounds, but realistically, it's just too astringent to be used as a food.

St. John's Wort
Clusiaceae/St. John's Wort Family

Hypericum perforatum L.
Klamathweed

Hypericum scouleri Hook.
Scouler's St. John's wort

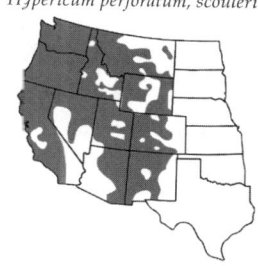

Hypericum perforatum, scouleri

Description
St. John's wort is an herbaceous perennial. The majority of species have opposite leaves, with each successive leaf set forming perpendicularly from the previous one. A bushy herb, Hypericum perforatum develops from a central taproot, whereas H. scouleri's stems are few. Both species' leaf margins (and select flower parts) are dotted with small black/red glands – the undersides are as well, but lesser so. The quarter–sized, 5–petaled, yellow flowers form in terminal cymes. H. perforatum has a greater flower display than H. scouleri. Both species have small seed capsules that contain numerous tiny seeds.

Distribution
Hypericum perforatum, a European native, is found throughout large sections of temperate North America. In the Pacific Northwest, it's considered an invasive weed. Look to disturbed areas, pastures, and field sides. H. scouleri is a plant native to the western United States. From Canada to Arizona and New Mexico, it's found along streamsides and around springs and wet meadows.

Chemistry
Naphthodianthrones: hypericin, pseudohypericin; phloroglucinols: adhyperforin, hyperforin; flavonoids: rutin, hyperoside, isoquercitrin, quercitrin, quercetin.

Medicinal Uses
Not only is St. John's wort an herbal medicine of long historical use, it also is an herb that is better understood today due to the clarifying lens of scientific research.

Externally, St. John's wort is well applied to ulcers, wounds, and cuts. Combined with fresh Aloe vera leaf pulp, it makes for a superb burn dressing. Sensitivity and inflammation are both reduced with its application. For injuries with some nerve tissue involvement, St. John's wort is specific. Topically applied, it assists in nerve repair and quiets related pain. The internally used tincture will favorably compound the topical treatment's effectiveness.

The plant is also quite beneficial when used as an internal/external approach for shingles, a unilateral nerve infection caused by VZV (varicella zoster virus)[79]. When topically combined with Larrea oil (and Skullcap internally), the combination is thought of by some to be remarkable. Topically and internally the plant is a good addition to any type 1 (oral) and/or type 2 (genital) herpes regiment, though introducing additional lysine–rich and alkalizing foods will have a more significant impact.

St. John's wort's sedative/mood altering qualities and effect on depressive states are well recorded. Abating to mild depression[80], the plant fits certain nuances more so than others: if insomnia is commingled with agitation and depression then try St. John's wort. It has a steadying influence on the psyche, particularly if there seems to be a rapid cycling of emotional states. Ultimately though, like other mood–lifting herbs, St. John's wort will best influence depressive states that seem to have no reasonable cause, unlike acute depression which often has a real–world event as an initiator (stress, loss, etc.). It combines well with Passionflower if a stronger sedative influence is needed, or Wild oats if emotional weariness is the main factor. I have also seen the plant do well in lifting the weight of depression that sometimes accompanies hypothyroidism.

Indications

- Ulcers/Wounds/Burns (external)
- Nerve damage/Neuralgias (external and internal)
- Herpes virus group (external and internal)
- Depression, mild–moderate

---

79 VZV belongs to the herpes virus group. Responsible for 'chicken pox' it often reactivates later in life causing 'shingles' and post–herpetic neuralgia.

80 It is generally agreed upon that St. John's wort is a mild MAO (monoamine oxidase) inhibitor. With St. John's wort, serotonin is allowed to linger in certain neuronal synapses. Serotonin's extended presence is what provides a degree of CNS stimulation, which then elevates the mood.

ST. JOHN'S WORT

Collection

If possible, gather the herb when in part–flower/part–seed. This peak stage is typical of the plant mid to late summer. Another sign of St. John's wort's potency, will be an abundance of flower/leaf glands. These small glands contain the pigments hypericin and pseudohypericin and are largely responsible for the plant's effect on the mood and possibly other areas.

Preparations

For internal use, the fresh plant tincture is preferred. Once dried, the plant loses some of its mood–altering qualities. For topical use, the traditional approach is to infuse the flowing tops in oil for a week or so while exposed to sunlight. Although this method is certainly time–tested, a better method, which keeps St. John's wort's fractions more intact, particularly hypericin, is as follows: take 1 part of fresh but wilted flowering tops and infuse them in 7 parts of olive oil. For 8 hours or so maintain the mixture's temperature at 120–130 degrees. This can be done in an oven that registers that low of a temperate, suspended above a stove, or even placed in the engine compartment of a vehicle over a day trip; get creative. After the flowers have been sufficiently infused, strain the oil from the flowers. There may be a small layer of water at the bottom of the container, if so, ladle the oil from the watery portion, then bottle and store. Discarding the watery segment insures the oil's preservation.

Dosage

» FPT/DPT (60% alcohol): 30–60 drops 2–3 times daily
» Herb infusion: 3–6 oz. 2–3 times daily
» Oil/Ointment/Salve: as needed

Cautions

There are a few cautions to be aware of when taking whole plant preparations of St. John's wort. Although remote, some of the plant's compounds have shown uterine stimulant activity, making its consistent use (occasional is fine) unwise during pregnancy.

Animals grazing heavily on the plant have been observed to develop sun–sensitivity dermatitis. However remote, this reaction is possible in Man with the ingestion of mega doses (more likely with the standardized extract). If this occurs, reduce the dose, switch to non–standardized preparations, or discontinue St. John's wort. Do not mix the standardized extract with pharmaceuticals due to St. John's wort stimulation of the liver's cytochrome P450 pathway. Drugs may be eliminated more quickly than intended, possibly causing dosing problems. This phenomenon has been particularly troublesome to patients taking chemotherapy and anti–rejection agents. And lastly, do not mix the plant, crude or standardized, with pharmaceutical antidepressants.

Stachys
Lamiaceae/Mint Family

Stachys pilosa Nutt. *(Stachys palustris subsp. pilosa)*
Hairy hedgenettle, Swamp hedgenettle, Marsh betony, Woundwort

Stachys pilosa

Description
Generally 1′–2′ feet tall, this herbaceous perennial has square hairy stems and opposite leaves. They reach 2″–3″ in length and have crenate–serrate margins. The flowers are arranged in interrupted spikes and are nestled in the leaf axils in radial groupings. The corollas are tubular, 2–lipped, and pale–rose; red to purple spots and/or veins are common. The calyx is 5–parted and about half the length of the floral tube. The seeds are small and dark brown.

Distribution
A common plant throughout the Rocky Mountains, boggy–moistened soil around streams and creeks, often next to nurse–shrubs, is its usual habitat. Marsh skullcap, Field mint, St. John's wort, and Nettle are some regular companions.

Chemistry
Stachys general: iridoids, flavonoids, phenolic acids, and diterpenoids.

Medicinal Uses
Stachys is a mild plant medicine. Its uses are congruent with related plants such as Self heal and Dragonhead. This species of Stachys has a consistent history of external application for simple complaints like insect stings and

bites, skin inflammations, and cuts and scrapes. In other words: use the plant as a basic vulnerary.

Soothing and mildly astringent, the tea made with the dried herb or the juice (diluted in water) is gargled for sore throats and general oral–esophageal irritations/inflammations. It's not particularly antimicrobial, but for simple tissue irritation, most find it effective. The same preparations, swallowed, are relieving to the inflammatory overtones of diarrhea and mild dysentery, be the origin from allergy or partly spoiled food.

Systemically, internal preparations of the tea, juice, or tincture are used as mild inflammation/free radical quenchers. Use Stachys to reduce liver excitability resulting in red–irritated eyes, headache, and the fatigue of allergen exposure, poor dietary choice, or alcohol use. Although not strong enough to block the pain of a skeletal/muscular arthritic episode, its use for the underling inflammation has merit. Its low–level qualities, for whatever situation, will be best harnessed by consistent daily use.

Indications
» As a vulnerary for stings, scrapes, cuts, etc. (external)
» Pharyngitis
» Diarrhea/Dysentery
» As a mild systemic antiinflammatory

Collection
Gather the herbal portions and use these fresh (tincture/juice) or dry (tea/dry plant tincture).

Preparations/Dosage
» Infusion: 4–8 oz. 2–3 times daily
» Fresh juice: ½–1 oz. 2–3 times daily or topically as needed
» FPT/DPT (50% alcohol): 30–60 drops 2–3 times daily
» Fresh plant poultice/Oil/Ointment/Salve: as needed

Cautions
There are no cautions for Stachys.

Sweet Cicely
Apiaceae/Carrot Family

Osmorhiza Raf.
Aniseroot, Sweetroot

Osmorhiza spp.

Description
Sweet cicely is an herbaceous perennial. Arising from a small to medium sized taproot, the leaves are either single, twice–pinnate, or thrice–pinnate. The white to yellowish flowers are inconspicuous. The small linear to oblong seeds are fairly aromatic when crushed.

Identification of the genus is not difficult (the Anise–like aromatics distinguishes it from most other Carrot family plants). However, identifying individual species can be next to impossible without the inspection of the flower/mature seed.

Distribution
A commonly encountered plant throughout most of the higher elevation/northern latitude mountain ranges, Sweet cicely is found in moist, but well–drained soils next to streams and draws. Both Baneberry and Ligusticum are common companion plants.

Chemistry
For osmorhiza chilensis: phenylpropanoids: anethole, estragole, 3,4–dimethoxyeugenol; polyacetylenes: falcarindiol, 3–o–methylfalcarindiol; monoterpenes; sesquiterpenes; coumarins; flavonoids.

Medicinal Uses
Little known today, Sweet cicely is best recognized by its sweetish taste and Anise–like aromatics. A strong cup of the root tea or dose of the root tincture in a hot cup of water is a useful diaphoretic. It is best used in dry fevers with stomach upset, possibly due to a wintertime viral infection affecting both the gastrointestinal and/or respiratory regions. An extra benefit is its pleasing taste – children typically are not repulsed by the tea.

Serving as a straight–forward aromatic carminative, it relieves trapped stomach/intestinal gas and is quieting to nausea. Some also find it less harsh and more agreeable than a strong cup of Peppermint as a post-vomiting soother. An additional plus for the gastrointestinal region is the plant's mild to moderate anesthetic influence. After holding the strongly made tea in the mouth for 10–15 seconds a slight numbing quality should be sensed. This same sensitivity reducing effect (though not as strong as Kava's) is responsible for its soothing gastrointestinal quality.

Use Sweet cicely as a mild expectorant. It especially fits if there is a sore throat and elevated temperature. Its effects will be heightened if combined with Ligusticum (though Ligusticum is the more stimulating of the two).

A number of the aromatic compounds in the plant have demonstrated moderate antifungal/antibacterial activity. Its topical application to poorly healing cuts and/or even skin-oriented fungal infections has merit.

Indications
» Fever, dry skin
» Bloating/Gas, gastrointestinal
» Nausea
» Pharyngitis
» As an expectorant
» Infections, bacterial/fungal (external)

Collection
Sweet cicely is found in deep forest litter, which makes collection not that difficult. With a small shovel or trowel gather the roots and clip and discard the stems and herb portions; however, if enough of the ripened seeds are available, they too can be used.

Preparations/Dosage
» FPT/DPT (60% alcohol): 60–90 drops 2–3 times daily
» Standard/Cold infusion: 4–6 oz. 2–3 times daily
» External preparations: as needed

Cautions
A random cup of tea during pregnancy will cause no issue; however, used daily Sweet cicely may be found too stimulating to be used without caution.

Other Uses
As a quarter-strength infusion, the tea makes a fine beverage.

Sweet Clover
Fabaceae/Pea Family

Melilotus albus Medik. *(Melilotus alba, M. leucanthus)*
White sweet clover, White melilot

Melilotus officinalis (L.) Pall. *(Melilotus graveolens, M. officinalis fo. suaveolens, M. suaveolens, Trifolium officinale)*
Yellow sweet clover, Yellow melilot, Ribbed melilot

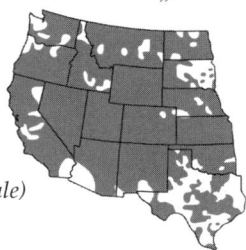

Melilotus albus, officinalis

Description
Some botanists consider these two plants to be of the same species. For our purposes, they will be kept separate due to flower color differences. However, both plants share a majority of other characteristics. Sweet clover reaches 3'–4' in height, although if found in optimal environments (moist soils of roadsides and streamsides) it can approach 6' or so. Herbaceous and weedy, both species have trifoliate leaf bundles, with each leaflet being oblanceolate and ½"–1" long. White flowers comprise White sweet clover's spike–like racemes, whereas yellow flower spikes make up Yellow sweet clover's. Small ovoid pods develop after flower pollination. Both are vanilla–scented and sweet–smelling (more so after drying).

Distribution
Both species are Eurasian natives. In the West, they are common and encountered in disturbed soils, trail shoulders, roadsides, and drainage areas where the soil stays moist from overflow.

Chemistry
Coumarin[81], melilotoside, melilotin, scopoletin, umbelliferone, kaempferol, quercetin.

[81] Coumarin found in Sweet clover is non–toxic and reasonably safe to consume. Dicumarol, a natural anticoagulant compound, does not occur in fresh (or properly dried) Sweet clover; however, this compound does manifest when Sweet clover is dried improperly (becomes moldy due to Penicillium and/or Aspergillus contamination). Dicumarol poisoning (Sweet clover disease) occurs when cattle feed on spoiled Sweet clover hay. It was problematic in America and Canada until the 1940s before its causation was fully understood. Soon after, the medical community began to test

Medicinal Uses

Since Sweet clover's medicinal beginnings, it has been employed towards a wide array of inflammatory conditions. The plant's effect is mainly due to its coumarin content, which becomes especially pronounced once dried (vanilla–scent). It's this group of compounds (and flavonoids) that is responsible for the plant's influence of pain, inflammation, and swelling.

Sufferers of CVI (chronic venous insufficiency) will certainly see benefit from Sweet clover. Venous congestion and related symptoms: varicosities, edema, pain, hyperpigmentation, fibrosis, and ulceration, will improve with the plant's consistent internal and external application. In these situations, it combines well with Horse chestnut and/or Butcher's broom. An ointment, with the fluidextract of Sweet clover replacing the water segment, is well–applied to hemorrhoids.

More broadly, Sweet clover reduces the swelling and edema associated with tissue injury, be it from an acute situation (burns and contusions) or chronic, such as arthritis or old injury flare–up. Even in abdominal–trunk–pelvic issues it should not be underestimated. Use a combination of bath soaks (or the sitz bath) along with the internal tea for ovarian/menstrual oriented pain and fluid retention, bloating/inflammation from a spastic intestinal episode, or really any body–core issue that has swelling and sensitivity as hallmarks. Even the soft tissue/duct pain of mastitis will be quieted with topical and internal doses. For wounds and ulcerations that have a lymphatic edema/tissue swelling aspect, consider Sweet clover a specific vulnerary.

It's generally agreed upon that the coumarin in Sweet clover diminishes swelling and lessens inflammation due to its strengthening effect on capillary bed (and venous tissue) walls. This activity of curbing protein–leakage edema is applicable to virtually any vessel injury, and is the reason why Sweet clover has been applied with success to so many varied and seemingly unrelated conditions.

Indications

- » Varicosities, with edema (external and internal)
- » Hemorrhoids (external and internal)
- » Injury, soft tissue, with swelling (external and internal)

and then develop dicumarol as an anticoagulant for the treatment of thrombosis. Warfarin (Coumadin), a synthetic derivative of dicumarol, was developed shortly after, initially as a rodent poison. By 1954 warfarin was introduced commercially as a pharmaceutical anticoagulant, replacing dicumarol. It is still used today.

- » Burns/Wounds/Ulcerations, poorly healing, with swelling (external and internal)
- » Mastitis (external and internal)

Collection
Due to its pleasant aroma, Sweet clover is an enjoyable herb to gather. Collect the flowering tops – flowers, leaves, and small stems. Be sure to dry them well spaced with adequate ventilation, or use a dehydrator.

Preparations/Dosage
- » Herb infusion: 4–8 ounces 2–3 times daily
- » Fluidextract (30% alcohol): 20–30 drops 2–3 times daily
- » Topical preparations: as needed

Cautions
There are no cautions for Sweet clover and the small quantities of coumarin which it contains. *See footnote on previous page.*

Other Uses
Sweet clover was used to protect wool clothes from moths – they are reportedly repelled by the dried herb. The herb was also once mixed with Tobacco in smoking mixtures due to its pleasant scent.

Toadflax
Plantaginaceae/Plantain Family

Linaria dalmatica (L.) Mill.
Dalmatian toadflax

Linaria vulgaris Hill (*Antirrhinum linaria*)
Butter and eggs

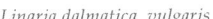
Linaria dalmatica, vulgaris

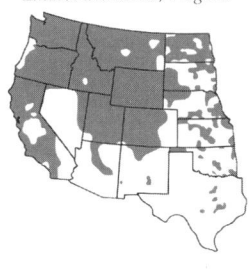

Description
Both species profiled here are 2'–3' tall herbaceous perennials with alternating leaves. Linaria dalmatica's tend to be ovate, clasp the stem, and overall have a tight, well–organized appearance. L. vulgaris's leaves are linear and do not clasp the stem. It is looser in appearance. The flowers for both species

are two-tone yellow, 5-lobed, 2-lipped, and end with a cone-like spur. The seed capsules are small and round. They develop extensive networks of colony-forming horizontal rhizomes.

Distribution

Both species are native to the Mediterranean region. Having escaped cultivation during the colonial period, they are now found throughout temperate regions of America and Canada. Though absent from most of the Southeast and Texas, Linaria dalmatica is well established in cooler, semi-arid western regions. L. vulgaris prefers moister soils and is extremely cold tolerant. Both plants are found in disturbed soils, pastures, roadsides, and open forest meadows.

Chemistry

Flavonoids: aureusin, bracteatin, cyanidin, linarin, pectolinarin; iridoids: aucubin, antirrinoside, antirride, procumbide.

Medicinal Uses

Toadflax is one of the stronger Figwort family (alternatively placed in the Plantain family) plant medicines of the West. More potent than related Penstemon and Figwort, yet not quite as harsh as the more eastern growing Culver's root (Leptandra), well dosed, Toadflax is able to modify a whole range of gastrointestinal and hepatic issues.

Toadflax's most basic application is as functional bitter tonic. Use it if suffering from chronic indigestion. Taken before meals, it serves as a broad visceral organ secretory stimulant. Stomach, liver, and intestinal secretions necessary for food digestion and assimilation will be augmented with its use.

Like other bitters it is well-combined with an aromatic herb (Field mint, Monarda, etc.) for a more complete stimulation of the gastric region. Some even notice a salivation-increasing effect when liquid preparations are swished in the mouth prior to swallowing. People whom are troubled by symptoms of poor lipid assimilation (gastrointestinal stasis, nausea, and headache) after consuming a rich meal, will do well with Toadflax.

If plagued by constitutionally dry and allergy-reactive skin, consider taking Toadflax daily. A wide range of liver activities are augmented by the plant, making it corrective for related functional problems of this organ. Those afflicted by chronic, non-active hepatitis, whether viral or otherwise, will often see a reduction in inflammatory/enzymatic markers such as bilirubin elevations, SGOT, and SGPT. For these situations and even associated jaundice, it combines well with Milk thistle, Turmeric, or Western mugwort. Toadflax tends to be more stimulating to the gastrointestinal tract than other chologogues. Even with moderate amounts it is not uncommon to experience a mild laxative effect.

Indications
- » Indigestion, asecretory
- » As a liver stimulant
- » Inflammation, liver, chronic

Collection
Gather the herbal portions, optimally when in flower. Dry the herb normally.

Preparations
The tea and dried plant tincture are the standard preparations. Toadflax is also a fine candidate for fluidextraction. Whatever preparation is decided upon, it should taste bitter, weakly saline, and weakly acrid.

Dosage
- » DPT (50% alcohol): 20–40 drops 2–3 times daily
- » Infusion: 2–4 oz. 2–3 times daily
- » Fluidextract: 10–15 drops 2–3 times daily

Cautions
Toadflax's main cautions are linked to its stimulant nature. Excess amounts are laxative, nauseating, and irritating to the liver (that which stimulates with proper dosage, irritates in excess). Moreover, it probably is best not to use Toadflax while pregnant or nursing.

Other Uses
The flowers were once used in Germany as a yellow dye.

Usnea
Parmeliaceae/Lichen Family

Usnea Dill. ex Adans.
Old man's beard, Beard lichen

Usnea spp.

Description
A lichen (an algae and fungi symbiosis), Usnea forms in tassel–like clumps on an array of living and dead trees and occasionally on artificial structures. The main body is greenish–gray–tan and comprised of an anchor point, pendulous strands (thallus) with a thin white myco core, and spore producing disk shaped fruiting bodies. It is thought that the majority of species are not destructive to their hosts and derive particulate matter and hydration solely from the air.

Distribution
Common throughout temperate zones world–wide, the only areas in the western United States to lack this lichen are the low elevation Southwest and Prairie/Grassland/Basin areas (that lack trees). Both conifers and hardwood trees host Usnea. It is usually most abundant on dead trees that receive a good amount of sunlight.

Chemistry
Sterols, diterpenoids, sesquiterpenoids, dibenzofurans: usnic acid, xanthones, anthraquinones, polysaccharides.

Medicinal Uses
Usnea's alignment of traditional use and modern research helps to shed light on its three best areas of influence: the lungs, urinary tract, and skin. The lichen's medicinal value is based on its mild immune stimulating polysaccharide and strongly antimicrobial usnic acid principles.

Applied to bronchitis, sore throats, and sinusitis, Usnea has a significant influence. Additionally, due to the tea's (or a small bunch well–chewed and swallowed) minor gelatinous quality, it's found particularly helpful when respiratory tissues are raw and inflamed. In fact, if caught early enough in their progressions (dry hacking cough), I've seen cases of soon–to–be bronchitis resolve without further incident.

Topical preparations of Usnea should be applied to problem wounds, cuts, and incisions where there is danger of growing infection. The ointment in conjunction with proper wound cleansing/dressing is the best way to proceed. Internal use of Usnea (or stronger immune stimulants such as Echinacea) combined with its topical use will be even more effective. Additionally, even low–level bacterial skin problems such as Acne vulgaris respond well to the tincture applied nightly to the problem area. My advice is, if it's a bacterial (fungal/yeast...lesser so) skin infection, try topically–applied Usnea. It most likely will help the condition.

Usnea has a sound record of addressing urinary tract infections that do not respond to Heath family plants (Uva–ursi, etc.). It also rarely causes renal irritation with over use, a caution that applies to most in the Heath family. Another option if the type of urinary infection is unknown, is to combine Usnea with Uva–ursi (or Madrone) in order to cover both bases – E. coli and non–E. coli types.

Some of the more common bacteria that Usnea (usnic acid) has shown activity against are Staphylococcus, Streptococcus, Bacteroides, and Mycobacteria strains. I don't recommend Usnea used as a stand–alone treatment for MRSA (methicillin–resistant Staphylococcus aureus) or MDR–TB (multi–drug–resistant tuberculosis) infections; however, its use alongside conventional antibiotics is theoretically promising.

Usnic acid demonstrates significant inhibitory activity against Trichomonas vaginalis, the parasite responsible for the Trichomoniasis or 'trich' infections. Try Usnea in these cases: the strong tea used as a douche along with the internal tincture or capsules (or for men, internal use alone) is potentially a good treatment.

Indications
- Bronchitis
- Sinusitis
- Infection, topical (external)
- Infection, urinary tract
- Vaginitis (external and internal)

Collection
Gather the low–hanging bunches. Usnea has a minuscule water content so additional drying time at most only has to be a week or so. In many cases

powdering Usnea for the dried 'plant' tincture or topical preparations can occur the same day as collection.

Preparations

Herbalists tend to spend a lot of time fussing about on how to prepare Usnea for internal use (boiling alcohol), this due to usnic acid and its difficultly of extraction. Given the potential toxicities of isolated usnic acid, preparations that yield lower amounts of this component may not be a bad thing. Primitive Man did fine with water–based preparations (or its crude ingestion). Taking from their example, I recommend the adoption of an iconic American saying that continues to serves me well – KISS (Keep It Simple Stupid).

When making Usnea oil, the alcohol intermediate technique is the preferred method. The oil's conversion into a potent ointment should include a strong Usnea tea as a replacement for the water fraction (See main Preparations section).

Dosage

» Capsule (00): 1–2, 1–3 times daily
» Fluidextract: 10–20 drops 2–3 times daily
» DPT (65% alcohol): 30–60 drops 2–3 times daily
» Decoction: 4–6 oz. 2–3 times daily

Cautions

Consider Usnea a short–term use medicinal lichen: 1–2 weeks of consecutive use at a time. The tea (and capsules) can sometimes be upsetting to the stomach. If this is the case, switch to tincture/fluidextract preparations. Dermatitis is rarely reported for individuals in daily contact with the lichen (forestry workers). If skin redness or irritation does develop with its topical use, it's best to switch to a different herbal treatment. Topical preparations during pregnancy, while nursing, or with children are fine, but I'm unable to confidently recommend its internal use.

Aside from an occasional upset stomach, reports of human Usnea (whole–lichen preparations) toxicity are few to none. However, isolated usnic acid or its salts, taken as an isolated substance may be problematic. A number of cases of hepatotoxicity have been reported for at least one weight loss supplement containing sodium usniate. Complicating the situation though is the supplement (Lipokinetix) also contained caffeine, Yohimbe, diiodothyronine, and norephedrine. Consumed in mega–doses (as diet supplements usually are) it's anyone guess as to what compound or combination thereof was problematic.

Uva–Ursi
Ericaceae/Heath Family

Arctostaphylos uva-ursi

Arctostaphylos uva–ursi (L.) Spreng.
Bearberry, Kinnikinnick

Description
Uva–ursi is a mat–like shrub with low–growing stems that reach heights of 1'–1½'. Rooting at stem nodes, older colonies can become well established and quite dense. The leaf blades are entire and oval to oblong. The upper leaf surfaces are glabrous and dark green. The lower surfaces are lighter green and somewhat puberulent, becoming glabrous with age. The small flowers form in racemes. They are distinctly urn–shaped and white to pinkish. The small berries are ⅓"–⅖" in diameter and bright red.

Distribution
Uva–ursi ranges through much of mountainous North America. It is found from Alaska, south to California, and throughout the interior western mountains. It extends as far south as Georgia and Arkansas. More broadly, it is a circumboreal species, equally found throughout Europe and Asia. It is considered a floristic indicator of the belted region between the Temperate Zone and Arctic. Look to coniferous forests, sandy soils, and rocky slopes.

Chemistry
Phenolic glycosides: arbutin, methylarbutin, hydroquinone; tannins: caffeic acid, gallic acid, catechol, ellagic acid; triterpenoids: uvaol, ursolic acid, lupeol, α–amyrin, β–amyrin, erythrodiol, oleanolic acid; anthocyanins/anthocyanidins: delphinidin, cyanidin; flavonoids: quercitrin, quercetin.

Medicinal Uses
Due to its circumboreal distribution and long recorded usage history, Uva–ursi is the best known and most widely employed of all the Heath family urinary astringents/disinfectants. It shares its basic therapeutic qualities

with two lesser known medicinal plants, Madrone and Manzanita. What makes Uva–ursi more used is its abundance and commercial availability and not necessarily any medicinal superiority.

Although many constituent groups within Uva–ursi have medicinal value, and likely add to the plant's net activity, it is arbutin and its conversion to hydroquinone that is generally accepted as the most important. Once Uva–ursi (or any arbutin–containing Heath family plant) is ingested, the arbutin (remaining at least partly intact due to the presence of hydrolyzable tannin complexes) exits the gut for the systemic system. Upon interaction with the kidneys, arbutin is cleaved to form hydroquinone, which is then excreted in the urine as hydroquinone glucuronide (and possibly hydroquinone sulfate). In the presence of alkaline urine, conjugated hydroquinone is once again liberated to a free form, and only then exerts its strong antiseptic effect. Interestingly, if urine pH is normal (slightly acidic), hydroquinone stays largely inactive (remaining as hydroquinone glucuronide/sulfate) and is of little infection–fighting value.

Another influence of Uva–ursi, apart from or at least only partly associated with hydroquinone, is its urine acidifying effect. This is important since the commonest urinary tract infection causing pathogen, Escherichia coli, is unable to successfully attach to cell walls and multiply in acidic urine[82].

Use Uva–ursi for non–complicated/non–organic urinary tract infections[83], either bladder or urethra oriented. If there is an active infection drink 2–3 cups a day, or at the slightest irritation, a single cup for maintenance purposes. If Cranberry juice has been found of value, chances are Uva–ursi will be found to have equal or greater value.

Like nearly all other Heath family medicinal plants, Uva–ursi is a urinary tract astringent. The leaves' tannin content is about the same as Manzanita's, yet more so than Madrone's, which points to its use for poor tone and

---

82 Healthy urine is slightly acidic. This helps to promote a more resilient urinary environment.

83 If plagued by on– and off– again UTIs, and basic hygiene (especially for women), dietary irritants (coffee or tea for instance), and structural issues have been ruled out, dietary habits may be a causative factor. High carbohydrate diets (vegan, vegetarian, and/or excessive consumption of refined sugars) tend to promote a more alkaline urinary environment and therefore a greater tendency for infection. Also, the simple addition of animal–source protein several times a week often reduces urinary infection prevalence.

laxity of the area. Most situations that exhibit chronic irritation, dribbling of urine, and cloudy urine will see benefit from Uva–ursi's tannin contingent.

As a postpartum sitz bath, Uva–ursi is useful in tonifying and soothing vaginal and cervical tissues. It can be relied upon to reduce passive hemorrhaging from birth canal abrasions. Also, since Uva–ursi is moderately inhibiting to Candida albicans (yeast infections) it is well worth combining sitz bath applications with the internal use of Thuja or Garlic.

Indications
» Cystitis/Urethritis, alkaline urine
» Vaginitis with or w/o Candida involvement
» As a postpartum sitz bath

Collection
Gather Uva–ursi leaves from late spring to summer after flowering when the ripe fruit is present. Its arbutin content is most concentrated at this time, but lesser so when the plant is in flower.

Preparations
If decocting the leaf be sure to first soak them for 3–4 hours in a small amount of water. This will better facilitate arbutin's conversion to hydroquinone.

Dosage
» Leaf decoction: 4–6 oz. 2–3 times daily
» DPT (40% alcohol, 10% glycerin): 30–60 drops 2–3 times daily
» Sitz bath: as needed

Cautions
If Uva–ursi is dosed sensibly and used for short to intermediate periods there will be little issue of side effect. Longer periods of use and greater than recommended amounts may cause renal and gastrointestinal irritations – common to most tannin (and arbutin) containing herbal medicines. For a longer–term use Heath family urinary astringent see Madrone.

Except for an occasional cup of tea, Uva–ursi should be avoided during pregnancy. The plant's tannin–related uterine lining effects combined with the reproductive unknowns of arbutin and hydroquinone, suggest it's not the wisest herbal medicine to be used during this time.

Other Uses
Mealy, seed-filled, and astringent, Uva-ursi's fruit are technically 'edible', but they are not especially pleasant tasting.

Valerian
Valerianaceae/Valerian Family

Valeriana officinalis L.
Garden valerian

Valeriana acutiloba Rydb. *(V. capitata ssp. acutiloba)*
Western valerian

Valeriana edulis Nutt. ex Torr. & A. Gray
Mexican valerian

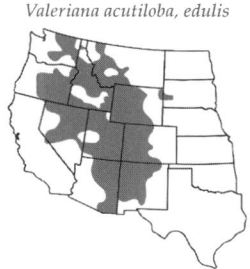

Valeriana acutiloba, edulis

Description
A large herbaceous perennial, Valeriana officinalis reaches heights of 5'-6'. The sizable pinnate leaves are oppositely arranged and composed of 3-25 leaflets. They are linear to elliptical and entire to toothed. The flowers form in compound panicles. Generally pink to white, each floral tube is about ¼" in length. Like many others within the genus, V. officinalis's roots are primarily sub-surface runners.

Compared to the other profiled species, Valeriana acutiloba is a small plant. Its long petioled basal leaves are spatulate, oblanceolate, or obovate. The flower stalk leaves are paired and entire to pinnately divided. The white-pink, ¼" long flowers form in dense panicles. The plant's creeping rhizomes are anchored just below the ground's surface by fine hair-like rootlets.

Valerian edulis is comprised of basal leaves for most of its growing season. Although they are highly variable in form, they are generally oblanceolate to divided. The small whitish flowers form in open panicles. Underground, V. edulis is a stout plant, sending down a robust and fleshy 1'-1½' tap root.

Distribution
Of Eurasian extraction, Valeriana officinalis is successful (considered invasive in Connecticut) throughout much of the Northeast. From Maryland and Iowa, it is found north into Canada. In the West, it is rarely encountered in the wild. It's apt to be found cultivated in an herb garden, or more reliably, encapsulated at the health food store. It's the main medicinal species of commerce.

Valeriana acutiloba is a plant of mountainous regions throughout the West. Look to coniferous forests, often with Douglas fir and almost always on a hillside with a drainage below. From the interior mountain states, such as Wyoming and Colorado, it is found south to Arizona and New Mexico. V. arizonica and V. occidentalis are an additional two species of note that share some physical and distribution characteristics with V. acutiloba. V. arizonica is common to the upper mountains of Arizona and New Mexico. V. occidentalis is found throughout the Rocky Mountains, where it often overlaps in distribution with V. acutiloba.

Valeriana edulis is encountered in some of the same places where V. acutiloba grows, but it's more tolerate of exposed meadows and grassy openings. The plant ranges from Montana south to Arizona.

Chemistry
Monoterpenoids; sesquiterpenoids: valerenic acid and its derivatives: valeranone, valeranal, kessyl esters; valepotriates: valtrate, didrovaltrate, acevaltrate, isovaleroxyhydroxyvaltrate; flavonoids: methyl apigenin, hesperidin, linarin; triterpenes, lignans, alkaloids.

Medicinal Uses
Like many medicinal plants, Valerian presents a number of therapeutic attributes, tending to better fit people with certain physiological tendencies, rather than simple conditions.

As a sedative, Valerian works best to bring sleep and relaxation to those with lowered innate vitality. The aged and individuals weakened from sickness, stress, or worry whom are having sleep problems, are good candidates for Valerian. When well–matched to the individual, it is not unusual for the plant to usher in a sense of clarity and peace of mind, as well as bring needed sleep.

If circulation is impaired (cold hands and feet, trouble adjusting to the cold), usually seen in the feeble, Valerian as a calming agent, is choice. Heart palpitations, from over–work and worry, especially combined with Passionflower, are lessened. Neuralgias with mild spasm or tremor are quieted as are headaches from excessive worry or mental effort.

Depression arising from long–term over–work and worry is often lifted by the fresh plant tincture, as is mental/emotional agitation and 'cerebral fog' arising from similar states. It is too occasionally lifting to the depression of hypothyroidism.

Valerian's carminative effects will be particularly well received by those whom suffer indigestion related to emotional agitation. The plant's volatile oil content is largely responsible for this activity. Gas and bloating are eased, as are headaches that are caused by imperfect upper gastric digestion.

Not all Valerian species or preparations act the same. For some people the fresh plant tincture tends to be a mild stimulant. Dried though, it is more reliably a sedative, especially the root infusion.

Valeriana officinalis is the strongest sedative, particularly if dried. The native species[84], although decent sedatives, are best used if there is obvious CNS (central nervous system) depression and debility. They have fair spinal/cerebral stimulatory properties.

As to how Valerian can produce these somewhat contradictory CNS effects and what group of constituents is responsible, is open to debate. It was originally thought that the plant's valepotriate content was largely responsible: this compound group inhibits GABA (γ–aminobutyric acid) re–uptake. Now though, other mechanisms are coming to light, which attribute altogether different compounds.

The plant's adenosine receptor influences may have something to do with the varying effects of different species and preparations. Alcohol preparations contain more lipophilic constituents, such as isovaltrate, and tend to serve as inverse agonists for adenosine A_1 receptors, causing CNS stimulation. Water based preparations stimulate adenosine A_1 receptors, bringing about CNS sedation.

Calcium channel blocking, serotoninergic, melatonergic, and dopaminergic effects have also been reported, making Valerian's CNS influence complex. Regardless of the intricacies, it is important to understand that Valerian is not the straight forward sedative that it is often touted to be.

---

84   Valeriana edulis has a high percentage of valepotriates and is often used as a base material for the extraction of these compounds.

Indications
- Insomnia/Restlessness
- Hysteria/Depression from weakness
- Heart palpitation, from nervous exhaustion
- Neuralgia/Spasm/Tremor
- Indigestion/Gas/Bloating

Collection
Valeriana officinalis is often cultivated as a garden plant. Its roots are easily unearthed due to their runner–type tendency. V. acutiloba has small roots that creep under the soil's surface. They cling to forest soils remarkably well. The herbage too of this species can be utilized. The leaves of V. edulis are nearly impotent, so only the roots of this species should be gathered and employed.

Preparations
Dried, water–based preparations of any species, but especially Valeriana officinalis, tend to be reliably sedative. The encapsulated dried plant (and the dried plant tincture) acts as a sedative, but less predictably. The fresh plant tincture of any species tends to be more stimulatory (the better preparation for depression). For some people, Valerian is a superb sedative, regardless of form, but for others it is equivalent to a cup of coffee before bed.

Forget standardized extracts. It's the whole plant which comprises Valerian's medicinal attributes and not one constituent or group.

Of course, no description of dried Valerian would be complete without mentioning its distinctive aroma. It's often described as smelling like odiferous feet/socks.

Dosage
- Root infusion: 3–6 oz. 1–3 times daily
- FPT/DPT (70% alcohol): 45–90 drops 1–3 times daily
- Fluidextract: 20–30 drops 2–3 times daily
- Capsule (00): 1–2, 1–3 times daily

Cautions
Valerian taken occasionally during pregnancy or while nursing will cause no problem; however, there may be an issue if used every day. Potentiation

may be an issue if it is combined with sedative pharmaceuticals (especially the benzodiazepine[85] class of drugs).

Verbena
Verbenaceae/Vervain Family

Verbena bracteata Lag. & Rodr.
Prostrate verbena, Bigbract verbena

Verbena macdougalii A. Heller
New Mexican verbena, MacDougal verbena

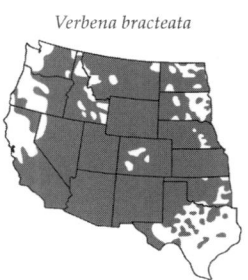

Verbena bracteata

Description
Verbena bracteata is a small, low-growing, spreading annual or short-lived perennial. The leaves are deeply lobed and form oppositely along ridged stems. The entire plant is hairy. The flower spikes are long and composed mostly of leaf-like bracts. The flowers are small and pinkish-purple.

Stately compared to others of the genus, Verbena macdougalii is a 2'-4' tall perennial. Its oblong-ovate shaped leaves are serrated, hairy, and arranged oppositely along the plant's ridged stems. The small and purplish flowers develop in spikes on the upper stem ends.

Distribution
At varying elevations, Verbena bracteata is distributed nearly throughout the entire country. Look to disturbed and moist soils: around cattle tanks, pond and lake edges, sumps, and bottomlands.

Verbena macdougalii is found from Wyoming to West Texas, Arizona, and New Mexico. Its core range is throughout the arid Southwest: here it is found at elevations of 5,000'–8,500'. On the edge of its range, in more northerly locals, it is encountered at lower elevations. Look to open Ponderosa pine forests and grassy meadows.

Chemistry
Anthocyanins/anthocyanidins; flavonoids: naringenin and eriodictyol; triterpenoids.

---

85 Valium is not derived from Valerian. This myth has been around for some time.

Medicinal Uses

Verbena is a sedative of mild strength. Its calming effect is useful in reducing nervousness and anxiety. Moreover, it is effective in relieving stress headaches with associated neck and upper back tension. It is a good herb for anxiety related indigestion: through the plant's countering of adrenaline–type stress, digestion and assimilation are enhanced, as are other parasympathetic functions.

If feverish and dry–skinned, Verbena stimulates diaphoresis. It is also stimulating to lactation (as are other Vervain family plants). Relatedly, it may have some influence of the neurotransmitter dopamine and hormone prolactin. Stressed mothers whom are unable to produce adequate quantities of milk often see good results from Verbena.

A number of species have small but inconsistent amounts of cardiac glycosides. In sensitive individuals, these compounds may influence the heart rate (slow and strengthen). The effect is rare but has been observed.

Indications

» Anxiety/Tension
» Headache, stress related
» Indigestion with poor circulation
» Fevers, dry
» Lactation, insufficient

Collection

Gather the upper herbaceous portions and lay these parts out to dry or alternatively tincture them fresh.

Preparations/Dosage

» FPT/DPT (60% alcohol): 30–60 drops 2–3 times daily[86]
» Herb infusion: 4–6 ounces 2–3 times daily

Cautions

Sensitive individuals may develop contact dermatitis from collection. Do not use excessive amounts during pregnancy due to the herb's potential effect on prolactin levels.

---

86 Verbena occasionally produces a fresh plant tincture that partly congeals. It's a cosmetic issue that vigorous shaking before dispensing usually solves.

Western Mugwort
Asteraceae/Sunflower Family

Artemisia ludoviciana Nutt. *(Artemisia mexicana, Artemisia vulgaris var. mexicana)*
Louisiana sagewort, Prairie sagewort, White sagewort, Estafiate

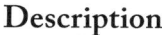
Artemisia ludoviciana

Description
A highly variable plant, Western mugwort's leaf size, shape, and color span the gamut: from entire to lobed, to blue–green and silver–gray, they are adept at adjusting size and structure in response to environmental conditions. Individually, the flowers are inconspicuous. However, in number, they form notable terminal spikes mixed with small leaves. Like other Artemisias, when crushed it emits a characteristic Sage–like aroma.

Distribution
A ubiquitous plant, Western mugwort is common throughout the West. Except for the Pacific Coast area, there are not many bioregions that mark the plant's absence.

Chemistry
Sesquiterpenes: arteannuin b, artemisinin, achillin, anthemidin, artedouglasia oxide, douglanine, ludovicin, tanaparthin–α–peroxide, tanapartholide b; monoterpenes: borneol, camphor, chrysanthemol, transchrysanthenol, α–pinene; flavonoids: butein, isoliquiritigenin, isorhamnetin, quercetin; coumarins: lacarol, scopoletin.

Medicinal Uses
Western mugwort ranks somewhere in the middle of the Artemisia continuum. Not as strong as Sagebrush with its thujone harshness, but more vigorous in effect than Mugwort (A. vulgaris), Western mugwort serves as a fine herbal medicine for a number of gastrointestinal, hepatic, and infectious problems.

As a bitter tonic, use Western mugwort for simple asecretory indigestion. The tea before meals broadly stimulates digestive secretion, which assists in food breakdown and therefore curbs feelings of gastric stasis and undue fullness.

Underlying Western mugwort's bitter tonic activity is its cytoprotective effect[87] on gastric (and intestinal) tissue, meaning the plant is adept at protecting and healing gastrointestinal tract mucosa from inflammatory responses and conditions. Furthermore, it also has some anti–Helicobacter pylori activity, making the herb useful if plagued by stomach–duodenal ulcers. Not only can it be used as a simple gastric stimulant, it also excels as a daily tea for inflammatory conditions such as peptic ulcer, gastritis, and ulcerative colitis.

Western mugwort is choleretic, serving to increase bile synthesis and release. If prone to gall stone formation, the plant will thin bile enough to diminish precipitants. More deeply, it has a cooling and antioxidant effect on hepatocyte function. These influences tend to reduce elevated liver enzyme levels – all stress markers evident in viral and general hepatitis. In addition, the plant inhibits glutathione depletion within hepatocytes. Its hepatoprotective effect can also be of benefit to individuals whom consume excess alcohol, rancid oils, and processed foods. Several ounces of the cool tea taken before bed is an excellent approach to next–morning frontal headaches, red–irritated eyes, and bad breath (all markers of general liver congestion).

Topically, Western mugwort is only mildly antibacterial and antifungal. It influences a wide array of microorganisms, but its effect is not strong (unlike Sagebrush). However, it is distinctly inhibiting to HSV (herpes simplex virus), type I and II. For cold sore treatment, the oil or salve in combination with Creosote bush is effective. With clients, I have observed herpes (genital and oral) outbreaks diminish with its internal and external application.

Like its larger cousin, Sagebrush, Western mugwort is successful against multiple intestinal organisms. Drink several cups of tea daily for the treatment of traveler's diarrhea (Entamoeba histolytica), giardiasis (Giardia lamblia), and pinworm infection. Do not underestimate it in these situations; the plant contains several compounds that are broadly anthelmintic.

The hot tea is a stimulating diaphoretic. Ingested cool with no elevated temperature, Western mugwort is diuretic. The plant tends also to stimulate menses, and is especially helpful if the pelvic area feels painful and congested.

---

[87] Providing cyclooxygenase inhibition, Western mugwort increases glycoprotein (mucus) synthesis, granulocyte degranulation inhibition, and transcription factor NF–KB inhibition.

Indications
- Dyspepsia/Gastritis
- Ulcer, gastric/duodenal
- Inflammation, intestinal
- Inflammation, liver, with no hepatic/biliary blockage
- Infection, bacterial/fungal (external)
- HSV, type I and II (internal and external)
- Diarrhea, amoeba/giardia
- Parasites, intestinal
- Fever, low–moderate temperature
- Amenorrhea, with pelvic rigidity

Collection
Depending on elevation and climate, Western mugwort's foliage is collectable from spring through fall. Gather it without the flowers as the pollen can occasionally trigger hayfever reactions in sensitive individuals.

Preparations/Dosage
- Herb infusion (cold or standard): 4–6 ounces 2–3 times daily
- FPT/DPT (50% alcohol): 20–40 drops 2–3 times daily
- DPT (100% vinegar): 20–40 drops 2–3 times daily
- Oil/Salve/Wash: as needed

Cautions
Do not use Western mugwort during pregnancy due to its dilating effect on uterine vasculature. Given the plant's cholagogue properties, it is not wisely used if there is a biliary blockage.

Wild Cherry
Rosaceae/Rose Family

Prunus seritona, virginiana

Prunus serotina var. rufula (Wooton & Standley) McVaugh *(Prunus serotina var. virens)*
Black cherry, Southwestern black cherry

Prunus virginiana var. demissa (Nutt.) Torr. *(Prunus virginiana var. melanocarpa)*
Western chokecherry, Black chokecherry

Description
Prunus serotina var. rufula is one of three varieties of Black cherry. This western grower is a small to medium sized tree (not a suckering shrub like Western chokecherry). The leaves are elliptic, obovate, to lanceolate with serrated margins. The young bark is covered with distinctive hash marks. The 5–petaled flowers are white and form in tubular racemes. The fleshy cherries are dark red to black and contain a large pit.

Reaching heights of 20′ (usually smaller), Prunus virginiana var. demissa grows to be a suckering large bush or small tree. On younger secondary branches the bark is smooth–grayish brown, and on this unfissured bark there are distinctive whitish hash marks. The older, lower trunk bark is usually fissured. The elliptic to obovate leaves have finely serrated margins. From shiny to slightly hairy, the leaves' undersides are variable. The flower clusters form in racemes at branch ends. Each white flower has 5 petals, 5 sepals, and is between ¼″–½″ in diameter. The dark red or nearly black fruit hang in drupes. Each cherry contains a large, smooth pit.

This variety of Chokecherry varies from the eastern variety (Prunus virginiana var. virginiana) by leaf shape. Variety demissa's largest leaves are at least twice as long as they are wide. Variety virginiana's largest leaves are more strongly elliptic and less than twice as long as wide.

Distribution
Prunus serotina var. rufula or Southwestern black cherry is found in the mid–mountains of Arizona, New Mexico, and West Texas and almost always along streams and drainages. Prunus virginiana var. demissa (Western chokecherry) is found from the Rocky Mountains to California; northern

Arizona to Washington. Usually thicket–forming, it prefers full exposures in and around stream banks, forest edges, and canyon bottoms. The easterly variety of Chokecherry (var. virginiana) is found mainly east of the Rockies. The two varieties do have some overlap in the northwestern states. However, var. demissa is the main Chokecherry of the West.

Chemistry

Cyanogenic glycosides: amygdalin, prunasin, prulaurasin; flavonoids; tannins.

Medicinal Uses

These days Wild cherry is most often thought of as simply a flavoring ingredient for OTC cough syrups and the like. However, there once was a time when it was the active component in similar formulations, and for good reason. Bark preparations are quelling to a dry–irritative cough. Whether associated with bronchitis, influenza, or other lung afflictions, Wild cherry works best as a cough suppressant in bronchial conditions with associated rapid pulse, quickened breathing, and fever. It is a sedative for bronchial mucus membrane irritation in relation to cardiac and vascular excitability. It often is the perfect fit for children whom exhibit these tendencies when sick with wintertime viruses. The plant should be considered a necessity when recovering from pleurisy or pneumonia with associated colliquative sweating. In this respect, Wild cherry acts Sage–like and is able to reduce fever–dependent perspiration.

The plant's particular cyanogenic glycoside content, a compound group common to many plants within the Rose family, is at least partly responsible for its sedative activity on the pneumal and cardiovascular systems. Even for straight–forward heart palpitations dependent on debility, psychosomatic responses to stress, or overexertion, Wild cherry is calming.

Whether related or not to the above cardio–pulmonary framework, the plant is also indicated in gastritis. Here it will be found soothing to inflamed mucosa.

Lastly, a potential use for Wild cherry: as a testosterone–dependent prostate–inflammation reducing treatment. In at least one in–vitro study[88], five species of Prunus were determined to have benign prostate hypertrophy reducing effects. Of the five, the bark of P. domestica (common Plum

[88] Jena, Ashish Kumar et al. Amelioration of testosterone induced benign prostatic hyperplasia by Prunus species. *Journal of Ethnopharmacology* 190 (2016) 33–45.

tree) was found to be comparable with Pygeum (Prunus africana or African cherry), a popular but over-exploited herbal treatment for prostate issues. Whether either species of Wild cherry profiled here shrinks the prostate remains to be seen. However, I believe there is enough parallel evidence to make experiments worthwhile.

Indications
» Cough, dry and hectic
» Bronchitis, with inflammation

Collection
Select a secondary branch with little or no older, fissured bark. Once removed, discard the smaller branchlets and leaves. With a knife, peel away the bark from the selected branch.

Preparations
Although drying the bark is important, heat degrades the value of Wild cherry. Once dry (fresh too) the bark should have an essence of Cherry fragrance. Even the quality of commercially purchased bark can be judged accordingly: if the bark has no subtle Cherry fragrance, it will be of little value.

For tea, the cold infusion method is choice. The syrup, if made without heat, is an excellent preparation. When making the dried plant tincture, be sure to include glycerin in the menstruum (See the main Preparation section). This addition will inhibit the plant's tannins from binding with other constituents.

Dosage
» Cold infusion: 4–6 oz. 2–3 times daily
» DPT (40% alcohol, 10% glycerin): 30–60 drops 2–3 times daily
» Syrup: 1–2 teaspoons 1–3 times daily

Cautions
Large amounts may theoretically cause bronchial and cardiovascular suppression[89]. There are no known cautions with normal usage.

89 Armchair internet 'experts' write to no end of Wild cherry's seeds and leaves, due to their cyanogenic glycoside content, as a deadly poison. Take this with a grain of salt: the recorded Prunus poisonings are from animals eating large amounts of the fresh/wilted leaves. Even if ingested in an active form, humans are physiologically

Other Uses

The bitter–sweet cherries can be eaten as is (minus the pit) or used as a jam/jelly base. Like other Cherry species, they are a rich source of antioxidant anthocyanin/anthocyanidin pigments. If they are found astringent, they have not fully ripened.

Most California Indians utilized the pits of various Wild cherry species for food at one time or another. In order to first neutralize their cyanogenic glycosides, drying, grinding, leaching, and/or roasting were common preparations. I suggest air–drying the pits first for a week or so, then roast them at 350 degrees for at least 45 minutes. Crack the outer shell and eat the kernel within. To be on the safe side, initially eat only a ½–dozen roasted kernels and then monitor yourself for gastrointestinal upset[90]. Let 30 minutes pass. If no problem is detected, then proceed with more.

Wild Iris
Iridaceae/Iris Family

Iris missouriensis Nutt. (*Iris arizonica, I. longipetala* var. *montana, I. montana, I. pariensis, I. pelogonus, I. tolmieana*)
Rocky mountain iris, Western blue flag

Iris missouriensis

Description

Wild iris is a 1'–1½' tall herbaceous perennial. Arising from a thickened rhizome, its leaves are sword–shaped and linear. 1–4 flowers form at stems ends. A showy arrangement, they are a combination of spreading sepals (white with purple lines and a yellow spot) and blue petals. The fruit is a thickened, elongated capsule.

---

capable of detoxifying low to moderate amounts of naturally occurring cyanogenic glycosides with no ill effect, given the individual is not anemic and/or protein–deficient. Drying degrades Prunus' glycosides making the bark (and other parts) safe to take internally (and it has been used safely this way for centuries). All the chatter about Prunus pits is an exaggeration too. After all many Indian tribes ate them as a supplemental food once processed to some degree.

90   Gastrointestinal upset is the first sign of naturally–occurring cyanogenic glycoside toxicity. I speak from experience.

Distribution

A plant of the western mountains, Wild iris is nearly always encountered in montane meadows and clearings or at least where tree cover is not that dense. Rare in Minnesota and the Dakotas, its most prominent range is throughout the Rocky Mountains. From Arizona and New Mexico and the Pacific Coast states, it is found abundantly into western Canada.

Chemistry

Quinones: irisoquin, deoxyirisoquin; triterpenoides: isoiridogermanal, zeorin; isoflavones: irisone a, irisone b; flavonoids.

Medicinal Uses

The application of Wild iris is essentially patterned after the official medicinal species, that of northeastern grower, Blue flag (Iris versicolor). For all intents and purposes, effects and indications (and botanical morphology) for the two plants are nearly identical.

Wild iris' effectiveness is due to its sub–irritant/stimulant influence. Properly dosed in small amounts, the plant's principle zone is the gastrointestinal tract and related organs. Gargle the tincture in a small amount of water as a sialagogue if plagued by dry mouth, receding gums, and generally poor oral health. Although Prickly ash bark tincture, swished in the mouth, will more quickly stimulate saliva production, Wild iris' consistent use will prove deeper affecting and longer lasting.

As a visceral organ enlivener the plant is significant. Its action is two–fold: superficially it stimulates the gastrointestinal tissues via topical contact, but more profoundly, Wild iris increases both pancreatic and hepatic secretions. This combination makes the plant specific for individuals suffering from poor fat digestion/assimilation with general nutrient malabsorption. Candidates for Wild iris are plagued by frontal headache, nausea, and even skin rashes after rich and fatty meals. Dietary–related liver/gallbladder tenderness, area fullness, and sporadic clay/light–colored stools are a number of other related symptoms that indicate its use.

Although there are few if any studies that report on Wild iris' thyroid effects, the plant should not be over looked as a constitutional medicine for hypo–tendencies, be the dysfunction autoimmune related or otherwise. The plant's glandular influences are likely not due to a direct thyroid effect, but rather a liver influence. It is possible that Wild iris augments tissue sensitivity to T_3 or T_4. What is known is that Wild iris' benefit is mostly seen in

WILD IRIS

individuals with a slowed metabolism, cool and dry skin, reduced digestive transit time, and general malaise – all hypothyroidal symptoms. For said issues it also combines well with Oregongrape.

The Eclectics considered Blue flag (Wild iris for our purposes) a core-influencing alterative and somewhat related to Poke root in use. But unlike Poke root, Wild iris' best indications as a systemic alterative are lymph node swelling, liver–centered dyspepsia, and poor fat digestion resulting in dietary related eczema.

Indications
» As a sialagogue
» Malabsorption
» Dyspepsia, especially from fats
» Hypothyroidism, sub–clinical
» Swelling, lymphatic, from poor visceral response

Collection
Wild iris is a root medicine. Preferably select a pre– or post– flowering stand in moistened soils. The rhizomes grow laterally several inches below the soil's surface, so digging to 1' in depth is usually adequate. In well–established stands the roots are intertwined and found in sizable amounts.

Preparations
Prior to tincturing, Wild iris roots should be processed to some degree. First, either when fresh or after the roots have dried, trim the anchoring tendrils from the main rhizome. Discard these small tendrils, as they are largely impotent. Second, the numerous brown scale–like sheaths covering the rhizome should be removed using either a wire brush, a knife blade, or a makeshift scraper. After processing, the rhizomes should be clean and whitish in color.

It is also important to dry the rhizomes and age them (sealed jar, away from sunlight) for 6 months. This lengthy process lessens the plant's gastrointestinal irritant qualities. When powdering the plant prior to tincturing try not to breath in the powder. Many find it irritating to the eyes, nose, and throat.

Dosage
» DPT (80% alcohol): 5–20 drops 2–3 times daily

Cautions

With over use Wild iris quickly turns from a gastrointestinal/visceral stimulant to irritant. Dull abdominal pain with accompanying diarrhea are the most common side effects from too high or frequent dosages. Severe gastroenteritis is possible with the ingestion of very large amounts. There is little to worry about if doses are kept to the prescribed range. Do not use Wild iris if suffering from acute gastrointestinal disease. It is a strongly acting plant medicine, but one that best remedies functional (not organic) problems. Wild iris is not recommended while pregnant or nursing.

Wild Rose
Rosaceae/Rose Family

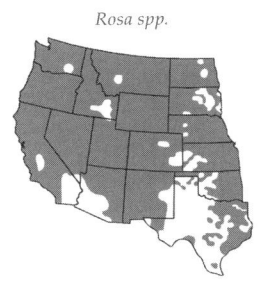

Rosa spp.

Rosa gymnocarpa Nutt.
Baldhip rose, Little wild rose

Rosa nutkana C. Presl
Nootka rose

Rosa woodsii Lindl.
Woods' rose, Mountain rose

Description

Wild rose is a small to medium sized, prickly, perennial shrub. The odd–pinnate leaves are comprised of 7–11 toothed leaflets. The leaf stipules are small and appear wing–like. As a good identifier for the genus, they are found at each leaf petiole's base. The flowers can be solitary or form in groups; they are 5–petaled and pink. Commonly called a 'hip' the fruit is red at maturity. Most native species readily hybridize making identification sometimes tedious.

1'–3' high and sparsely prickly, Rosa gymnocarpa's leaf is comprised of 5–9 elliptic, toothed, gland–dotted leaflets. R. nutkana, a slightly larger shrub and occasionally thicket–forming, can reach heights of 5'. The plant's largest prickles are obvious and form just below the leaf nodes. R. woodsii also reaches heights of 5'. Look for gland–tipped leaflet teeth and prickle sets just below each leaf.

Distribution

Rosa gymnocarpa ranges from British Columbia, then south throughout much of Washington, Oregon, and northern/coastal California. A number of isolated stands exist in San Diego County. Idaho and western Montana also host the plant. Found in a variety of woodlands and shrublands, it's abundant from sea level to mid–elevations.

Rosa nutkana is encountered from southern Alaska and the Pacific Coast states (to northern California), east to Montana, ending its range in northern New Mexico. Look to forest openings and moist flats. The widest ranging species profiled here, R. woodsii, stretches from Alaska, south to California, and east to Wisconsin and Texas. It is common to forest openings, mountain grasslands, and even the disturbed soils of logged areas and mountain roadsides.

Chemistry

Like cultivated Rose, Wild rose contains an array of natural compounds that tend to collect in varying concentrations within three main parts. Leaves: primarily phenolic acids (tannins), flavonoids (mainly quercitin and kaempferol), and sesquiterpenes (if glandular). Flowers: phenolic acids, flavonoids, monoterpenes, and anthocyanins/anthocyanidins. Hips (with seeds): phenolic acids, flavonoids, anthocyanins/anthocyanidins, tocopherols (vitamin E), carotenoids (carotenes, zeaxanthin, lutein), ascorbic acid (vitamin C), fatty acids (linoleic, etc.).

Medicinal Uses

Because Wild rose is therapeutically diverse, I've separated its medicinal uses into two sections. The first section covers leaf/flower preparations. A 50/50 leaf to flower ratio is optimal for the following conditions.

Use the tea as a sore throat gargle. Repeated every hour or so, this application will soothe[91] reddened and painful tissues. Sinusitis and rhinitis sufferers will see benefit in the tea as an isotonic nasal wash. Most find it superior to using a saline solution alone, especially if there is nasal discharge and sinus membrane irritation.

Like Red raspberry and Wild strawberry, women find the tea used as a sitz bath reducing to the redness and inflammation of vaginitis and cervicitis. If there is a microbial or viral component (there often is) combine

[91] Not only do tannins/phenolic acids have mild antimicrobial influences, their topical effect also reduces inflammatory mediators responsible for tissue sensitivity.

Wild rose with equal parts of Sagebrush, Thuja, or Cypress. If suffering from excessive menstruation, due to no particular organic problem, the tea (internal) will be found lessening. Mid–cycle spotting should too respond well to several cups a day. Some women entering into perimenopause find the tea abating to excessive/erratic menstruation. The internal tea combined with the wash or sitz bath is soothing and tonifying to post–partum traumatized tissues.

For mild cases of cystitis and urethritis most will find Wild rose soothing and antiinflammatory. Though not strong enough to counter an acute bacterial infection, try 2–3 cups a day for on–again–off–again urinary irritability.

Another common application for Wild rose is its topical use towards rashes, scrapes, minor cuts, and insect bites. Due to the plant's array of tannins, a tea–soaked towel applied to skin irritation and minor injury will be found beneficial. Relatedly, the poulticed fresh herb or ointment made with the herb tea (instead of water) is of similar use.

Although the tea and/or syrup of the hip (fruit) has value, its optimal preparation is the coarse power, encapsulated or simply mixed with water, taken internally. Consider the hips a concentrated superfood with medicinal overtones, rather than strictly an herbal medicine. Taken for its nutritional aspects, with no medicinal orientation, the hips are an excellent natural source of vitamins (especially vitamin C), minerals, and health–promoting lipids.

Virtually any condition that exhibits inflammation and oxidative stress will benefit from hip supplementation. Reactive and/or poorly healing skin conditions will improve with Wild rose hips: dermatitis, eczema, psoriasis and lingering ulcers, sores, and wounds to name a few. Vascular conditions such as varicose veins and hemorrhoids, whether linked to CVI (chronic venous insufficiency) or otherwise will improve.

Additionally, systemic–oriented autoimmune condition with inflammatory signatures (i.e. Lupus, rheumatoid arthritis, asthma, allergies, etc.) will show betterment with Wild rose hips. As a cancer–preventative it combines well with Turmeric. As a ward against cardiovascular inflammation, use it with Hawthorn. Or if suffering from chronic hepatitis (viral related for example) or cirrhosis its mixture with Western mugwort, Milk thistle, or Tumeric has merit. Really, the sky's the limit with the hips' application.

Indications

herb
- » Pharyngitis
- » Sinusitis/Rhinitis
- » Vaginitis/Cervicitis (external)
- » Menstruation, heavy
- » Irritability, urinary tract
- » Rashes/Cuts/Scrapes (external)

hips
- » As a general nutritional supplement
- » Skin conditions
- » Inflammatory conditions

Collection

With gloves or pruners, strip/snip Wild rose's leaves. If in bloom, collect the flowers too. Not only will they add some color to the leaves but the constituents found in the petals stimulate tissue healing more so than the leaves alone. Dry these parts normally away from direct sunlight.

Gather the hips in the late summer to early fall when they are fully mature (they'll be red and faintly sweet at this point). If gathered early they are overly astringent and lacking in many important compounds. Use a dehydrator to dry the fresh hips. A second option is to purchase dried whole Rose hips in bulk (or the cut–and–sifted grade) and powder them as needed.

Preparations/Dosage

- » Herb infusion: 4–8 oz. 1–3 times daily
- » Sitz bath: 1–2 times daily
- » Ointment/Oil/Salve/Poultice: as needed
- » Rose hip powder: 2–4 capsules (00) 2–3 times daily or 1 teaspoon in water 2–3 times daily

Cautions

Aside from overconsumption leading to constipation, there are no cautions for Wild rose.

Other Uses
Although they're not the best tasting wild fruit (seed–filled/insipid), the hips can be eaten fresh. As a jelly, preserve, or syrup base (and alcoholic beverage), various species are still extensively used.

Wild Strawberry
Rosaceae/Rose Family

Fragaria vesca L
Woodland strawberry

Fragaria virginiana Duchesne
Virginia strawberry

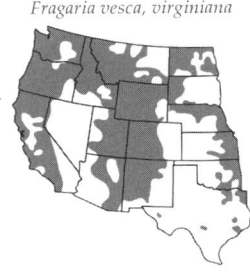

Fragaria vesca, virginiana

Description
Herbaceous, perennial, and ground–creeping, Wild strawberry forms long–petioled leaves and abundant runners. Each leaf is comprised of three toothed leaflets. The 5–petaled flowers are white to cream and uniformly cup–shaped. The mature fruit is ovoid, red, more or less juicy, and ½" or so in diameter.

Distribution
Both species of Wild strawberry have extensive ranges throughout temperate North America and the West. Although largely absent from the deserts, they are abundant in higher mountainous regions. Look to open forest meadows, grassy areas, and along forest margins.

Chemistry
Flavonoids: catechin, epicatechin, kaempferol, quercetin; ellagitannins: castalagin, vescalagin; anthocyanins/anthocyanidins.

Medicinal Uses
As a Rose family astringent, Wild strawberry's application is predictable: use it as a mild, low–level tissue–tightener best applied to reduce surface inflammation. Used in this way, externally or internally, for gastrointestinal, reproductive, or topical issues, this little herb has a wide influence.

Its topical use as a sitz bath/douche will reduce the redness, inflammation, and discharge of vaginitis and cervicitis. Although Wild strawberry is not strongly antibacterial or antifungal, these tissues will nonetheless positively respond to the herb's application. For idiosyncratic heavy menstruation, due to no particular organic problem, the tea, like Red Raspberry, will prove lessening. Specifically, mid–cycle spotting and lingering menses should respond to Wild strawberry's internal use.

The plant's flavonoid–tannin complexes are specific to the reproductive area; in fact, consider Wild strawberry a fair replacement for Red raspberry. 1 cup of tea daily as a last–trimester uterine tonic is a practical dosage/application. Even as a soothing and tonifying postpartum wash/sitz bath, the plant is nearly identical in use to Red raspberry.

For mild cystitis, urethritis, and general urinary tract irritation, the tea is nicely soothing. 2–3 cups a day is especially useful for irritabilities and mucus–tinged urine dependent upon shifts in urinary pH, diet, and other transitory non–infectious factors.

Indications
- Vaginitis/Cervicitis, idiosyncratic (external)
- Menstruation, heavy
- As a last–trimester tonic
- As a postpartum tonic (external)
- Irritability, urinary tract

Collection
Wild strawberry can be tedious to collect, and frankly, it is usually gathered only when other Rose family plants (Red raspberry, Cinquefoil, etc.) are not readily available. Simply snip the leaves (and flowers) from the plant's stem–like runners. Dry these parts normally[92].

Preparations/Dosage
- Herb infusion: 4–8 oz. 1–3 times daily
- Sitz bath: 1–2 times daily

---

92   The herb of cultivated Strawberry can be used the same as wild species.

Cautions
There are few to no cautions for Wild strawberry. Excessive use may lead to some stomach upset – but for this to happen ingested qualities need to be large.

Other Uses
In the wild, berry (aggregate fruit) production can be erratic and is smaller than that of cultivars. However, if discovered ripe and healthy, they will not disappoint.

Wild Violet
Violaceae/Violet Family

Viola spp.

Viola L
Blue violet, Canadian violet, Dog violet, etc.

Description
Most native Viola species of the West are small perennial herbs. The leaves are primarily basal, heart–shaped (occasionally lanced shaped), and have serrated margins. The long–stemmed flowers are composed of 5 sepals and 5 petals. The lower three petals are attached to a sac–like spur. The upper two are banner–like and erect. The flower color varies from species to species: blue, cream, and yellow are common. The 3–sectioned seed capsules are filled with small seeds.

Distribution
The majority of western–growing native species are found in temperate forest or grassland areas. Many are mountain dwellers associated with Aspen and conifers. Viola adunca, V. canadensis, and V. nephrophylla are just several species common to the West. Nearly 120 species are recorded for America. It's a wide–ranging and circumpolar genus.

Chemistry
Viola (general): coumarins; carotenoids; cyclotides; mucilages; saponins; salicylic acid derivatives; polyphenols: flavonoids, polyphenol carboxylic acids, anthocyanins/anthocyanidins.

Medicinal Uses

Wild violet tends to go in and out of favor, taking a generation or two to complete a cycle. Like Scarlet pimpernel, as of this writing, we're somewhere within the ebb phase, but knowing the fickleness of herbal groupthink, this could all change overnight.

The herbage should be mildly mucilaginous and bitter when chewed, this giving a sensory preview of the plant's uses. The infusion is laxative. It's gentle in activity and child-safe. Not quite approaching the strength of Buckthorn or Bitter aloe, there's no need to mix it with an aromatic carminative (to limit anthraquinone griping). Simply drink a strong cup before bed. This is often enough to stimulate gastrointestinal secretions for a bowel movement the next morning.

1–2 teaspoons of the tincture reduces asthmatic/allergy-oriented bronchial inflammation. Alone or mixed with Turmeric tincture, most sufferers find it opening to the area. The plant's diminishing effect on airway inflammation and mucus hypersecretion is reportedly due to its mild suppressant effect on the common offenders: IgE antibodies, cytokines, and eosinophils, among other immunological factors.

Topically, use Wild violet as an ointment, oil, or salve on cuts, scrapes, ulcerations, and burns. Mildly antibacterial, its application fits any condition that needs a soothing vulnerary.

Indications
» Constipation
» Bronchial inflammation, asthma/allergy-oriented
» Injury, tissue (external)

Collection

Gather the above ground portions of Wild violet, if possible when in flower. The roots too can be included (but are not necessary).

Preparations/Dosage
» Herb infusion: 4–8 oz. 2–3 times daily
» FPT/DPT (50% alcohol): 30–60 drops 2–3 times daily
» Topical preparations: as needed

Cautions

There are no cautions for Wild violet.

Willow
Salicaceae/Willow Family

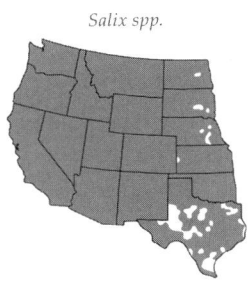
Salix spp.

Salix amygdaloides Andersson
Peachleaf willow

Salix bebbiana Sarg.
Bebb willow, Beaked willow, Diamond willow

Salix exigua Nutt.
Coyote willow, narrowleaf willow, Sandbar willow

Description
Salix amygdaloides grows to be a fair-sized tree. Reaching heights of 35', it displays narrowly lanceolate leaves that are finely serrated when mature. They are green above and paler beneath. The twigs are yellow to grayish. The female catkins are longer than the male catkins.

Both Salix bebbiana and S. exigua are bush willows. They generally grow to sizes of 15'. S. bebbiana's branchlets are purplish to brown and fuzzy. The leaves are obovate to elliptic and reach sizes of 5" long and 2" wide. The female catkins are twice as large as the male catkins. At maturity, the leaves of S. exigua are 4"–5" in length and ½"–1" wide, but when young they are smaller and silver-pubescent. The female catkins are slightly larger than the male catkins.

Distribution
Except for the Southeast, low-elevation Southwest, California, and coastal Oregon and Washington, Salix amygdaloides is common throughout much of the country. It is particularly fond of the moist soils of streamsides. S. bebbiana, also common throughout much of country, is absent from Texas/Oklahoma east to the Atlantic Coast. More adaptive to poor soils, look for it in and around wetlands and next to streamsides. S. exigua, yet another streamside grower, is a dominant western species. From Saskatchewan, Montana, and Texas, it is distributed west to the Pacific Coast states.

Chemistry
Phenolic glycosides: salicin, fragilin, salicortin.

Medicinal Uses

Willow offers its main medicinal attribute, that of a pain reliever, by way of its phenolic glycoside content. The bark tea addresses both the pain of chronic inflammation and acute/recent issues.

Besides its use as a broadly-acting pain remedy, internally the fresh plant tincture made with the immature buds is quieting to irritative conditions of the genitourinary tract[93]. Like Cottonwood, Willow buds soothe urethral and bladder irritation as well as mild prostatitis dependent upon chronic laxity of involved tissues. It particularly excels at diminishing irritation that triggers spermatorrhea; and in both men and women, heightened sexual preoccupation from urogenital irritation/sensitivity (there often is an underlying infection in these cases). During the 1800s it was one of several popular anaphrodisiac (opposite of aphrodisiac) for men.

Indications

bark
» Pain/Inflammation, chronic and acute

leaf buds
» Irritation, chronic, urinary tract
» Prostatitis
» Spermatorrhea
» Sexual preoccupation from genital irritation

Collection

Gather the leaf buds in the early spring. For the bark: find a secondary branch with light, non-fissured, smooth bark. Cut the branch from its attaching point, then clip and discard all of the small branchlets (less than a finger's width). Once started the bark should strip easily. Dry the bark with adequate ventilation out of direct sunlight.

Preparations/Dosage

» Bark decoction: 4 oz. 2–3 times daily or externally as needed
» FPT/DPT (75% alcohol) of leaf buds: 30–60 drops 3–4 times daily

---

93   I apply here to willow what the Eclectic physicians used Black willow (Salix nigra) for over one hundred years ago.

Cautions

Due to a possible synergism with Willow's glycosides, use caution when mixing it with blood thinning pharmaceuticals. The chance of Willow triggering Reye's syndrome in feverish children is incredibly remote. However, I'm mentioning it as a theoretical possibility.

Yarrow
Asteraceae/Sunflower Family

Achillea millefolium

Achillea millefolium
Milfoil, Western yarrow, Plumajillo

Description

As an herbaceous perennial, Yarrow displays finely dissected and feather–like leaves. The flower clusters form in dense panicles. Each inflorescence (white to pink) is composed of both ray and disk flowers. The entire plant is aromatic when crushed, particularly the leaves and flowers.

Distribution

Except for Texas, the western Plains, and low elevation Southwest, Yarrow's distribution is vast. Almost as common as Dandelion or Plantain, it's found in an array of divergent habitats, though disturbed soils, forest openings, and meadows are some of its more preferred places.

Chemistry

Partial list for Achillea millefolium: flavonoids: casticin, santin, apigenin, luteolin, rutin, quercetin; hydrocarbons: n–hexadecane, p–cymene; monoterpenes: camphor, tricyclene, α–thujene, α–pinene, β–pinene, camphene, myrcene, γ–terpinene, terpinolene; 1,8–cineole, linalool, β–terpineol, borneol, terpinen–4–ol, α–terpineol; monterpenyl esters: bornyl acetate, sabinyl acetate, α–terpinyl acetate; sesquiterpene hydrocarbons: α–copaene, β–caryophyllene, γ–cadinene; sesquiterpene lactones: guaianolides, eudesmanolides, longipinenes, germacrane derivatives; proazulene.

Medicinal Uses

Effectively combining elements of an astringent, stimulant, and antiinflammatory, Yarrow serves as a multi-faceted application for an array of problems. The plant's best overall use is as a tonic in conditions where there is tissue laxity due to low regional vitality. In whatever area (urinary, reproductive, or gastrointestinal) this tendency of deficiency that Yarrow best addresses often results in unchecked, yet minor, hemorrhage or discharge.

As an herb for the urinary tract, it best influences chronic conditions. Try the tea or tincture if there is a lingering bladder (or urethra/ureter) infection that seems on the verge of resolving, but only renews at the slightest stress or dietary relapse. Relatedly, Yarrow is specific for mucus tinged urine (usually due to infection) and/or hematuria (blood in the urine) with accompanying pain and irritation.

For women, if menorrhagia is due to atony, be it too lengthy periods or mid-cycle spotting, the plant usually lessens blood flow. Several of Yarrow's flavonoids do have at least some influence over estrogen receptor sites; along with the plant's phenolic glycoside-based astringency, this could partly explain its influence of the reproductive environment. Although not as strong as other plants with spasmolytic qualities, i.e. Baneberry or Western peony, Yarrow used when there is dysmenorrhea will prove pain relieving. For chronic vaginitis, both as a sitz bath and internally, it's a simple yet effective remedy.

The plant's antiinflammatory properties well-accent its tissue stimulant activities. At first glance it appears that Yarrow is a medicinal conundrum. However, many other herbal medicines are a combination of tissue stimulant/sedative, i.e. Yerba mansa, Bayberry, and Goldenseal. For Yarrow and other plants, this is due to an abundance of aromatic volatiles (stimulant qualities) and antiinflammatory phenolic glycosides (tissue sedation). This means that Yarrow makes a choice application when applied topically to poorly healing wounds or imbibed as a tea for chronic gastrointestinal inflammation.

For ulcerative colitis, it's a better tea for the atonic phases rather than the acute flare-ups. However, taking into account Yarrow's astringent and antispasmodic effects, small to moderate amounts of tea will too be of benefit even in acute episodes. Not only does Yarrow address the spasm, hemorrhage, and ulceration of this painful condition, it also lends a protective and healing influence to gastric mucosa. Additionally, if suffering from chronic gastritis and/or ulcer formation, consider the tea specific.

As an aromatic bitter tonic, taken before meals, the tea or diluted tincture dispels atonic indigestion and quiets gas pains. The plant is also a moderate choleretic. Its stimulating effect on bile release assists in small intestinal fat digestion and assimilation.

Thanks to the plant's volatile oil content the hot tea helps to break a stubborn dry fever. Like other stimulating diaphoretics care should be taken if the temperature is dangerously high – Yarrow may cause a slight increase in temperate before promoting diaphoresis. In these cases, the professional use of Aconite, Veratrum, or Gelsemium may be more appropriate.

For toothache pain a shredded fresh piece of the root should be applied to the area and kept along the offending tooth (like tobacco chew). A cottonball soaked with the fresh plant tincture of the root can also be applied to the area, but be careful if there is exposed nerve tissue.

Indications
- Hematuria
- Menorrhagia
- Dysmenorrhea
- Vaginitis (external and internal)
- Wounds, poorly healing (external)
- Ulcerative colitis/Inflammation, gastrointestinal
- Indigestion with gas pains
- Fever, dry skin
- Toothache (external)

Collection
Because the stems lack substantial astringency and aromatics, discard them after the essential parts (roots, leaves, and flowers) have been stripped away.

Preparations/Dosage
- FPT/DPT (50% alcohol): 30–60 drops 2–3 times daily
- Herbal infusion: 3–6 oz. 2–3 times daily
- External preparations: as needed
- Sitz bath: 1–2 times daily, or as needed

Cautions

An occasional cup of tea or dose of tincture poses no issue during pregnancy, but Yarrow used consistently as a daily herb during this time may cause a problem due to its influence of reproductive tissue.

Proceed with caution when using the tea as a diaphoretic in children with high fevers – there may be a temperature spike before sweating commences. In acute gastrointestinal inflammations too much Yarrow may aggravate the situation.

Yellow Pond Lily
Nymphaeaceae/Water Lily Family

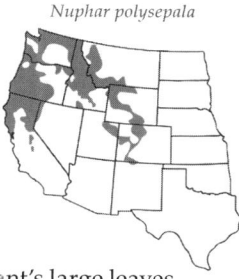

Nuphar polysepala

Nuphar polysepala Engelm. *(Nuphar lutea subsp. polysepala, Nymphaea polysepala)*
Yellow water lily, Cow lily, Rocky mountain pond lily

Description
Yellow pond lily is a water thriving perennial. The plant's large leaves are cordate to oval and usually found floating on the water's surface. They are attached to submerged rhizomes by long thickened petioles. The solitary yellow flowers rise above the water by 1' or so on long sub-surface stalks. They are composed of 5–12 sepals, which surround the smaller, yet more numerous, inner petals. The fruit is a many-seeded capsule. The underwater rhizomes are its most interesting characteristic – at least from a collector's point of view. They rest on the pond's bottom like thickened submerged branches.

Distribution
From northern New Mexico to Alaska, Yellow pond lily is common throughout the Rocky Mountains. Oregon, Washington, and California additionally host the plant. Look to mountain ponds – but any quiet and generally shallow body of fresh water potentially supports the plant.

Chemistry

(Rhizomes): fatty acids: arachidic acid, behenic acid, palmitic acid; trans–cinnamic acid; alkaloids: nupharolidine, nuphacristine, nupharidine, nupharamine; polyphenols: gallotannins, ellagitannins.

Medicinal Uses

Yellow pond lily belongs to an extremely ancient family with near identical relatives once existing tens–of–millions of years ago. That it has gone unchanged for so long may have something to do with its interesting sulphur–containing alkaloidal composition[94].

For women, Yellow pond lily addresses reproductive inflammation and related pain. Good results will be seen with its application to ovarian pain of varying origins: general cycle–related ovulation sensitivity and polycystic ovarian syndrome are two examples. It also gives positive results if used for menstrual cramps, especially if combined with Western peony.

For men, Yellow pond lily also affects reproductive tissues. It is best applied to the dull ache of epididymitis, prostatitis, and other tubular irritations of the region. In times past, this plant (and Nymphaea) was considered an anaphrodisiac (the opposite of an aphrodisiac) to be used if there was an underlying irritation or inflammation that was linked to excessive arousal. Consider its use here (for men and women) if there appears to be an underlying physical disturbance (such as a low–level infection or even a structural abnormality) commingled with a sexual obsession.

As a remedy for urinary complaints, use Yellow pond lily[95] if the passage of urine takes on a burning/scalding quality – usually hallmarks of a lower urinary tract infection. Even though it often reduces both the tissue sensitivity and infection, the addition of any Cypress family plant (Juniper) will further increase the plant's positive influence.

Use it to calm irritative diarrhea (often from stress or poor food choices). Too many chilies, curries, spices, or certain alcohols often elicit what feels like anal/intestinal 'burning'. If plagued by this, use Yellow pond lily as needed. Other intestinal episodes that produce sensations of lower

---

94 Some studies place the alkaloid content of the dried rhizome at .5% – no small amount.

95 Medicinal similarities between White waterlily (Nymphaea odorata), N. alba (European white waterlily), and Yellow pond lily are difficult to ignore. They all have therapeutic histories of reducing urogenital and intestinal irritations/inflammations. Minor differences aside, they all can be treated more or less alike in application.

abdominal sensitivity and pain (spastic diarrhea, colitis, etc.) will respond well to the tea. Additionally, use the tea for diarrhea and related intestinal pain/upset from food poisoning. Here it combines very well with Monarda or even conifer (Pine, Spruce, or Fir) spirit (add 5–10 drops per cup of tea).

The tea makes a soothing and antimicrobial gargle for sore throats. As a sitz bath, use it as an antiinflammatory astringent for cervical and vaginal irritations. If there is a bacterial or fungal element (Candidiasis) consider Yellow pond lily a specific treatment. Here it is best used both internally and externally.

One well known disease–causing strain the plant has some inhibitory influence over is Staphylococcus aureus, a common and virulent bacterium, responsible for an array of local and systemic suppurative (pus–forming) infections. Even Yellow pond lily's inhibition (in vitro) of fungal microorganisms rivals the antifungal pharmaceutical amphotericin b (ambisome or amphotec) in effectiveness.

Although researchers have largely moved on, up until the last part of the 20th century there was a consistent amount of interest in Nuphar's chemistry and pharmacological activity, at least in relation to how the rhizome affects pathogenic microorganisms. Its unique sulphur–oriented alkaloids were a magnet for researchers interested in pharmaceutical development. Even though the results are now in some cases decades old, the findings continue to inform us on the use of this special aquatic plant.

Indications
- » Inflammation/Pain, reproductive
- » Dysmenorrhea
- » Irritation, genitourinary
- » Irritation/Inflammation, urinary
- » Diarrhea, inflammatory/bacterial
- » Pharyngitis (gargle)
- » Vaginitis (internal and external)
- » Candidiasis (internal and external)

Collection
Gathering Yellow pond lily is an unforgettable experience. First, a clean body of water should be selected. This may be difficult due to Yellow pond lily's fondness of stagnant sections of lakes/ponds and the abundance of croplands and runoff in some areas. A small mountain pond is usually the

best choice. Once a site is selected, prepare to get wet. Summertime collection is optimal due to fair water temperatures.

Enter the water from the bank into a cluster of floating leaves. Keep moving until the thickened log–like rhizomes are stepped upon. The rhizomes often form lattice–like arrangements resting on the pond's murky bottom. In mature Yellow pond lily patches the collector can sometimes balance on the log–like rhizomes to keep from slipping into the mushy pond bottom. While supported by the rhizomes, reach into the water and use a hand saw to cut through a section. Once cut, the rhizome part can be broken off by hand, or it can be sawed off with a second cut.

Miscellaneous factors to be considered by the meek are water snakes, all types of insects resting on the pads, leeches, and a seemingly bottomless pit of pond mire beneath the supporting rhizomes. For the diehard wildcrafters out there – this one's for you.

Preparations

Remove the smaller tendrils (anchoring rootlets), dead material, and anything else that may be adhering to the log–like rhizomes. Chop, slice, or dice them into small pieces before tincturing fresh. If drying the rhizome, be sure to cut it into small pieces, or else mold growth can be a problem. Leaving the rhizome in larger pieces is fine if a dehydrator is being used.

Similar to Spikenard, the rhizome resins/aromatics tend to linger on the skin for several days despite washing. If anything, the smell (swampy–sulphur) will serve as a reminder of the past collecting trip.

Dosage

» FPT/DPT (60% alcohol): 20–40 drops 2–3 times daily
» Decoction: 4–6 oz. 2–3 times daily

Cautions

Yellow pond lily is probably not the best plant to be used during pregnancy due to its influence of the reproductive area. Its unique sulfur–containing alkaloid composition is still not entirely understood, at least in regards to how a prepartum baby may be affected. Its use while nursing or with children, in small amounts, is fine.

This plant, particularly the rhizome, tends to be a heavy metal accumulator, therefore harvesters should be aware of local environmental conditions. A pristine mountain lake with no surrounding mining/agricultural activity is a choice situation.

Other Uses

The seeds serve as a fair wild food. Prepared as a ground meal, popped in a little oil, or roasted they contain good lipid and protein quantities.

THERAPEUTIC INDEX

Gastrointestinal

Amebiasis (Barberry, Oregongrape, Sagebrush, Western mugwort)
Candidiasis (Barberry, Hops, Monarda, Oregongrape, Scarlet pimpernel, Uva–ursi, Yellow pond lily)
Constipation (Buckthorn, Green gentian, Wild violet)
Cramps, intestinal (Angelica, Henbane, Monarda, Sagebrush, Silk tassel, Yellow pond lily)
Diarrhea (Alumroot, Apache plume, Bilberry, Birch, Bistort, Fireweed, Fragrant sumac, Geranium, Oak, Ribes, Self heal, Squawroot, Stachys, Western mugwort)
Dyspepsia, asecretory (Aspen, Balsam poplar, Barberry, Bitterbrush, Bogbean, Chicory, Cottonwood, Dandelion, Gentian, Green gentian, Hops, Hoptree, Oregongrape, Pulsatilla, Sagebrush, Toadflax, Western mugwort, Wild iris)
Dyspepsia, with bloating (Agastache, Field mint, Hedeoma, Hoptree, Monarda, Monardella, Sagebrush, Spearmint, Sweet cicely, Valerian, Western mugwort, Yarrow)
Food poisoning (Barberry, Hoptree, Monarda, Oregongrape, Sagebrush)
Gastritis (Agastache, Angelica, Bistort, False Solomon's seal, Geranium, Hops, Rattlesnake plantain, Western mugwort)
Giardiasis (Barberry, Oregongrape)
Hiccups (Field mint, Monarda, Spearmint)
Infection, intestinal (Barberry, Fir, Monarda, Oregongrape, Pine, Sagebrush, Spruce)
Inflammation, intestinal (Alumroot, Birch, Fireweed, Plantain, Rattlesnake plantain, Ribes, Self heal, Western mugwort)
Malabsorption, nutrient/lipid (Alfalfa, Chicory, Dock, Nettle, Wild iris)
Nausea (Angelica, Bistort, Field mint, Geranium, Henbane, Spearmint, Sweet cicely)
Ulcer, duodenal/gastric (Checker mallow, Hollyhock, Hops, Western mugwort)
Ulceration, intestinal (Western mugwort, Yarrow)
Ulceration, intestinal, bleeding, passive (Shepherd's purse, Yarrow)
Vomiting (Henbane)
Worms (Barberry, Hoptree, Oregongrape, Sagebrush, Western mugwort)

Heart

Angina pectoris (Hawthorn)
Arrhythmia (Dogbane, Hawthorn)
Cardiac weakness, with edema (Dogbane)
Hypertension, general (Hawthorn)
Inflammation, vascular (Agastache, Hawthorn, Wild rose)
Palpitations, stress involvement (Bugleweed, Hawthorn, Valerian)
Tachycardia (Dogbane, Hawthorn)
Tachycardia, thyroid involvement (Bugleweed)
Valvular regurgitation (Dogbane, Hawthorn)

Liver–Gallbladder

Deficiency, liver (Buckthorn, Green gentian, Sagebrush, Scarlet pimpernel, Toadflax)
Inflammation, liver (Barberry, Chicory, Dandelion, Oregongrape, Red root, Toadflax, Western mugwort)
Spasm, gall bladder (Silk tassel)

Lymph–Immune–Spleen
Enlargements, lymph node (Red root, Wild iris)
Splenitis (Red root, Wild iris)

Men
Benign prostatic hypertrophy (Nettle)
Debility, genital (Pulsatilla)
Epididymitis (Pulsatilla, Yellow pond lily)
Herpes simplex virus (St. John's wort, Western mugwort)
Irritation, genital (Pulsatilla, Willow, Yellow pond lily)
Orchitis (Pulsatilla, Yellow pond lily)
Prostatitis (Aspen, Balsam poplar, Cottonwood, Nettle, Pipsissewa, Pyrola, Willow, Yellow pond lily)
Seminal vesicle and/or Cowper's gland inflammation (Pulsatilla, Shepherd's purse, Yellow pond lily)
Spermatorrhea (Pulsatilla, Willow)

Metabolic
Acidosis, mild (Alfalfa, Nettle)
Diabetes (NIDDM)/Hyperglycemia (Bogbean, Gentian, Green gentian, Nettle)
Diabetic neuropathy (Bilberry)
Gout (Asparagus, Dandelion)

Mouth and Throat
Gingivitis (Barberry, Monarda, Oregongrape)
Gums, spongy and bleeding (Alumroot, Fragrant sumac, Oak, Ribes)
Periodontitis (Barberry, Monarda, Oregongrape)
Saliva, to stimulate (Wild iris)
Sore throat, general (Alumroot, Apache plume, Arnica, Balsam poplar, Barberry, Bistort, Checker mallow, False Solomon's seal, Fragrant sumac, Geranium, Ligusticum, Lomatium, Oak, Oregongrape, Rattlesnake plantain, Red root, Ribes, Squawroot, Stachys, Sweet cicely, Wild rose, Yellow pond lily)
Sores, mouth (Bistort, Geranium, Oak, Plantain, Rattlesnake plantain, Ribes)
Strep throat (Barberry, Monarda, Oregongrape)
Thrush (Barberry, Hops, Monarda, Oregongrape, Scarlet pimpernel, Uva–ursi, Yellow pond lily)
Tonsillitis (Red root, Wild iris)
Toothache (Yarrow)
Vocal cores, stressed (Ligusticum)

Nervous System
Alzheimer's disease (Angelica, Field mint)
Depression (Baneberry, Pulsatilla, St. John's wort, Valerian)
Herpes simplex virus (St. John's wort, Western mugwort)
Insomnia/anxiety (Agastache, Coral root, Cow parsnip, Hops, Pedicularis, Pulsatilla, Skullcap, Valerian, Verbena)
Insomnia/anxiety with muscular tension (Cow parsnip, Pedicularis, Valerian, Verbena)
Memory loss/Poor cognition (Angelica, Field mint)

Nerve damage (Cow parsnip, St. John's wort)
Neuralgia (Cow parsnip, Skullcap, St. John's wort)
Parasympathetic/cholinergic functions, to suppress (Henbane)
Seizure activity/Tremors/Tics (Cow parsnip, Skullcap, Valerian)
Stress, with cardio involvement (Bugleweed, Valerian)
Stress, with hyperthyroid tendencies (Bugleweed)

Pain

Arthritis, as a counter–irritant (Marsh marigold, Pulsatilla)
Arthritis, general (Aspen, Balsam poplar, Baneberry, Cottonwood, Nettle, Willow, Wild rose)
Arthritis, with constipation (Buckthorn)
Fibromyalgia/Inflammation, with constipation (Buckthorn)
Injury, acute, with pain (Aspen, Balsam poplar, Cottonwood, Willow)
Injury, pain and unbroken skin (Arnica, Aspen, Balsam poplar, Cottonwood, Field mint, Henbane, Willow)
Muscular pain, chronic (Arnica, Baneberry)
Headache, general (Aspen, Balsam poplar, Cottonwood, Field mint, Henbane, Stachys, Willow)
Headache, migraine, acute pain (Aspen, Balsam poplar, Cottonwood, Field mint, Henbane, Willow)
Headache, migraine, beginning stages (Baneberry, Pulsatilla)
Headache, stress (Pedicularis, Stachys, Valerian, Verbena)
Spasm, muscle, from injury (Henbane, Valerian)

Renal–Urinary

Albuminuria (Pipsissewa, Pyrola)
Colic, renal (Henbane)
Cystitis, general (Agrimony, Alumroot, Balsam poplar, Balsamroot, Birch, Checker mallow, Cinquefoil, Cleavers, Fir, Fragrant sumac, Grindelia, Hollyhock, Horsetail, Juniper, Madrone, Mullein, Nettle, Pine, Pipsissewa, Pyrola, Red raspberry, Spruce, Uva–ursi, Wild rose, Wild strawberry)
Fluid retention, cardio involvement (Dogbane)
Fluid retention, general (Asparagus, Dandelion)
Hematuria (Agrimony, Alumroot, Apache plume, Avens, Cinquefoil, Fragrant sumac, Horsetail, Madrone, Shepherd's purse, Uva–ursi, Wild rose, Wild strawberry, Yarrow)
Incontinence/bed wetting (Agrimony, Avens, Cinquefoil, Fragrant sumac, Mullein)
Infection, alkaline urine (Madrone, Pipsissewa, Pyrola, Uva–ursi)
Inflammation, lower urinary tract, weakened tissues (Apache plume, Aspen, Avens, Balsam poplar, Cinquefoil, Cottonwood, Fragrant sumac, Juniper, Mullein, Wild rose, Willow)
Kidney stones, general (Agrimony, Checker mallow, Hollyhock, Horsetail)
Kidney stones, uric acid (Asparagus, Dandelion)
Nephritis, chronic (Agrimony, Aspen, Balsam poplar, Bilberry, Checker mallow, Cinquefoil, Cottonwood, Hollyhock, Juniper, Pipsissewa, Pyrola, Willow)
Pyelitis (Pipsissewa, Pyrola)
Ureteritis/Urethritis (Agrimony, Balsam poplar, Balsamroot, Cinquefoil, Cleavers, Madrone, Pipsissewa, Pyrola, Red raspberry)

Respiratory (Lower)

Asthma, copious phlegm (Henbane)
Asthma, dry, non–spasmodic (Grindelia)
Asthma, general (Angelica, Hoptree, Wild rose, Wild violet)
Bronchitis with copious phlegm (Henbane, Ox–eye daisy)
Bronchitis with difficult expectoration (Angelica, Balsam poplar, Balsamroot, Cow parsnip, Fir, Ligusticum, Lomatium, Marsh marigold, Pine, Spruce, Sweet cicely)
Bronchitis with dry cough (Bitterbrush, Checker mallow, Coral root, False Solomon's seal, Grindelia, Henbane, Hollyhock, Mullein, Plantain, Pussytoes, Wild cherry)
Bronchitis with dry fever (Angelica, Balsamroot, Coral root, Cow parsnip, Ligusticum, Lomatium, Sagebrush)
Bronchitis with flu/virus (Ligusticum, Lomatium)
Cough, dry and painful (Balsamroot, Bitterbrush, Checker mallow, Hollyhock, Mullein, Wild cherry)
Cough, spasmodic (Henbane)
Inflammation, bronchial (Pussytoes, Wild rose, Wild violet)

Respiratory (Upper), Eyes, and Ears

As a general antioxidant, eyes (Bilberry, Wild rose)
Conjunctivitis (Barberry, Oregongrape, Pulsatilla)
Ear ache (Mullein)
Night vision, to improve (Bilberry)
Rhinitis (Agrimony, Cinquefoil, Nettle, Wild rose)
Sinusitis (Barberry, Bistort, Geranium, Oregongrape, Wild rose)
Styes (Pulsatilla)

Thyroid

Hyperthyroidism, mild (Bugleweed)
Hypothyroidism, mild (Barberry, Oregongrape, Wild iris)

Topical

Abscess (Barberry, Checker mallow, Hollyhock, Oregongrape, Sagebrush)
Bedsores (Barberry, Birch, Oak, Oregongrape, Wild rose, Yarrow)
Bites/Stings, insect, general (Alumroot, Apache plume, Bistort, False Solomon's seal, Figwort, Fragrant sumac, Geranium, Plantain, Rattlesnake plantain)
Boils (Barberry, Oregongrape, Sagebrush)
Burns, heat/sunburn (Alumroot, Apache plume, Checker mallow, Figwort, Geranium, Henbane, Hollyhock, Hound's tongue, Plantain, Rattlesnake plantain, Squawroot, St. John's wort, Sweet clover, Wild violet)
Chicken pox (St. John's wort)
Contusions (Arnica, Aspen, Balsam popular, Cottonwood, Henbane, Field mint, Sagebrush, Sneezeweed)
Dermatitis/Eczema (Barberry, Birch, Cleavers, Dandelion, Dock, Figwort, Grindelia, Juniper, Oregongrape, Toadflax, Wild rose)
Herpes simplex virus (St. John's wort, Western mugwort)
Hives/Rashes (Dock, Figwort, Plantain, Rattlesnake plantain, Squawroot, Wild rose, Wild violet)

Infections, bacterial (Balsam poplar, Balsamroot, Barberry, Cow parsnip, Elder, Fir, Gentian, Hedeoma, Hops, Lomatium, Monarda, Monardella, Oregongrape, Pine, Sagebrush, Scarlet pimpernel, Spruce, Sweet cicely, Western mugwort)

Infections, Candida (Barberry, Hops, Oregongrape, Scarlet pimpernel, Sweet cicely, Yellow pond lily)

Infections, fungal, general (Barberry, Cow parsnip, Gentian, Hops, Lomatium, Monarda, Oregongrape, Sagebrush, Scarlet pimpernel, Sweet cicely, Western mugwort)

Lice (Larkspur)

Pain/Inflammation, general (Aspen, Cottonwood, Cow parsnip, Henbane, Willow)

Poison ivy rash (Grindelia)

Psoriasis (Barberry, Birch, Cleavers, Dandelion, Juniper, Oregongrape, Toadflax, Wild rose)

Scrapes/Abrasions/Cuts (Alumroot, Apache plume, Balsam poplar, Balsamroot, Barberry, Bistort, Bitterbrush, Chicory, Cottonwood, False solomon's seal, Figwort, Fragrant sumac, Hops, Oak, Plantain, Rattlesnake plantain, Ribes, Self heal, Squawroot, Stachys, Wild rose, Wild violet)

Shingles (Skullcap, St. John's wort)

Skin/Hair/Nails, supportive (Horsetail)

Soft tissue injury/Swelling (Henbane, Sweet clover, Wild rose)

Ulcers, poorly healing (Barberry, Birch, Elder, Grindelia, Red osier dogwood, St. John's wort, Sweet clover, Wild rose)

Varicosities/Spider veins (Hawthorn, Sweet clover, Wild rose)

Wounds (Barberry, Bilberry, Birch, Chicory, Elder, Figwort, Horsetail, Hound's tongue, Marsh marigold, Oregongrape, Plantain, Red osier dogwood, St. John's wort, Sweet clover, Wild rose, Wild violet, Yarrow)

Vascular

Atherosclerosis (Hawthorn)

Hemorrhaging, passive, general (Bugleweed)

Hemorrhoids (Sweet clover, Wild rose)

Hemorrhoids, bleeding (Shepherd's purse, Wild rose)

Leg heaviness, fatigue, and fluid retention (Bilberry, Dogbane)

Nosebleeds, chronic (Bugleweed, Wild rose)

Raynaud's syndrome (Bilberry, Wild rose)

Varicosities (Hawthorn, Sweet clover, Wild rose)

Women

Candidiasis (Barberry, Hops, Monarda, Oregongrape, Scarlet pimpernel, Uva–ursi, Yellow pond lily)

Cramps, ovarian (Angelica, Baneberry, Henbane, Pulsatilla, Silk tassel, Yellow pond lily)

Cramps, uterine (Agastache, Angelica, Baneberry, Henbane, Pulsatilla, Sagebrush, Silk tassel, Western mugwort, Yarrow, Yellow pond lily)

Debility, genital (Pulsatilla)

Fibroids, breast and uterine (Red root)

Herpes simplex virus (St. John's wort, Western mugwort)

Inflammation/Irritation, genital (Pulsatilla, Yellow pond lily)

Lactation, insufficient (Verbena)

Mastitis (Red root, Sweet clover)
Menstruation, heavy (Agrimony, Apache plume, Avens, Cinquefoil, Red raspberry, Shepherd's purse, Squawroot, Wild rose, Wild strawberry, Yarrow)
Menstruation, slowed (Agastache, Baneberry, Coral root, Hedeoma, Monarda, Monardella, Pulsatilla, Sagebrush, Western mugwort)
Miscarriage, potential with spotting (Shepherd's purse)
Perimenopause (Baneberry, Bugleweed, Hops)
Prepartum tonic (Red raspberry, Wild strawberry)
Postpartum hemorrhage, passive (Alumroot, Bistort, Geranium, Shepherd's purse, Squawroot, Uva-ursi)
Postpartum tonic (Agrimony, Avens, Cinquefoil, Madrone, Pussytoes, Red raspberry, Wild rose, Wild strawberry)
Vaginitis (Agrimony, Alumroot, Apache plume, Avens, Bistort, Cinquefoil, Geranium, Ox-eye daisy, Red raspberry, Uva-ursi, Wild rose, Wild strawberry, Yarrow, Yellow pond lily)

Miscellaneous

Anorexia (Alfalfa, Bogbean, Gentian, Hoptree)
Connective tissues, hair, nails, skin, and bones, weakened (Horsetail)
Deficiency, nutritional (Alfalfa, Horsetail, Nettle, Red raspberry, Wild rose)
Fever, dry skin, low-moderate temperature (Agastache, Angelica, Elder, Field mint, Goldenrod, Hedeoma, Monarda, Monardella, Sagebrush, Skullcap, Spearmint, Sweet cicely, Verbena, Western mugwort, Yarrow)
Fever with autoimmune inflammation (Barberry, Oregongrape)
Fever with flu (Ligusticum, Lomatium)
Fever with moderately high temperature (Aspen, Balsam poplar, Cottonwood, Willow)
Sweating, colliquative (Ox-eye daisy, Red osier dogwood)

GLOSSARY

Abscess
An accumulation of pus (defunct leukocytes, damaged tissue cells, and cellular wastes) within tissues or organs either resolving by coming to 'a head' or diminishing internally.

Acetylcholine
Serves as a neurotransmitter throughout the central and peripheral nervous systems, though it is most closely associated with the parasympathetic branch of the autonomic nervous system.

Acetylcholinesterase (AChE)
An enzyme of the central nervous system that breaks down acetylcholine into choline and acetate.

Achene
A term used to describe a seed common to the Sunflower family.

Adaptogen
A somewhat vague term used widely in the herbal medicine field to describe a plant which is capable of increasing an individual's tolerance to stress. Actions of these plants often seem contradictory, at times providing stimulation and at others, sedation. Ginseng is considered a classic adaptogen.

Addison's disease
A life threatening disease caused by tuberculosis or autoimmune involvement. Symptoms of hypotension, abnormal skin pigmentation, weight loss, and weakness are caused by diminished levels of adrenal cortex hormones, cortisol and aldosterone.

Adrenal cortex
The outer layer of the adrenal gland; secretes mineralocorticoids and glucocorticoids.

Adrenal medulla
Inner layer of the adrenal gland; secrets catecholamines epinephrine and norepinephrine.

Adrenaline
(Epinephrine) Both a catecholamine hormone and a neurotransmitter. It is secreted by the adrenal medulla and is used by the sympathetic branch of the central nervous system. It is a prominent physiologic agent in fight or flight reactions and low-grade stress states.

Albumin
A plasma protein crucial in transporting many organic substances – bile acids, hormones, and fatty acids. It is also important in maintaining proper plasma osmotic pressure. Plasma albumin levels diminish in certain renal and hepatic diseases, and if dietary levels of protein are insufficient.

Aldosterone
A mineralocorticoid secreted by the adrenal cortex. It is involved in sodium/potassium dynamics and blood pressure.

Allopathic
Pertaining to present day conventional medicine when solely used to suppress or oppose symptoms, such as steroids for inflammation, analgesics for pain, etc.

Alterative
Pertaining to the quality, or a substance (usually an herbal medicine) that positively alters organs or functions of elimination, detoxification, or immunity.

Alveoli
(Pulmonary alveoli) Small sacs within the lungs where carbon dioxide and oxygen exchange takes place.

Alzheimer's disease
A progressive brain disease with a number of potential causative factors. Senile plaques, neurofibrillary tangles, and loss of acetyltransferase activity are common. Progressed effects are dementia and personality change.

Amebiasis
(Montezuma's revenge or Traveler's diarrhea) An intestinal infection involving Entamoeba histolytica from contaminated food or water. Usually the large intestine is affected but in severe cases infection can migrate to the liver, spleen, brain, lungs, and other areas.

Amenorrhea
The abnormal cessation of menses, often due to extreme weight loss, physical–emotional stress, or the alteration of ovarian hormones.

Amylase
Present in saliva and pancreatic juice, this enzyme breaks down starches into simple sugars.

Anaphrodisiac
That which curbs libido.

Anaphylaxis
A potentially life threatening allergic reaction. Shock and respiratory distress usually accompanies an episode.

Androgen
Any substance, but usually hormonal, that promotes masculinization. Testosterone and androstenedione are examples.

Anesthetic
An agent that causes numbness or reduces/eliminates pain sensations.

GLOSSARY

Angina pectoris
A particular spasmodic, suffocative pain due to heart tissue ischemia. Radiating left arm pain is a common symptom. An episode may be precipitated by physical exertion and is caused by coronary artery obstruction from plaque buildup.

Annual
Any plant that germinates, then sets seed and dies in one year.

Anorexia
Simply the lack of appetite for food. Anorexia nervosa, more complex than a simple loss of appetite, is considered a mental disorder.

Anovulatory cycle
A menstrual cycle without ovulation.

Antibody
(See Immunoglobulin)

Anticholinergic
Inhibiting to the parasympathetic nervous system. Pertaining to any substance whether pharmaceutical, herbal, or otherwise that lessens gastrointestinal tract, mucosal, and skin secretion and excretion.

Antigen
A substance capable of stimulating a specific acquired immune response. Bacteria and foreign particles are prime examples.

Antiseptic
Inhibiting to the growth and spread of microorganisms.

Antiviral
Inhibiting to virus reproduction or its cellular attachment.

Aphrodisiac
A sexual excitant.

Aphthous stomatitis
(Canker sore) A small white ulcer of the oral mucosa. Stress, immune deficiency, and allergic reaction are common underlying factors.

Apoptosis
The innate process of programed cell death. When operating properly this function is a key cancer inhibitor. Many illnesses are linked to an excess or lack of apoptosis.

Arachidonic acid (AA)
An essential fatty acid intrinsic to prostaglandin, leukotriene, and thromboxane synthesis. It holds a place in both normal cellular process and disease development.

Arrhythmia
Irregular rhythm of the heartbeat.

Asthenic
Weakness; deficiency.

Asthma
A condition of bronchial constriction due to spasm or autoimmune inflammation.

Asthma, humid
Asthma with copious expectoration.

Atherosclerosis
Arterial inflammation in conjunction with plaque deposits. Also known as 'hardening of the arteries'.

Atonic
Lacking normal tone.

Autonomic nervous system
Composed of the sympathetic and parasympathetic nervous systems; mainly involved with visceral function.

Ayurveda
Traditional Indian medicine. Thought to predate Traditional Chinese Medicine, the system describes herbs as having energetic qualities and people being of different constitutional types.

Basophil
A granular leukocyte involved in innate immunity.

Bedsore
Ulcer development from bed confinement. Lack of circulation and continual pressure are factors in development.

Benign prostate hypertrophy (BPH)
Prostate enlargement associated with age and corresponding DHT levels.

Bifidobacteria
One of a number of gram–positive, anaerobic bacteria belonging to the Bifidobacterium genus. Common species found in the large bowel are B. adolescentis, B. eriksonii, and B. infantis.

Bile
An alkaline liquid secreted by the liver composed of cholesterol, bile salts, phospholipids, bilirubin diglucuronide, and electrolytes. It is essential for fat digestion.

Boil
(Furuncle) A painful, subcutaneous nodule with an enclosed core. Usually caused

by Staphylococci entering through hair follicles. Liver and immune deficiencies are common constitutional factors.

Bract
A modified leaf situated at the base of a flower.

Bradycardia
A slowed heart rate, usually slower than 60 beat per minute (although this is considered normal for athletes and young adults).

Bronchitis
Mechanical, bacterial, viral, or allergy induced inflammation of one or more bronchi.

Bronchorrhoea
Excessive lung airway discharge.

Canker sores
(See Aphthous stomatitis)

Cardiac glycoside
Glycosides found in some Cactus, Figwort, Dogbane, and Lily family plants. In therapeutic doses, they are slowing and strengthening to the heart.

Carminative
A term used to describe a medicine that relieves gas pains and bloating.

Catkin
(Ament) A compact male or female, spike–like inflorescence, typically found in Willow or Birch family plants.

Central nervous system
The segment of the nervous system consisting of the brain and spinal cord.

Cervical dysplasia
Cellular changes in the epithelium of the cervix. It is regarded as a precursor to carcinoma. HPV infection is thought to be the main inducer of cervical dysplasia.

Cervicitis
Inflammation of the cervix, either due to infection or injury.

Chicken pox
(Varicella–zoster) A contagious herpes–type virus causing reddened and itching vesicles.

Cholecystokinin (CCK)
Both a hormone secreted by the upper small intestine and by the hypothalamus as a neurotransmitter. It stimulates gallbladder contraction, secretion of pancreatic enzymes, and in response to food it is involved in feelings of satiety and fullness.

Cholesterol
A common sterol produced by the liver and obtained from the diet. It is involved in cell–membrane structure, is a base for steroidal hormones, and is the precursor in bile formation. It is a contributing factor in arterial plaques and in some gallstones.

Choleretic
Either an activity or an agent that stimulates bile production by the liver.

Cholinergic
(Parasympathomimetic) Referring to autonomic nerve fibers that use acetylcholine as a neurotransmitter.

Chologogue
Any substance that stimulates bile release from the gallbladder. Most herbal chologogues are choleretics as well.

Coccidioides immitis
The fungus responsible for Coccidioidomycosis or Valley fever.

Coccidioidomycosis
(Valley fever) The disease caused by Coccidioides immitis. Primary manifestations are cough, fever, and joint pain. The infection is usually self–resolving but can be serious in some racial groups and immune compromised individuals.

Collagenation
The process of collagen formation in cartilage or other tissues.

Colonic flora
Bacterial strains existing in the large intestine, many of which are necessary for gastrointestinal and systemic health.

Condyloma acuminatum
(Venereal or genital warts) caused by Human papillomavirus (HPV). Infectious and sexually transmitted, infection predisposes women to cervical dysplasia.

Conjunctivitis
An inflammation of the conjunctiva, typically involving redness, swelling, and discharge. There can be bacterial, viral, mechanical, or allergic involvement.

Corpus luteum
A temporary glandular mass located in the ovary; secretes progesterone during pregnancy and throughout part of the menstrual cycle.

Corticosteroids
Two groups of hormones secreted by the adrenal cortex: glucocorticoids (cortisol) and mineralocorticoids (aldosterone).

Cortisol
The main glucocorticoid secreted by the adrenal cortex. It is involved in glucose,

protein, and fat metabolism, stress response, and immunity.

Cyclooxygenase
An enzyme or activity involved in prostaglandin synthesis, particularly the inflammatory processes.

Cystitis
Inflammation of the urinary bladder.

Deciduous
Describing a plant that is not evergreen; herbage falling from the plant seasonally.

Dehydroepiandrosterone (DHEA)
An adrenal cortex steroid hormone. It plays a large role as an androgen precursor in premenopausal women and as a major androgen in postmenopausal women. Supplementation in women can be masculinizing.

Dementia
Loss of cognitive ability, memory, and judgement. Alzheimer's disease, stroke, or a variety of neurological diseases are common causes.

Demulcent
A quality or an agent that is soothing and allays irritation of surface tissues. Most in this class are mucilaginous or oily.

Diaphoresis
Perspiration or sweating.

Diaphoretic
A substance that promotes sweating (diaphoresis) or the activity of something that promotes sweating.

5–α–dihydrotestosterone (DHT)
Formed through 5–α–reductase's activity on testosterone, DHT is both an important androgen and one of the main causes of BPH and male pattern baldness.

Dioecious
Imperfect male and female flowers borne on different plants.

Diuretic
A substance that promotes urine excretion or the activity of increasing urine excretion.

Doctrine of Signatures
A philosophy of resemblance applied to herbal medicine popular up until the 17th century. Example: if in some way a plant resembles a heart then it is a medicine for that organ.

Dopamine
A catecholamine–type neurotransmitter, widely acting throughout the central nervous system.

Duodenal ulcer
An ulcer of the upper small intestine or duodenum.

Dust cell
(Alveolar macrophage or Alveolar phagocyte) A phagocyte that resides within the lung's alveoli. They ingest inhaled particulate matter and are important in pulmonary immunity.

Dysmenorrhea
Painful menstruation.

Dyspepsia
Faulty digestion, resulting in discomfort, gas, and sometimes, gastrointestinal tract stasis.

Eclectics
A school of medicine existing up until the mid–20th century, devoted to potentiated plant medicines and the treatment of the individual (not just the symptom).

Edema
Increased intercellular fluid buildup from numerous causes, but typically from kidney or heart dysfunction, or venous or lymphatic obstruction.

Emmenagogue
Something that induces menstruation.

Endometriosis
A condition where endometrial tissue develops in other than normal areas (ex. pelvic cavity). Cyclic pain and inflammation are common symptoms.

Endometrium
Inner mucus membrane layer of the uterus.

Entamoeba histolytica
A common ameboid protozoa; the cause of amebiasis. Severe infections may affect the lungs, liver, spleen, and other organs.

Enteric
Of the small intestine.

Enteric coated
A coating applied to a tablet or capsule specially designed to breakdown in the small intestine.

GLOSSARY

Entire
Referring to the margin of a leaf; not toothed, lobed, or divided, but continuous.

Eosinophil
A granular leukocyte involved in innate immunity; it is specific to parasite defense.

Erythrocyte
(Red blood cell) A main component of blood; responsible for oxygen transport.

Escherichia coli
A gram negative, anaerobic bacterium normally found in the large intestine. The organism typically causes urinary tract infections. Colonization often takes place through poor hygiene and alkaline urine.

Essential oil
The non–polar, volatile oil content of an aromatic plant. Commonly extracted through distillation. Mint family plants are typical subjects.

Essential hypertension
(Idiopathic or primary hypertension) Elevated blood pressure without organic causes. It is largely a functional problem with sodium intake, weight, and stress as the primary causes.

Estrogen
A hormone found in both sexes; necessary for proper female sexual development, reproductive health, and pregnancy.

Eupatory tribe
A division of the Sunflower family. Plants in this division are apt to contain either toxic or non–toxic pyrrolizidine alkaloids. The Brickellia and Eupatorium genera are both in this tribe.

Extracellular fluid
Pertaining to fluid outside of a cell, such as lymphatic fluid.

Fibroid
(Uterine leiomyoma) A benign tumor composed of smooth muscle usually developing in the myometrium of the uterus during a women's 30s or 40s.

Flavonoids
A group of phenolic compounds closely related to tannins; many have therapeutic effects on cell/tissue structure.

Follicle stimulating hormone (FSH)
A pituitary hormone necessary for women's follicle maturation and in men, proper spermatogenesis.

Fusarium
A genus of fungi; a number of species are pathogenic to man.

Gamma–aminobutyric acid (GABA)
A key inhibitory neurotransmitter found throughout the central nervous system.

Gastritis
Inflammation of the stomach often caused from stress, poor diet, mechanical insults, or pharmaceutical side effects.

Gastroenteritis
Inflammation of the stomach and intestinal lining. It can be viral or bacterial initiated, and in some cases, is triggered by intense adrenergic reaction. It is most commonly the result of food poisoning.

Genital warts
(See Condyloma acuminatum)

Giardia
A parasite in humans and in other vertebrates, commonly spread by contaminated food, water, and direct human/animal contact. Giardia lamblia is the most notorious species. The organism attaches itself to the microvilli of the intestinal walls causing diarrhea, nausea, weight loss, and fatigue among other symptoms.

Gingivitis
An acute or chronic inflammation of the gingivae or gums.

Glaucoma
A group of eye diseases caused by increased intraocular pressure. Changes in the optic disk and ultimately blindness occur if left untreated.

Glomerulonephritis
Inflammation of the capillary structures in the glomeruli of the kidney from a residual hemolytic infection or an autoimmune involvement.

Glucose–6–phosphate–dehydrogenase deficiency (G6PD)
A genetic deficiency causing, to varying degrees, hemolytic anemia.

Glutathione
An important naturally occurring tripeptide involved in detoxification and antioxidant functions.

Glycogen
The primary storage carbohydrate found in liver and muscle tissue. It is broken down to glucose.

Gout, primary
Affecting 30–50 year old men and post–menopausal women, symptoms are due to improper purine metabolism resulting in urate crystals forming around the joints and as urinary deposits. If left unchecked it can be painful and debilitating.

Granulocyte
Typically a neutrophil, basophil, or eosinophil that contains immunologic granules that when released heighten inflammatory–defense processes.

Helicobacter pylori
(Campylobacter pylori) A gram–negative bacterium involved in gastric ulcer formation and gastritis.

Hematuria
Blood in the urine.

Hemolysis
The collapse of red blood cell membranes resulting in the liberation of hemoglobin. This can be caused from a myriad of factors but most predominantly, it is triggered by autoimmune reaction, snake venom, microorganisms, and some plant saponins.

Hemolysis, intravascular
Severe red blood cell breakdown within blood vessels.

Hemorrhoids
A varicosity affecting the anal region.

Hemostatic
An activity or something that slows or stops blood flow; typically astringents or other substances that have a localized or systemic vasoconstrictive effect.

Hepatitis C
Inflammation of the liver caused by the hepatitis C virus. This chronic infection is typically the result of contaminated blood transfusions or intravenous drug use.

Hepatocyte
A liver cell.

Herbaceous
Herb–like. Describing a plant or a portion of a plant that is non–woody.

Herpes zoster
(See Shingles)

Homeopathy
A system of medicine founded by Samuel Hahnemann. 'Like treats like' and infinitesimal doses are hallmarks of this system.

Human papillomavirus (HPV)
A significant group of viruses responsible for common and genital warts, cervical dysplasia, and most cases of cervical cancer.

Hyaluronidase
A class of enzymes that breakdown hyaluronic acid. They occur naturally in

various tissues and in bee and snake venoms. It is surmised one reason Echinacea is useful in limiting some of the deleterious effects of snakebite is through its antihyaluronidase activity.

Hydrochloric acid (HCL)
Solutions of hydrogen chloride secreted by gastric parietal cells in response to hormonal, local, or nervous system stimulation; necessary for initial protein breakdown in the stomach.

Hydrophilic
(See hygroscopic)

Hydrophobic
Insoluble in water; lacking polar constituents.

Hygroscopic
Absorbing water or having water–interacting polar groups.

Hyperglycemia
Elevated blood glucose levels.

Hyperglycemia, post–prandial
Elevated blood glucose levels after meals.

Hypertension
(See Essential hypertension)

Hypoglycemia
Lowered blood glucose levels.

Immunoglobulin
A specific immune system molecule (IgM, IgG, IgA, IgD, and IgE) that interacts only with a particular antigen. They are classed by individual function.

Immunoglobulin E (IgE)
An antibody that has a significant role in the allergic process.

Influenza
(Flu) A highly variable group of RNA viruses belonging to a single sub–type. They affect both people (usually the young and old) and animals.

Insomnia
Inability to sleep.

Insulin dependent diabetes mellitus (IDDM)
(Juvenile onset or Type I) Onset usually occurs in late childhood or in the early teens and is characterized by the destruction of the pancreatic beta cells by viral infection or autoimmune reaction. There is some genetic predisposition as well. Lack of endogenous insulin is the hallmark of IDDM. Reliance upon exogenous insulin is

necessary, otherwise hyperglycemia and corresponding problems result. IDDM is difficult to treat solely with natural therapies.

Interleukin
A broad group of immunologic compounds (cytokines), of which many are produced by T–lymphocytes and macrophages. They are involved in an array of immunologic activities, including inflammatory responses.

Intermittent claudication
Usually dependent upon atherosclerosis and/or smoking, this lack of circulation to the extremities causes pain, cramping, and numbness.

Interstitial cystitis
Chronic inflammation of urinary/bladder tissue. Research points to bladder wall dysfunction/damage.

Interstitial fluid
Fluid between cells or tissue, as opposed to intracellular fluid.

Intraocular pressure
Pressure within the eye. When elevated it is associated with glaucoma.

Involucre
A whorl of bracts at the base of a flower.

Ischemia
Lack of blood in an area. Often due to blood vessel constriction or damage (atherosclerosis).

Isotonic
A solution that has the same tonicity as the tissues that are exposed to the solution. Most notable are eyewash solutions that have roughly the same tonicity/salinity as ocular membranes or tears.

Keratin
The main protein group that forms the skin, hair, and nails.

Keratinocyte
(Malpighian cell) A keratin producing epidermal cell.

Kupffer cell
A line of phagocytic cells residing in the liver.

Lactobacillus
A genus of naturally occurring bacteria found in the mouth, intestine, and vagina. In proper concentrations the bacteria plays a role in surrounding tissue health.

Lanceolate
Widest below the middle; narrow and tapering to the tip.

Latex
A milky sap from a plant.

Leukocyte
(White blood cell) A granular or non–granular type cell, largely involved in immunologic processes.

Leukotriene
A group of immunologically active compounds responsible for leucocyte movement and inflammatory responses.

Lipolysis
The breakdown of fat.

Lithiasis
The formation of urinary tract deposits/concretions.

Litholysis
The breakdown of urinary tract deposits.

Low density lipoprotein (LDL)
A group of lipoproteins involved in the transport of cholesterol from the liver to peripheral tissues. Elevated levels usually reflect poorly on cardiovascular health.

Luteinizing hormone (LH)
A pituitary hormone that promotes ovulation and progesterone secretion. In men, it is important in the formation of the teste's Leydig cells.

Lymphocyte
Divided into T–lymphocytes and B–lymphocytes they are responsible for humoral and cellular immunity. Closely associated with acquired immunity.

Macrophage
A mononuclear phagocyte widely distributed throughout varying tissues. It comprises one of the first lines of defense in response to pathogens; part of the body's innate cellular immunity.

Malaria
An infectious disease caused by the protozoa genus Plasmodium. It is transmitted through mosquito bites.

Mast cell
Intrinsic to the inflammatory–allergic response, these cells release histamine and heparin containing granules.

Melanocyte
Surface skin cells that synthesize the pigment melanin.

GLOSSARY

Menopause
The cessation of menstruation due to insufficient reproductive hormones. Naturally occurring in the 4th or 5th decade.

Menorrhagia
Excessive menstruation.

Menorrhalgia
(See Dysmenorrhea)

Menorrhea
Normal menstruation.

Micrococcus
A genus of gram–positive bacterial; found in soil, water, and dairy products.

Microsporum
A genus of ringworm–type fungi causing skin and hair infections.

Microvasculature
The finer circulatory vessels of the body.

Mineralocorticoids
Mainly aldosterone secreted by the adrenal cortex necessary in proper water and electrolyte balance. This group of adrenal hormones causes water and sodium retention and potassium loss.

Monoamine oxidase
Enzymes responsible for the breakdown of an array neurotransmitters or similar agents, i.e. serotonin, norepinephrine.

Monocyte
These phagocytic leukocytes are formed within bone marrow and eventually migrate to tissues where they develop into macrophages.

Monoecious
Separate male and female flowers borne on the same plant.

Montezuma's revenge
(See Amebiasis)

Mucin
The main component of mucus; composed of glycoproteins, glycolipids, and polysaccharides.

Mucor
A genus of fungi. Many species form on decaying bread; some are pathogenic to humans.

Mucus
Composed of mucin, inorganic salts, and leukocytes. Secreted by mucus membranes and is necessary for proper functioning of many organs and tissue groups.

Multiple sclerosis
A disease where demyelination of white (sometimes gray as well) matter in the central nervous system causes weakness, incoordination, and other CNS disturbances. There is a significant autoimmune component.

Mutagenic
Causing genetic change. A description applied especially to cancer–causing agents.

Myasthenia gravis
An autoimmune disorder affecting acetylcholine receptor sites. Symptoms of fatigue and muscular weakness, especially affecting the eyes, face, and throat are common.

Mycobacterium
A large family of gram–positive bacteria. A number of species are pathogenic, causing diseases such as tuberculosis and leprosy.

Natural killer cells (NK cells)
Large, granular lymphocytes which play a significant part in innate immunity.

Nephritis
Inflammation of the kidneys.

Nephron
A functional unit of the kidney. The majority of renal activities are carried out by nephrons.

Nightshade alkaloids
Alkaloids found in the Nightshade family. Many of these compounds have profound anticholinergic effects. Atropine and scopolamine are two of these compounds that are still used in conventional medicine.

Nocturnal emission
(See Spermatorrhea)

Non–insulin dependent diabetes mellitus (NIDDM)
(Adult onset or Type II) Chronic hyperglycemia as a result of a sedentary lifestyle, poor dietary choices, and genetics. Typically, insulin levels are normal or even elevated. The situation is closely related to the notorious 'Syndrome X'. If insulin sensitivity is left impaired, cardiovascular and peripheral nervous system disturbances can ensue.

Norepinephrine
(Noradrenaline) A catecholamine acting as a hormone and neurotransmitter. Secreted by the adrenal medulla and the sympathetic nervous system, it is largely involved in stress (fight or flight) reactions.

GLOSSARY

Oblanceolate
Lance shaped, but slightly rounded towards the end of the leaf and narrower towards the leaf stem.

Obovate
Egg–shaped.

Oncotic pressure
The force that counterbalances capillary blood pressure.

Orthostatic hypotension
A fall in blood pressure and associated sensations when quickly standing or moving from a static position.

Panicles
Flowers maturing in branched groupings from the bottom of the cluster, up.

Parasympathetic
The cholinergic branch of the autonomic nervous system involved in rest, repair, and nutritive functions of the body.

Parenchymal cells
Functional cells of an organ or group of tissues, as opposed to structural cells.

Pelvic inflammatory disease (PID)
A description of general inflammation of the reproductive area in women. STDs are the most common cause. Associated with endometriosis and infertility.

Pepsin
A proteolytic enzyme derived from pepsinogen by hydrochloric acid. It is responsible for the bulk of gastric protein breakdown.

Perennial
A plant that lives three years or more.

Perimenopause
The period before menopause when reproductive hormones and their effects within the body become irregular.

Periodontitis
Inflammation of the tissues surrounding the teeth. Often a progression of chronic gingivitis, it can ultimately cause tooth and bone loss.

Peripheral
Away from the center.

Peripheral vascular disease
Vascular disturbance of the larger non–trunk circulatory vessels. Usually associated with atherosclerosis, ischemia, and thrombosis

Peristalsis
The wave-like contraction of the alimentary canal and other tubular organs/ducts which serve to move contents.

Petiole
A leaf stalk.

Phagocytosis
A process by which white blood cells – macrophages and neutrophils – engulf and eliminate particulate material or microorganisms deemed harmful to the internal environment.

Pharyngitis
Inflammation of the pharynx.

Pimple
A pustule usually on the upper parts of the body, commonly a result of Acne vulgaris.

Pinnae
(Pinna) a leaflet of a pinnate leaf.

Pinnate
A compound leaf with leaflets arranged on both sides of the axis.

Pinnatifid
Pinnately cleft, narrow lobes of a leaf not reaching the mid–vein.

Pinworms
(Enterobius vermicularis, formally called Ascaris vermicularis or Oxyuris vermicularis) Nematode type worms that can colonize the upper large intestine. Common in children and causes anal itching. Infection can occasionally spread to female genitals and bladder.

Pistillate
Used to describe a female flower. A flower lacking stamens.

Placenta
A temporary organ that forms between the mother and fetus. It provides blood borne nutrients, hormones, and other necessary substances for the fetus's development.

Plasmodium falciparum
The main protozoa that causes malaria.

Platelet activating factor (PAF)
A compound produced by an array of immunologic and tissue cells designed to stimulate certain immune functions, platelet aggregation, inflammation, and allergic response.

Platelet aggregation
The clumping together of platelets often triggered by injury or a number of metabolic syndromes.

Pleurisy
An acute or chronic inflammation of the lung and thoracic cavity's serous membrane or pleura. Fever, dry cough, and stitch in the side are common symptoms.

Portal vein
The vein that carries enriched blood from the digestive organs to the liver.

Postpartum
(Postnatal) The period following birth. During this time (4–6 weeks) the mother's body is returning to pre–pregnancy conditions while the newborn adapts to external life.

Progesterone
A reproductive hormone secreted by the corpus luteum, placenta, and in small quantities, by the adrenal cortex. Aside from uterine preparatory and pregnancy sustaining effects, altered circulating levels of the hormone is a factor in premenstrual discomforts and menstrual cycle irregularities.

Prolactin
Traditionally defined as a hormone secreted by the anterior pituitary responsible for lactation. Research suggests the hormone has a broader role in chronic stress states.

Prostaglandin
A diverse group of naturally occurring compounds involved in a wide array of physiological responses. Many are pro–inflammatory, cellular excitants.

Prostatitis
Inflammation of the prostate.

Proteolytic enzyme
An enzyme that breaks down protein into smaller polypeptides by splitting peptide bonds. In supplement form they are used as digestive aids and as antiinflammatories.

Protozoa
Simple, single celled organisms; many are parasitic.

Psoriasis
A syndrome of inflammation and excessive cellular production affecting the skin, joints, and even nails. Red and scaly patches of skin called psoriatic plaques are common. Cause of the disease is an issue of debate. Both autoimmune reaction and excessive growth of skin cells have been implicated as possible factors.

Psychosomatic
Having physical symptoms that originate from the mind or emotions.

Pubescent
Hair–like quality.

Pyorrhea
(See Periodontitis)

Pyrrolizidine alkaloids
A group of compounds common in the Sunflower and Borage families responsible for liver inflammation and subsequent hepatocyte breakdown.

Raceme
An unbranched, elongated group of flowers with pedicels.

Raynaud's syndrome and disease
Severity seems to be the main dividing line between the two types. Vasoconstriction of the smaller vessels in the extremities, resulting in discolored, painful, and cold fingers and/or toes. In severe cases ulceration and infection can develop. Smoking and stress are the main aggravators.

5–α–reductase
The enzyme responsible for the conversion of testosterone to DHT.

Reye's syndrome
Usually occurring as a result of an acute viral infection (often respiratory centered or associated with chicken pox). Fever, vomiting, elevated liver enzyme levels, and brain swelling are common. This childhood syndrome is rare, but can result in seizures and death. Aspirin use in febrile conditions has been linked as a possible factor.

Rheumatoid arthritis
Chronic joint inflammation usually affecting the hands and feet. It is autoimmune mediated and if left untreated leads to lack of mobility and joint deformation.

Rhinitis
Inflammation of nasal mucus membranes; a typical hayfever response.

Ringworm
A non–specific term for a fungal infection affecting the skin. Often developing in a ring–like pattern, numerous fungal strains are causative agents.

Roundworm
(Nematode) An organism from the nematode class; many are intestinal parasites.

Rubefacient
Something that reddens the skin, usually through vasodilation.

Salmonella
A genus of gram–negative bacteria. Many species cause food poisoning.

Samara
A winged fruit, common in the Fraxinus and Ailanthus genera.

Scrofula (Scrofuloderma)
A tuberculous or similar infection affecting the skin and underlying lymph nodes particularly of the neck area.

Scrofulous
A somewhat antiquated term; afflicted with scrofula or having a scrofula–like appearance.

Seborrheic dermatitis
(Cradle cap, seborrheic eczema, or seborrhea) A chronic skin condition characterized by redness and yellow scaly patches on the trunk, groin, face, and/or scalp. Allergic and constitutional factors are involved.

Seminal vesicle
A pair of glands situated next to the urinary bladder; their secretions comprise approximately 60% of semen.

Sequela
A complication or condition arising from an initial disease or injury.

Serrate
Designating a toothed margin; saw–like.

Shigella
A gram–negative bacteria in the Enterobacteria family. Many cause severe diarrhea/dysentery.

Shingles
(Herpes zoster) More common in the elderly and immune compromised individuals, shingles manifests as nerve pain and corresponding vesicles over affected dermatomes. Occurrence is normally on one side of the body and is thought to involve expression of latent varicella–zoster virus – called Herpes ophthalmicus when the virus affects the trigeminal nerve.

Simple
An undivided leaf that is not separated into leaflets. Describing an herb used singly, not in formula.

Sinusitis
Inflammation of the sinuses. Typical causes are allergic reaction or bacterial, viral, or fungal infections. Poor tissue health and local immunity are predisposing factors.

Spasmolytic
Antispasmodic.

Spermatorrhea
Involuntary and excessive discharge of semen without copulation; excessive wet dreams or nocturnal emission.

Spikelet
The flower cluster of grasses and sedges, or a secondary spike.

Staminate
Used to describe a male flower. A flower bearing only stamens, not pistils.

Staphylococcus
A genus of gram–positive, anaerobic bacteria; many are pathogenic.

Strep throat
Streptococcus infection affecting the throat.

Streptococcus
A gram–positive genus of bacteria. Most species are pathogenic, notably S. pyogenes.

Streptomycetes
A genus of fungus–like aerobic bacteria. Many conventional antibiotics are derived from this group. A number of species are pathogenic.

Succus entericus
Secretions of the small intestine containing enzymes, hormones, and mucus.

Sudorific
Diaphoretic; an agent that causes sweating.

Sympathetic nervous system
A branch of the autonomic nervous system closely associated with fight or flight/stress responses.

Sympathomimetic
(Adrenergic) Having sympathetic nervous system–like effects (postganglionic fibers).

Tachycardia
Accelerated heartbeat; usually greater than 100 beat per minute.

Taiga
Meaning forest in Russian. A circumboreal forest zone existing below the tundra.

Tepal
A specialized sepal or petal; common in the Passionflower family.

Testosterone
A major male sex hormone produced in the testes. It is crucial for bone and muscle

growth and sperm formation in the male.

Thyroid stimulating hormone (TSH)
(Thyrotropin) a pituitary hormone that is necessary in the thyroid's normal functioning. Low levels can be an indicator of hyperthyroidism.

Thyroxine (T_4)
A pro–hormone secreted by the thyroid gland. It is transformed into T_3 at tissue sites.

Thromboxane
An eicosanoid responsible for platelet aggregation and vasoconstriction.

Thrush
(Candidiasis or yeast infection) Called oral thrush when limited to the mouth region.

Tinnitus
Ringing in the ear. Causes range from local injury to cardiovascular disease.

Tobacco heart
Cardiovascular weakness caused from years of smoking.

Tomentose
Covered by soft, matted hair.

Tonsillitis
Inflammation of the small rounded masses of lymph tissue (palatine tonsils) located near the back of the tongue. This normally occurs through heightened leukocyte activity.

Traveler's diarrhea
(See Amebiasis)

Trichophyton
A genus of fungi known to cause skin, nail, and hair infections.

Trifoliate
Three–leaved.

Triiodothyronine (T_3)
A thyroid hormone responsible for the majority of that gland's cellular effects.

Ulcerative colitis
(Crone's disease) Chronic inflammation affecting the mucosa and submucosa of the colon wall. Symptoms are abdominal pain, diarrhea, and ulceration. Autoimmune involvement is typical.

Ureter
The urinary tube arising from the kidney leading to the bladder.

Ureteritis
Inflammation of the ureter.

Urethra
The urinary tube leading from the bladder to the body's exterior.

Urethritis
Inflammation of the urethra.

Uric acid
The end result of purine (RNA–DNA) catabolism in primates. Gout is a disorder of excess uric acid.

Vaginitis
Inflammation of the vagina. There is usually a bacterial/fungal/viral component.

Vagus nerve
A key parasympathetic cranial nerve involved in viscera innervation. It affects the digestive tract, lungs, heart, liver, and other areas. Certain herbs (Asclepias) stimulate vagus nerve function, particularly when digestive function is depressed by stress.

Vasoconstriction
Blood vessel constriction.

Vasodilation
Blood vessel dilation.

Vermifuge
An agent that kills or expels parasites.

Verruca vulgaris
Common wart. A member of the larger HPV group.

Vertigo
The illusionary sensation of (the body or surroundings) revolving. Often associated with inner ear or CNS disorders.

Very low density lipoprotein (VLDL)
Transports triglycerides from the intestine and liver to adipose and muscle tissues. High levels of VLDLs are associated with atherosclerosis.

Vitiligo
A chronic pigmentary disorder resulting in depigmented skin. A hyperpigmented border may surround these white patches. It is possibly autoimmune mediated with some genetic predisposition.

Volatile oil
Non-polar aromatics that disperse easily through sun exposure or through other forms of heat such as boiling.

Vulnerary
An agent that encourages wound healing.

White blood cell
(See leukocyte)

BIBLIOGRAPHY

Agastache

Estrada–Reyes, Rosa et al. Comparative chemical composition of Agastache mexicana subsp. mexicana and A. mexicana subsp. xolocotziana. *Biochemical Systematics and Ecology* 32 (2004) 685–694.

Hernandez–Abreu, Oswaldo et al. Antihypertensive and vasorelaxant effects of tilianin isolated from Agastache mexicana are mediated by NO/cGMP pathway and potassium channel opening. *Biochemical Pharmacology* 78 (2009) 54–61.

Hong, Jung–Joo et al. Inhibition of cytokine–induced vascular cell adhesion molecule–1 expression; possible mechanism for anti–atherogenic effect of Agastache rugosa. *FEBS Letters* 495 (2001) 142–147.

Lawrence, B.M. et al. Gill. Terpenoid composition of some Canadian Labiatae. *Phytochemistry* 11 (1972) 2638–2639.

Vogelmann, James E. Flavonoids of Agastache section Agastache. *Biochemical Systematics and Ecology* 12, 4 (1984) 363–366.

Agrimony

Copland, A. et al. Antibacterial and Free Radical Scavenging Activity of the Seeds of Agrimonia Eupatoria. *Fitoterapia* 74 (2003) 133–135.

Venskutonis, P.R., M. Škėmaitė, and B. Sivik. Assessment of Radical Scavenging Capacity of Agrimonia Extracts Isolated by Supercritical Carbon Dioxide. *J. of Supercritical Fluids* 45 (2008) 231–237.

Venskutonis, P.R., M. Škėmaitė, and O. Ragažinskienė. Radical Scavenging Capacity of Agrimonia Eupatoria and Agrimonia Procera. *Fitoterapia* 78 (2007) 166–168.

Alumroot

Wilkins, Cornelius. Galloyl glucose derivatives from Heuchera cylindrica. *Phytochemistry* 27, 7 (1988) 2317–2318.

Angelica

Doneanu, Catalin and Gheorghe Anitescu. Supercritical carbon dioxide extraction of Angelica archangelica L. root oil. *Journal of Supercritical Fluids* 12 (1998) 59–67.

Kanaya, K. et al. Effect of food supplement F containing ferulic acid and angelica archangelica on behavioral disorder of dementia. *Dementia and neurological disorders – Dementia* xx (xxxx) 552.

Kumar, Dinesh et al. Coumarins from Angelica archangelica Linn. and their effects on anxiety–like behavior. *Progress in Neuro–Psychopharmacology & Biological Psychiatry* 40 (2013) 180–186.

Lee, Mee–Young et al. Anti–asthmatic effects of Angelica dahurica against ovalbumin–induced airway inflammation via up–regulation of heme oxygenase–1. *Food and Chemical Toxicology* 49 (2011) 829–837.

Lim, Hun Jai et al. Inhibition of air way inflammation by the roots of Angelica decursiva and its constituent, columbianadin. *Journal of Ethnopharmacology* 155 (2014) 1353–1361.

Senol, Fatma Sezer et al. An in vitro and in silico approach to cholinesterase inhibitory and antioxidant effects of the methanol extract, furanocoumarin fraction, and major coumarins of Angelica officinalis L. fruits. *Phytochemistry Letters* 4 (2011) 462–467.

Seoa, Woo Duck et al. Identification and characterisation of coumarins from the roots of Angelica dahurica and their inhibitory effects against cholinesterase.

Journal of Functional Foods 5 (2013) 1421–1431.

Sigurdsson, Steinthor and Sigmundur Gudbjarnason. Effect of oral imperatorin on memory in mice. *Biochemical and Biophysical Research Communications* 441 (2013) 318–320.

Wang, Junzhi et al. The anti–ulcer activities of bisabolangelone from Angelica polymorpha. *Journal of Ethnopharmacology* 123 (2009) 343–346.

Wang, Yu–Wen et al. Inhibitory effects of imperatorin on voltage–gated K+ channels and ATP–sensitive K+ channels. *Pharmacological Reports* 67 (2015) 134–139.

Arnica

Gertsch, Jurg et al. Influence of Helenanolide–Type Sesquiterpene Lactones on Gene Transcription Profiles in Jurkat T Cells and Human Peripheral Blood Cells Anti–Inflammatory and Cytotoxic Effects. *Biochemical Pharmacology* 66 (2003) 2141–2153.

Kennedy, J.F et al. White. Analysis of the Oligosaccharides from the Roots of Arnica Montana L., Artemisia Absinthium L., and Artemisia Dracunculus L. *Carbohydrate Polymers* 9 (1988) 277–285.

Koo, H., B.P.F.A. et al. In Vitro Antimicrobial Activity of Propolis and Arnica Montana Against Oral Pathogens. *Archives of Oral Biology* 45 (2000) 141–148.

Merfort, I. and D. Wendisch. Sesquiterpene Lactones of Arnica Cordifolia, Subgenus Austromotana. *Phytochemistry* 34, 5 (1993) 1436–1437.

Puhlmann, J., M.H. Zenk, and H. Wagner. Immunologically Active Polysaccharides of Arnica Montana Cell Cultures. *Phytochemistry* 30, 4 (1991) 1141–1145.

Wagner, Steffen and I. Merfort. Skin Penetration Behavior of Sesquiterpene Lactones from Different Arnica Preparations Using a Validated GC–MSD Method. *Journal of Pharmaceutical and Biomedical Analysis* 43 (2007) 32–38.

Asparagus

Adams, Michael et al. Medicinal herbs for the treatment of rheumatic disorders—A survey of European herbals from the 16th and 17th century. *Journal of Ethnopharmacology* 121 (2009) 343–359.

Sakaguchi, Yumi et al. Major anthocyanins from purple asparagus (Asparagus officinalis). *Phytochemistry* 69 (2008) 1763–1766.

Shiomi, Norio. Two novel hexasaccharides from the roots of Asparagus officinalis. *Phytochemistry*, 20, 11 (1981) 2581–2583.

Sun, Zhouxuan, Xuefeng Huang, and Lingyi Kong. A new steroidal saponin from the dried stems of Asparagus officinalis L. *Fitoterapia* 81 (2010) 210–213.

Aspen

Pearl, Irwin A. and Stephen F. Darling. Hot Water Phenolic Extractives of the Bark and Leaves of Diploid Populus Tremuloides. *Phytochemistry* 10 (1971) 483–484.

Avens

Granica, Sebastian et al. Effects of Geum urbanum L. root extracts and its constituents on polymorphonuclear leucocytes functions. Significance in periodontal diseases. *Journal of Ethnopharmacology* 188 (2016) 1–12.

Yoshida, Takashi et al. Gemins D, E, and F, ellagitannins from Geum japonicum. *Phytochemistry*, 24, 5 (1985) 1041–1046.

Balsam Popular

Mattes, Benjamin R. et al. Volatile constituents of Balsam poplar: The phenol glycoside connection. *Phytochemistry* 26, 5 (1987) 1361–1366.

Pearl, Irwin A. and Stephen F. Darling. Investigation of the hot water extracts of Populus balsamifera bark. *Phytochemistry* 8 (1969) 2393–2396.

Pearl, Irwin A. and Stephen F. Darling. Studies on the barks of the family Salicaceae–XVII. Trichoside, a new glucoside from the bark of Populus trichocarpa. *Phytochemistry* 7 (1968) 825–829.

Simard, François et al. Balsacones D–I, dihydrocinnamoyl flavans from Populus balsamifera buds. *Phytochemistry* 100 (2014) 141–149.

Balsamroot

Bohlmann, Ferdinand et al. Guaianolides, heliangolides, diterpenes, and cycloartenol derivative from Balsamorhiza sagittaria. *Phytochemistry* 24, 9 (1985) 2029–2036.

Mullin, W.J. et al. Macronutrients content of Yellow Glacier Lily and Balsamroot; root vegetables used by indigenous peoples of northwestern North America. *Food Research International* 30, 10 (1997) 769–775.

Barberry

Ivanovska, N. and S. Philipov. Study on the Anti–Inflammatory Action of Berberis Vulgaris Root Extract, Alkaloid Fractions and Pure Alkaloids. *International Journal Of Immunopharmacology* 18, 10 (1996) 553–561.

Janbaz, K.H. and A.H. Gilani. Studies on Preventive and Curative Effects of Berberine on Chemical–Induced Hepatotoxicity in Rodents. *Fitoterapia* 71 (2000) 25–33.

Ji, Xiuhong et al. Determination of the Alkaloid Content in Different Parts of some Mahonia Plants by HPCE. *Pharmaceutica Acta Helvetiae* 74 (2000) 387–391.

Kostalova, D., A. Kardosova, and V. Hajnicka. Effect of Mahonia Aquifolium Stem Bark Crude Extract and One of its Polysaccharide Components on Production of IL–8. *Fitoterapia* 72 (2001) 802–806.

Maung–U, Khin and Nwe–Nwe–Wai. Effect of Berberine on Enterotoxin–Induced Intestinal Fluid Accumulation in Rats. *J Diarrhoeal Dis Res* 10, 4 (1992) 201–204.

Sack, R.B. and J.L. Froehlich. Berberine Inhibits Intestinal Secretory Response of Vibrio Cholerae and Escherichia Coli Enterotoxins. *Infect Immun* 35, 2 (1982) 471–475.

Shamsa, F., A. Ahmadiani, and R. Khosrokhavar. Antihistaminic and Anticholinergic Activity of Barberry Fruit (Berberis Vulgaris) in the Guinea–Pig Ileum. *Journal of Ethnopharmacology* 64 (1999) 161–166

Sohni, Y.R., P. Kaimal, and R.M. Bhatt. The Antiamoebic Effect of a Crude Drug Formulation of Herbal Extracts Against Entamoeba Histolytica In Vitro and in Vivo. *Journal of Ethnopharmacology* 45, 1 (1995) 43–52.

Sohni, Youvraj R. and Ranjan M. Bhatt. Activity of a Crude Extract Formulation in Experimental Hepatic Amoebiasis and in Immunomodulation Studies. *Journal of Ethnopharmacology* 54 (1996) 119–124.

Stermitz, F.R. et al. 5'–Methoxyhydnocarpin–D and Pheophorbide A Berberis Species Components that Potentiate Berberine Growth Inhibition of Resistant Staphylococcus Aureus. *Journal of Natural Products* 63, 8 (2000) 1146–1149.

Stermitz, Frank R. et al. Staphylococcus Aureus MDR Efflux Pump Inhibitors from a Berberis and a Mahonia (Sensu Strictu) Species. *Biochemical Systematics and*

Ecology 29 (2001) 793–798.
Yesilada, Erdem and Esra Küpeli. Berberis Crataegina DC. Root Exhibits Potent Anti–Inflammatory, Analgesic and Febrifuge Effects in Mice and Rats. *Journal of Ethnopharmacology* 79 (2002) 237–248.

Bilberry
Canter, Peter H. and Edzard Ernst. Anthocyanosides of Vaccinium Myrtillus (Bilberry) for Night Vision—A Systematic Review of Placebo–Controlled Trials. *Survey of Ophthalmology* 49, 1 (2004) 38–50.
Seeram, N. P. et al. Cyclooxygenase Inhibitory and Antioxidant Cyanidin Glycosides in Cherries and Berries. *Phytomedicine* 8, 5 (2001) 362–369.
Yao, Yu and Amandio Vieira. Protective Activities of Vaccinium Antioxidants with Potential Relevance to Mitochondrial Dysfunction and Neurotoxicity. *NeuroToxicology* 28 (2007) 93–100.

Birch
Mshvildadze, Vakhtang et al. Anticancer diarylheptanoid glycosides from the inner bark of Betula papyrifera. *Phytochemistry* 68 (2007) 2531–2536.
O'Connell, Margaret M. et al. Betulin and lupeol in bark from four white–barked Birches. *Phytochemistry* 27, 7 (1988) 2175–2176.
Seshardi, T.R. et al. Chemical examination of the barks and heartwoods of Betula species of American origin. *Phytochemistry* 10 (1971) 897–898.
Williams, David E. et al. Triterpene constituents of the Dwarf birch, Betula glandulosa. *Phytochemistry* 31, 7 (1992) 2321–2324.

Bitterbrush
Dreyer, David L. et al. Cucurbitacins in Purshia tridentata. *Phytochemistry* 17 (1978) 325–326.
Nakanishi, Tsutomu et al. Structures of New and Known Cyanoglucosides from a North American Plant, Purshia tridentata DC. *Chem. Pharm. Bull.* 42, 11 (1994) 2251–2255.

Bogbean
Janeczko, Zbigniew et al. A triterpenoid glycoside from Menyanthes trifoliata. *Phytochemistry* 29, 12 (1990) 3885–3887.
Weckesser, S. et al. Screening of plant extracts for antimicrobial activity against bacteria and yeasts with dermatological relevance. *Phytomedicine* 14 (2007) 508–516.

Buckthorn
Kremer, D. Anthraquinone profiles, antioxidant and antimicrobial properties of Frangula rupestris (Scop.) Schur and Frangula alnus Mill. bark. *Food Chemistry* 131 (2012) 1174–1180.
Lacornbe, Norman R. and Herber W. Youngken. Studies on the Anatomy of Rhamnus lanceolata Pursh and Rhamnus Frangula L. *Journal of the American Pharmaceutical Association* 32 (1943) 193–202.
Leistner, E. A second pathway leading to anthraquinones in higher plants. *Phytochemistry* 10 (1971) 3015–3020.

Bugleweed

Beer, A.-M. et al. Lycopus europaeus (Gypsywort) effects on the thyroidal parameters and symptoms associated with thyroid function. *Phytomedicine* 15 (2008) 16–22.

Román, Gustavo C. Autism Transient in utero hypothyroxinemia related to maternal flavonoid ingestion during pregnancy and to other environmental antithyroid agents. *Journal of the Neurological Sciences* 262 (2007) 15–26.

Vonhoff, Christian et al. Extract of Lycopus europaeus L. reduces cardiac signs of hyperthyroidism in rats. *Life Sciences* 78 (2006) 1063 – 1070.

Xie, Junbo et al. Rapid identification and determination of 11 polyphenols in Herba lycopi by HPLC–MS/MS with multiple reactions monitoring mode (MRM). *Journal of Food Composition and Analysis* 24 (2011) 1069–1072.

Chicory

Ahmed, Bahar et al. Antihepatotoxic activity of seeds of Cichorium intybus. *Journal of Ethnopharmacology* 87 (2003) 237–240.

Gadgoli, Chhaya and S.H. Mishra Antihepatotoxic activity of Cichorium intybus. *Journal of Ethnopharmacology* 58 (1997) 131–134.

Gilani, A.H. and K.H. Janbaz. Evaluation of the liver protective potential of Cichorium intybus seed extract on Acetaminophen and CCl4–induced damage. *Phytomedicine* 1 (1994) 193–197.

Petrovic, J. et al. Antibacterial activity of Cichorium intybus. *Fitoterapia* 75 (2004) 737– 739.

Nørbæk, Rikke et al. Anthocyanins from flowers of Cichorium intybus. *Phytochemistry* 60 (2002) 357–359.

Rehman, Ali et al. Antibacterial and antifungal study of Cichorium intybus. *Asian Pacific Journal of Tropical Disease* 4, 2 (2014) 943–945.

Suntar, Ipek et al. Comparative evaluation of traditional prescriptions from Cichorium intybus L. for wound healing Step wise isolation of an active component by invivo bioassay and its mode of activity. *Journal of Ethnopharmacology* 143 (2012) 299–309.

Zafar, Rasheeduz and S. Mujahid Ali. Anti–hepatotoxic effects of root and root callus extracts of Cichorium intybus L. *Journal of Ethnopharmacology* 63 (1998) 227–231.

Cleavers

Atmaca, Harika et al. Effects of Galium aparine extract on the cell viability, cell cycle and cell death in breast cancer cell lines. *Journal of Ethnopharmacology* 186 (2016) 305–310.

Bolivar, Paulina et al. Antimicrobial, anti–inflammatory, antiparasitic, and cytotoxic activities of Galium mexicanum. Journal of Ethnopharmacology 137 (2011) 141– 147.

Cottonwood

English, S, W. et al. Analysis of Phenolics in the Bud Exudates of Populus Deltoides, P. Fremontii, P. Sargentii and P. Wislizenii by GC–MS. *Phytochemistry* 31, 4 (1992) 1255–1260.

Greenaway, W. and F.R. Whatley. Analysis of phenolics of bud exudate of Populus angustifolia by GC–MS. *Phytochemistry* 29, 8 (1990) 2551–2554.

Tiitto, Julkunen Riitta. A Chemotaxonomic Survey of Phenolic in Leaves of Northern Salicaceae Species. *Phytochemistry* 25, 3 (1986) 663–667.

Cow Parsnip

Adams, Michael et al. Epilepsy in the Renaissance A survey of remedies from 16th and 17th century German herbals. *Journal of Ethnopharmacology* 143 (2012) 1–13.

Hajhashem, Valiollah et al.. Anti–inflammatory and analgesic properties of Heracleum persicum essential oil and hydroalcoholic extract in animal models. *Journal of Ethnopharmacology* 124 (2009) 475–480.

O'Neill, Taryn et al. The Canadian medicinal plant Heracleum maximum contains antimycobacterial diynes and furanocoumarins. *Journal of Ethnopharmacology* 147 (2013) 232–237.

Sayyah, Mohammad et al. Anticonvulsant activity of Heracleum persicum seed. *Journal of Ethnopharmacology* 98 (2005) 209–211.

Steck, Wareen. Leaf furanocoumarins of Heracleum lanatum. *Phytochemistry* 9 (1970) 1145–1146.

Webster, Duncan et al. Immunostimulant properties of Heracleum maximum Bartr. *Journal of Ethnopharmacology* 106 (2006) 360–363.

Dandelion

Grases, F. et al. Urolithiasis and Phytotherapy. *International Urology and Nephrology* 26, 5 (1994) 507–511.

Kisiel, W. and B. Barszcz. Further Sesquiterpenoids and Phenolics from Taraxacum Officinale. *Fitoterapia* 71 (2000) 269–273.

Rauwald, Hans–Willi and Jai–Tung Huang. Taraxacoside, A Type of Acylated Gamma–Butyrolactone Glycoside from Taraxacum officinale. *Photochemistry* 24, 7 (1985) 1557–1559.

Williams, Christine A., Fiona Goldstone, and Jenny Greenham. Flavonoids, Cinnamic Acids, and Coumarins from the Different Tissues and Medicinal Preparations of Taraxacum Officinale. *Phytochemistry* 42, 1 (1996) 121–127.

Dock

Fairbairn, J. W. and F.J. El–Muhtadi. Chemotaxonomy of Anthraquinones in Rumex. *Phytochemistry* 11 (1972) 263–268.

Saleh, Nabiel A.M. et al. Flavonoids and Anthraquinones of some Egyptian Rumex Species (Polygonaceae). *Biochemical Systematics and Ecology* 21, 2 (1993) 301–303.

Vasas, Andrea et al. The Genus Rumex: Review of traditional uses, phytochemistry and pharmacology. *Journal of Ethnopharmacology* 175 (2015) 198–228.

Dogbane

Duprey, A.J.B. A case of mitral incompetency and ascites treated with Apocynum cannabinum. *The Lancet* (1905) 955.

Kim, Dong–Wook et al. Effects of aqueous extracts of Apocynum venetum leaves on spontaneously hypertensive, renal hypertensive and NaCl–fed–hypertensive rats. *Journal of Ethnopharmacology* 72 (2000) 53–59.

Wright, C.I. et al. Herbal medicines as diuretics A review of the scientific evidence. *Journal of Ethnopharmacology* 114 (2007) 1–31.

Walker, Thomas James. Apocynum cannabinum – To the editors of The Lancet. *The Lancet* (1904) 895.

Elder

Ahmadiani, A. et al. Antinociceptive and Anti-inflammatory Effects of Sambucus Ebulus Rhizome Extract in Rats. *Journal of Ethnopharmacology* 61 (1998) 229–235.

Bergner, Paul. Elderberry (Sambucus Nigra, Canadensis). *Medical Herbalism* 8, 4 (1996–1997).

Buhrmester, Rex A. et al. Sambunigrin and Cyanogenic Variability in Populations of Sambucus Canadensis L. (Caprifoliaceae). *Biochemical Systematics and Ecology* 28 (2000) 689–695.

Caceres, Armando et al. Plants Used in Guatemala for the Treatment of Dermatophytic Infections. 1. Screening for Antimycotic Activity of 44 Plant Extracts. *Journal of Ethnopharmacology* 31 (1991) 263–276.

Caceres, Armando et al. Plants Used in Guatemala for the Treatment of Gastrointestinal Disorders. 1. Screening of 84 Plants Against Enterobacteria. *Journal of Ethnopharmacology* 30 (1990) 55–73.

Hernández, Nancy E. et al. Antimicrobial Activity of Flavonoids in Medicinal Plants from Tafí del Valle (Tucumán, Argentina). *Journal of Ethnopharmacology* 73 (2000) 317–322.

Losey, Robert J. et al. Exploring the Use of Red Elderberry (Sambucus Racemosa) Fruit on the Southern Northwest Coast of North America. *Journal of Archaeological Science* 30 (2003) 695–707.

McCutcheon, A.R. et al. Towers. Antiviral Screening of British Columbian Medicinal Plants. *Journal of Ethnopharmacology* 49 (1995) 101–110.

Evening Primrose

Howard, Geraldine and T.J. Mabry. Distribution of flavonoids in twenty one species of Oenothera. *Phytochemistry* 11 (1972) 289–291.

Zinsmeister, H.D. and W. Biering. Flavonoids–glycosides in Oenothera hookeri. *Phytochemistry* 12 (1973) 234.

False Solomon's Seal

Yang, Shun-Li et al. Steroidal saponins and cytoxicity of the wild edible vegetable—Smilacina atropurpurea. *Steroids* 74 (2009) 7–12.

Field Mint

Oinonen, Päivi P. et al. Linarin, a selective acetylcholinesterase inhibitor from Mentha arvensis. *Fitoterapia* 77 (2006) 429–434.

Rao, B.R. Rajeswara. Biomass and essential oil yields of cornmint (Mentha arvensis L. f. piperascens Malinvaud ex Holmes) planted in different months in semi-arid tropical climate. *Industrial Crops and Products* 10 (1999) 107–113.

Tiwari, Pragya. Recent advances and challenges in trichome research and essential oil biosynthesis in Mentha arvensis L. *Industrial Crops and Products* 82 (2016) 141–148.

Fir

Keeling, Christopher I. and Jorg Bohlmann. Diterpene resin acids in conifers. *Phytochemistry* 67 (2006) 2415–2423.

Manville, John F. and Alan S. Tracy. Chemical differences between alpine Firs of British Columbia. *Phytochemistry* 28, 10 (1989) 2681–2986.

Tumena, Ibrahim et al. Wound repair and anti-inflammatory potential of essential oils from cones of Pinaceae Preclinical experimental research in animal models. *Journal of Ethnopharmacology* 137 (2011) 1215–1220.

Wagner, Michael R. et al. Maturational variation in needle essentil oils from Pseudotsuga Menzieii, Abies concolor and Picea engelmannii. *Phytochemistry* 28, 3 (1989) 765–770.

Zavarin, Eugene. Chemotaxonomy of the genus Abies II. Within tree variation of the terpenes in cortical oleoresin. *Phytochemistry* 7 (1968) 92–107.

Zavarin, Eugene and Karel Snajberk. Chemotaxonomy of the genus Abies I. Survey of the terpenes present in the Abies balsams. *Phytochemistry* 4 (1965) 141–148.

Zavarin, Eugene and Karel Snajberk. Geographical variability of monoterpenes from Abies balsamea and A. Fraseri. *Phytochemistry* 11 (1972) 1407–1421.

Fireweed

Granica, Sebastian et al. Phytochemistry, pharmacology and traditional uses of different Epilobium species (Onagraceae): A review. *Journal of Ethnopharmacology* 156 (2014) 316–346.

Hiermann, A. et al. Influence of Epilobium extracts on prostaglandin biosynthesis and carrageenin induced of the raw paw. *Journal of Ethnopharmacology* 17 (1986) 161–169.

Maruska, Audrius et al. Flavonoids of willow herb (Chamerion angustifolium (L.) Holub) and their radical scavenging activity during vegetation. *Advances in Medical Sciences* 59 (2014) 136–141.

Vitali, Federica et al. Inhibition of intestinal motility and secretion by extracts of Epilobium spp. in mice. *Journal of Ethnopharmacology* 107 (2006) 342–348.

Fragrant Sumac

Homer, K.A., F. Manji, and D. Beighton. Inhibition of Protease Activities of Periodontopathic Bacteria by Extracts of Plants Used in Kenya as Chewing Sticks (Mswaki). *Archives of Oral Biology* 35, 6 (1990) 421–424.

Saxena, G., A.R. McCutcheon, S. Farmer, G.H.N. Towers, and R.E.W. Hancock. Antimicrobial Constituents of Rhus Glabra. *Journal of Ethnopharmacology* 42 (1994) 95–99.

Wu, Tao et al. Evaluation of antioxidant activities and chemical characterisation of staghorn sumac fruit (Rhus hirta L.). *Food Chemistry* 138 (2013) 1333–1340.

Zalacain, A., M. Prodanov, M. Carmona, and G.L. Alonso. Optimization of Extraction and Identification of Gallotannins from Sumac Leaves. *Biosystems Engineering* 84, 2 (2003) 211–216.

Gentian

Aktay, Goknur et al. Hepatoprotective effects of Turkish folk remedies on experimental liver injury. *Journal of Ethnopharmacology* 73 (2000) 121–129.

Hostettmann–Kaldas, Maryse et al. Xanthones, flavones and secoiridoids of American Gentiana species. *Phytochemistry* 20 (1981) 443–446.

Jia, Na et al. Iridoid glycosides from the flowers of Gentiana macrophylla Pall. ameliorate collagen–induced arthritis in rats. *Journal of Ethnopharmacology* 189 (2016) 1–9.

McMullen, Michael K. et al. Bitter tastants alter gastric–phase postprandial haemodynamics. *Journal of Ethnopharmacology* 154 (2014) 719–727.

Ozturk, N. et al. Choleretic Activity of Gentiana lutea ssp. symphyandra in rats.

Phytomedicine 5, 4 (1998) 283–288.
Suh, Hyo–Weon et al. A bitter herbal medicine Gentiana scabra root extract stimulates glucagon–like peptide–1 secretion and regulates blood glucose in db/db mouse. *Journal of Ethnopharmacology* 172 (2015) 219–226.
Weckesser, S. et al. Screening of plant extracts for antimicrobial activity against bacteria and yeasts with dermatological relevance. *Phytomedicine* 14 (2007) 508–516.
Wu, Min et al. Iridoids from Gentiana loureirii. *Phytochemistry* 70 (2009) 746–750.

Geranium

Amabeoku, G.J. Antidiarrhoeal activity of Geranium incanum Burm. f. (Geraniaceae) leaf aqueous extract in mice. *Journal of Ethnopharmacology* 123 (2009) 190–193.
Calzada, Fernando et al. In vitro antiprotozoal activity from the roots of Geranium mexicanum and its constituents on Entamoeba histolytica and Giardia lamblia. *Journal of Ethnopharmacology* 98 (2005) 191–193.
Shim, Jae–Uoong et al. Anti–inflammatory activity of ethanol extract from Geranium sibiricum Linne. *Journal of Ethnopharmacology* 126 (2009) 90–95.
Tuominen, Anu et al. Defensive strategies in Geranium sylvaticum. Part 1 Organ-specific distribution of water–soluble tannins, flavonoids and phenolic acids. *Phytochemistry* 95 (2013) 394–407.
Zhang, Xi–Quan et al. Anti–Helicobacter pylori compounds from the ethano lextracts of Geranium wilfordii. *Journal of Ethnopharmacology* 147 (2013) 204–207.

Goldenrod

Starks, Courtney M. et al. Antibacterial clerodane diterpenes from Goldenrod (Solidago virgaurea). *Phytochemistry* 71 (2010) 104–109.
Tamura, Eduardo Koji et al. Inhibitory effects of Solidago chilensis Meyen hydroalcoholic extract on acute inflammation. *Journal of Ethnopharmacology* 122 (2009) 478–485.
Tori, Motoo et al. Nine new clerodane diterpenoids from rhizomes of Solidago altissima. *Phytochemistry* 52 (1999) 487–493.

Green Gentian

Cao, Tuan–Wu et al. Chemical constituents of Swertia yunnanensis and their anti–hepatitis B virus activity. *Fitoterapia* 89 (2013) 175–182.
Dreyer, David L. and James H. Bourell. Xanthones from Frasera albomarginata and F. speciosa. *Phytochemistry* 20, (1981) 493–495.
Reen, R.K. et al. Screening of various Swertia species extracts in primary monolayer cultures of rat hepatocytes against carbon tetrachloride– and paracetamol–induced toxicity. *Journal of Ethnopharmacology* 75 (2001) 239–247.
Zheng, Xi–Yuan et al. Two xanthones from Swertia punicea with hepatoprotective activities in vitro and in vivo. *Journal of Ethnopharmacology* 153 (2014) 854–863.

Grindelia

Ferreres, Federico et al. HPLC–DAD–ESI/MSn analysis of phenolic compounds for quality control of Grindelia robusta Nutt. and bioactivities. *Journal of Pharmaceutical and Biomedical Analysis* 94 (2014) 163–172.
Fraternale, Daniele et al. Essential oil composition and antioxidant activity of aerial parts of Grindelia robusta from Central Italy. *Fitoterapia* 78 (2007) 443–445.
Krenn, Liselotte et al. Contribution of methylated exudate flavonoids to the

anti–inflammatory activity of Grindelia robusta. *Fitoterapia* 80 (2009) 267–269.
Timmermann, Bardara N. et al. Grindelane diterpenoids from Grindela squarrosa and G. camporum. *Phytochemistry* 24, 5 (1985) 1031–1034.

Hawthorn

Degenring, F. H. et al. A Randomised Double Blind Placebo Controlled Clinical Trial of a Standardised Extract of Fresh Crataegus Berries (Crataegisan®) in the Treatment of Patients with Congestive Heart Failure NYHA II. *Phytomedicine* 10 (2003) 363–369.

Ozcan, Musa, Haydar Hacıseferogulları, Tamer Marakoglu, and Derya Arslan. Hawthorn (Crataegus spp.) Fruit Some Physical and Chemical Properties. *Journal of Food Engineering* 69 (2005) 409–413.

Svedstrom, Ulla et al. Into Laakso, Raimo Hiltunen. Isolation and Identification of Oligomeric Procyanidins from Crataegus Leaves and Flowers. *Phytochemistry* 60 (2002) 821–825.

Veveris, Maris et al. Crataegus Special Extract WSR 1442 Improves Cardiac Function and Reduces Infarct Size in a Rat Model of Prolonged Coronary Ischemia and Reperfusion. *Life Sciences* 74 (2004) 1945–1955.

Zick, Suzanna M. et al. The Effect of Crataegus Oxycantha Special Extract WS 1442 on Clinical Progression in Patients with Mild to Moderate Symptoms of Heart Failure. *European Journal of Heart Failure* 10 (2008) 587–593.

Hedeoma

Conway, George A. and John C. Slocumb. Plants used as abortifacients and emmenagogues by Spanish New Mexicans. *Journal of Ethnopharmacology* 1 (1979) 241–261.

David, T.J. and S.C. Randall. Fetal malformations: A hazard of attempted abortion. *Forensic Science* 4 (1974) 71–73.

Firmage, David H. and Robert Irving. Effect of development on monoterpene composition of Hedeoma drummondii. *Phytochemistry* 18 (1979) 1827–1829.

Henbane

Christen, P. Tropane alkaloids: old drugs used in modern medicine. *Studies in Natural Products Chemistry* 22 (2000) 717–749.

Jaziri, Mondher et al. Tropane alkaloids production by hairy root cultures of Datura stramonium and Hyoscyamus niger. *Phytochemistry* 27, 2 (1988) 419–420.

White, Edmund. Poisoning by Hyoscyamus. *The Lancet* xx (1873) xxx.

Hops

Chadwick, L.R., G.F. Pauli, and N.R. Farnsworth. The Pharmacognosy of Humulus Lupulus L. (Hops) with an Emphasis on Estrogenic Properties. *Phytomedicine* 13 (2006) 119–131.

Delmulle, L. et al. Anti–Proliferative Properties of Prenylated Flavonoids from Hops (Humulus Lupulus L.) in Human Prostate Cancer Cell Lines. *Phytomedicine* 13 (2006) 732–734.

Gerhauser, Clarissa. Beer Constituents as Potential Cancer Chemopreventive Agents. *European Journal of Cancer* 41 (2005) 1941–1954.

Heyerick, Arne et al. A First Prospective, Randomized, Double–Blind, Placebo–Controlled Study on the Use of a Standardized Hop Extract to Alleviate

Menopausal Discomforts. *Maturitas* 54 (2006) 164–175.

Monteiro, Rosario et al. Modulation of Breast Cancer Cell Survival by Aromatase Inhibiting Hop (Humulus Lupulus L.) Flavonoids. *Journal of Steroid Biochemistry & Molecular Biology* 105 (2007) 124–130.

Overk, Cassia R. et al. In Vivo Estrogenic Comparisons of Trifolium Pratense (Red Clover) Humulus Lupulus (Hops), and the Pure Compounds Isoxanthohumol and 8–Prenylnaringenin. *Chemico–Biological Interactions* 176, 1 (2008) 30–39.

Schiller, H. et al. Sedating Effects of Humulus Lupulus L. Extracts. *Phytomedicine* 13 (2006) 535–541.

Viesti, Vittoria Di et al. Ethnopharmacological communication Increased sexual motivation in female rats treated with Humulus lupulus L. extract. *Journal of Ethnopharmacology* 134 (2011) 514–517.

Zanoli, P. et al. Experimental evidence of the anaphrodisiac activity of Humulus lupulus L. in naïve male rats. *Journal of Ethnopharmacology* 125 (2009) 36–40.

Zanoli, Paola and Manuela Zavatti. Pharmacognostic and Pharmacological Profile of Humulus Lupulus L. *Journal of Ethnopharmacology* 116 (2008) 383–396.

Zanoli, P. et al. Evidence that the β–Acids Fraction of Hops Reduces Central GAB-Aergic Neurotransmission. *Journal of Ethnopharmacology* 109 (2007) 87–92.

Hoptree

Dreyer, David L. Citrus and bitter principles–V. Botanical distribution and chemotaxonomy in the Rutaceae. *Phytochemistry* 66, 5 (1966) 367–378.

Dreyer, David L. Coumarins and alkaloids of the genus Ptelea. *Phytochemistry* 8 (1969) 1013–1020.

Gray, Alexander R. Coumarins in the Rutaceae. *Phytochemistry* 17 (1978) 845–864.

Horsetail

Amarowicz, R. et al. Free–Radical Scavenging Capacity and Antioxidant Activity of Selected Plant Species from the Canadian Prairies. *Food Chemistry* 84 (2004) 551–562.

Grases, F. et al. Urolithiasis and Phytotherapy. *International Urology and Nephrology* 26, 5 (1994) 507–11.

Gurbuz, Iÿlhan. et al. In Vivo Gastroprotective Effects of Five Turkish Folk Remedies Against Ethanol–Induced Lesions. *Journal of Ethnopharmacology* 83 (2002) 241–244.

Harrison, C.C. Evidence for Intramineral Macromolecules Containing Protein from Plant Silicas. *Phytochemistry* 41, 1 (1996) 37–42.

Veit, Markus et al. Interspecific and Intraspecific Variation of Phenolics in the Genus Equisetum Subgenus Equisetum. *Phytochemistry* 38, 4 (1995) 881–891.

Hound's Tongue

Cordell, Geoffrey A. Fifty years of alkaloid biosynthesis in Phytochemistry. *Phytochemistry* 91 (2013) 29–51.

Reinbothe, H. and K. Mothes. Ureide biosynthesis in higher plants. *Tetrahedron Letters* 25 (1960) 32–36.

Van Dam, Nicole M. et al. Distribution, biosynthesis and turnover of pyrrolizidine alkaloids in Cynoglossum officinale. *Phytochemistry* 39 (1995) 287–292.

Juniper

Adams, Robert P. Systematics of the One Seeded Juniperus of the Eastern Hemisphere Based on Leaf Essential Oils and Random Amplified Polymorphic DNAs (RAPDs). *Biochemical Systematics and Ecology* 28 (2000) 529–543.

Adams, Robert P., Ernst Von Rudloff, and Lawrence Hogge. Chemosystematic Studies of the Western North American Junipers Based on their Volatile Oils. *Biochemical Systematics and Ecology* 11, 3 (1983) 189–193.

Adams, Robert P., Thomas A. Zanoni, and Lawrence Hogge. Analyses of the Volatile Leaf Oils of Juniperus Deppeana and its Infraspecific Taxa Chemosystematic Implications. *Biochemical Systemics and Ecoclogy* 12, 1 (1984) 23–27.

Adams, Robert P. et al. The South–Western USA and Northern Mexico One–seeded Junipers their Volatile Oils and Evolution. *Biochemical Systematics and Ecology* 9, 2/3 (1981) 93–96.

Karaman, I. et al. Antimicrobial Activity of Aqueous and Methanol Extracts of Juniperus Oxycedrus L. *Journal of Ethnopharmacology* 85 (2003) 231–235.

San Feliciano, A. et al. Antineoplastic and Antiviral Activities of some Cyclolignans. *Planta Med* 59, 3 (1993) 246–249.

Tunón, H., C. Olavsdotter, and L. Bohlin. Evaluation of Anti–Inflammatory Activity of some Swedish Medicinal Plants. Inhibition of Prostaglandin biosynthesis and PAF–Induced Exocytosis. *Journal of Ethnopharmacology* 48 (1995) 61–76.

Larkspur

Batbayar, Nyamdari et al. Norditerpenoid alkaloids from Delphinium species. *Phytochemistry* 62 (2003) 543–550.

Burgess, Ian F. Human Lice and Their Management. *Adances In Parasitology* 36 (1995) 272–342.

Cook, David et al. The relative toxicity of Delphinium stachydeum in mice and cattle. *Toxicon* 99 (2015) 36–43.

Ligusticum

Appelt, Glenn D. Pharmacological Aspects of Selected Herbs Employed in Hispanic Folk Medicine in the San Luis Valley of Colorado, USA I. Ligusticum Porteri (Osha) and Matricaria Chamomellia (Manzanilla). *Journal of Ethnopharmacology* 13 (1985) 51–55.

Del–Ángel, Mayela et al. Anti–inflammatory effect of natural and semi–synthetic phthalides. *European Journal of Pharmacology* 752 (2015) 40–48.

Linares, Edelmira and Bye, Robert A. A Study of Four Medicinal Plant Complexes of Mexico and Adjacent United States. *Journal of Ethnopharmacology* 19 (1987) 153–183.

Lomatium

Asuming, Winna A. et al. Essential oil composition of four Lomatium Raf. species and their chemotaxonomy. *Biochemical Systematics and Ecology* 33 (2005) 17–26.

McCutcheon, A.R. et al. Antifungal Screening of Medicinal Plants of British Columbian Native Peoples. *Journal of Ethnopharmacology* 44, 3 (1994) 157–169.

McCutcheon, A.R. et al. Antiviral Screening of British Columbian Medicinal Plants. *Journal of Ethnopharmacology* 49 (1995) 101–110.

Madrone

Robinson, Frank P. and Hernri Martel. Betulinic acid from Arbutus menziesii. *Phytochemistry* 970 (1969) 907–909.

Robinson, Frank P. and Thomas N. McCaig. Lupeol and B–sitosterol in Arbutus menziesii. *Phytochemistry* 10 (1971) 3307–3308.

Wittig, Jorg, Sabine Wittemer, and Markus Veit. Validated method for the determination of hydroquinone in human urine by high–performance liquid chromatography–coulometric–array detection. *Journal of Chromatography B* 761 (2001) 125–132.

Marsh Marigold

Baykal, T. et al. Two oleanene glycosides from the aerial parts of Caltha polypetala. *Phytochemistry* 51 (1999) 1059–1063.

Stermitz, Frank R. and John A. Adamovics. Alkaloids of Caltha Leptosepala and Caltha biflora. *Phytochemistry* 16 (1977) 500.

Suszko, Agnieszka and Bozena Obminska–Mrukowicz. Influence of polysaccharide fractions isolated from Caltha palustris L. on the cellular immune response in collagen–induced arthritis (CIA) in mice. A comparison with methotrexate. *Journal of Ethnopharmacology* 145 (2013) 109–117.

Turner, Nancy J. Counter–irritant and other medicinal uses of plants in Ranunculaceae by native peoples in British Columbia and neighboring areas. *Journal of Ethnopharmacology* 11 (1984) 181–201.

Monarda

Chen, W. and A.M. Viljoen. Geraniol — A review of a commercially important fragrance material. *South African Journal of Botany* 76 (2010) 643–651.

Feng, Wu, Jiaping Chen, Xiaodong Zheng, and Qing Liu. Thyme oil to control Alternaria alternata in vitro and in vivo as fumigant and contact treatments. *Food Control* 22 (2011) 78–81.

Gwinn, Kimberly D. et al. Role of Essential Oils in Control of Rhizoctonia Damping–Off in Tomato with Bioactive Monarda Herbage. *The American Phytopathological Society* 100, 5 (2010) 493–201.

Hart, Jeffrey A. The ethnobotany of the northern Cheyenne Indians of Montana. *Journal of Ethnopharmacology* 4 (1981) 1–55.

Tin, W., N.R. Farnsworth, and H.H.S. Fono. Isolation and inentification of alkanes from three taxa of Monarda. *Lloydia* 32 (1969) 509.

Monardella

Bräuchler, Christian, Harald Meimberg, and Günther Heubl. Molecular phylogeny of Menthinae (Lamiaceae, Nepetoideae, Mentheae) – Taxonomy, biogeography and conflicts. *Molecular Phylogenetics and Evolution* 55 (2010) 501–523.

Tanowitz, Barry D., Dale M. Smith, and Steven A. Junak. Terpenoid constituents of three taxa of Monardella. *Phytochemistry* 26, 10 (1987) 2751–2752.

Mullein

Khuroo, M.A. et al. Sterones, Iridoids and a Sesquiterpene from Verbascum Thapsus. *Phytochemistry* 27, 11 (1988) 3541–3544.

Turker, Arzu Ucar and N.D. Camper. Biological Activity of Common Mullein, a Medicinal Plant. *Journal of Ethnopharmacology* 82 (2002) 117–125.

Warashina, Tsutomu, Toshio Miyase, and Akira Ueno. Phenylethanoid and Lignan Glycosides from Verbascum Thapsus. *Phytochemistry* 31, 3 (1992) 961–965.

Nettle

Bnouham, Mohamed et al. Antihyperglycemic Activity of the Aqueous Extract of Urtica Dioica. *Fitoterapia* 74 (2003) 677–681.

Bondarenko, Boris et al. Long–Term Efficacy and Safety of PRO 160/120 (A Combination of Sabal and Urtica Extract) in Patients with Lower Urinary Tract Symptoms (LUTS). *Phytomedicine* 10 (2003) 53–55.

Guarrera, Paolo Maria. Traditional Phytotherapy in Central Italy (Marche, Abruzzo, and Latium). *Fitoterapia* 76 (2005) 1–25.

Guerrero, Guil J.L. et al. Fatty Acids and Carotenoids from Stinging Nettle (Urtica dioica L.). *Journal of Food Composition and Analysis* 16 (2003) 111–119.

Gülçin, Ùllhami et al. Antioxidant, Antimicrobial, Antiulcer and Analgesic Activities of Nettle (Urtica Dioica L.). *Journal of Ethnopharmacology* 90 (2004) 205–215.

Lowe, Franklin C. and Elliot Fagelman. Phytotherapy in the Treatment of Benign Prostatic Hyperplasia An Update. *Urology* 53 (1999) 671–678.

Madersbacher, Stephan. et al. Medical Management of BPH Role of Plant Extracts. *Eau–Ebu Update Series* 5 (2007) 197–205.

Ozcan, Mehmet Musa et al. Mineral Content of Some Herbs and Herbal Teas by Infusion and Decoction. *Food Chemistry* 106 (2008) 1120–1127.

Sajfrtova, M. et al. Near–Critical Extraction of Sitosterol and Scopoletin from Stinging Nettle Roots. *Journal of Supercritical Fluids* 35 (2005) 111–118.

Testai, Lara. et al. Cardiovascular Effects of Urtica Dioica L. (Urticaceae) Roots Extracts In Vitro and In Vivo Pharmacological Studies. *Journal of Ethnopharmacology* 81 (2002) 105–109.

Oak

Chen, C.L. Constituents of Quercus alba. *Phytochemistry* 9 (1970) 1149.

Feeny, P.P. and H. Bostock. Seasonal changes in the tannin content of Oak leaves. *Phytochemistry* 7 (1968) 871–880.

Masson, Gilles et al. Localization of the ellagitannins in the tissues of Quercus robur and Quercus petraea woods. *Phytochemistry* 37, 5 (1994) 1245–1249.

Scalbert, Augustin. Polyphenols and chemical defence of Quercus robur. *Phytochemistry* 26, 12 (1987) 3191–3195.

Oregongrape

Ivanovska, N. and S. Philipov. Study on the Anti–Inflammatory Action of Berberis Vulgaris Root Extract, Alkaloid Fractions and Pure Alkaloids. *International Journal Of Immunopharmacology* 18, 10 (1996) 553–561.

Janbaz, K.H. and A.H. Gilani. Studies on Preventive and Curative Effects of Berberine on Chemical–Induced Hepatotoxicity in Rodents. *Fitoterapia* 71 (2000) 25–33.

Ji, Xiuhong et al. Determination of the Alkaloid Content in Different Parts of some Mahonia Plants by HPCE. *Pharmaceutica Acta Helvetiae* 74 (2000) 387–391.

Khin–Maung–U and Nwe–Nwe–Wai. Effect of Berberine on Enterotoxin–Induced Intestinal Fluid Accumulation in Rats. *J Diarrhoeal Dis Res* 10, 4 (1992) 201–204.

Kostalova, D., A. Kardosova, and V. Hajnicka. Effect of Mahonia Aquifolium Stem Bark Crude Extract and One of its Polysaccharide Components on Production of IL–8. *Fitoterapia* 72 (2001) 802–806.

Sack, R.B. and J.L. Froehlich. Berberine Inhibits Intestinal Secretory Response of Vibrio Cholerae and Escherichia Coli Enterotoxins. *Infect Immun* 35, 2 (1982) 471–475.
Shamsa, F., A. Ahmadiani, and R. Khosrokhavar. Antihistaminic and Anticholinergic Activity of Barberry Fruit (Berberis Vulgaris) in the Guinea–Pig Ileum. *Journal of Ethnopharmacology* 64 (1999) 161–166
Sohni, Y.R., P. Kaimal, and R.M. Bhatt. The Antiamoebic Effect of a Crude Drug Formulation of Herbal Extracts Against Entamoeba Histolytica In Vitro and In Vivo. *Journal of Ethnopharmacology* 45, 1 (1995) 43–52.
Sohni, Youvraj R. and Ranjan M. Bhatt. Activity of a Crude Extract Formulation in Experimental Hepatic Amoebiasis and in Immunomodulation Studies. *Journal of Ethnopharmacology* 54 (1996) 119–124.
Stermitz, F.R. et al. 5′–Methoxyhydnocarpin–D and Pheophorbide A Berberis Species Components That Potentiate Berberine Growth Inhibition of Resistant Staphylococcusaureus. *Journal of Natural Products* 63, 8 (2000) 1146–1149.
Stermitz, Frank R. et al. Staphylococcus Aureus MDR Effux Pump Inhibitors from a Berberis and a Mahonia (Sensu Strictu) Species. *Biochemical Systematics and Ecology* 29 (2001) 793–798.
Yesilada, Erdem and Esra Küpeli. Berberis Crataegina DC. Root Exhibits Potent Anti–Inflammatory, Analgesic and Febrifuge Effects in Mice and Rats. *Journal of Ethnopharmacology* 79 (2002) 237–248.

Ox–Eye Daisy

Wilcox, Balafama H.R. Favonoid Distribution Patterns in Leucanthemum and Related Species from North Africa. *Biochemical Systematics and Ecology* 1, 4 (1984) 357–361.
Wrang, Per A. and Jorgen Lam. Polyacetylenes from Chrysanthemum leucanthemum. *Phytochemistry* 14 (1975) 1027–1035.

Pedicularis

Berg, Thomas et al. Iridoid glucosides from Pedicularis. *Phytochemistry* 24, 3 (1985) 491–493.
Bao–Ning, Su et al. Neolignan, phenylpropanoid and iridoid glycosides from Pedicularis verticillata. *Phytochemistry* 45, 6 (1997) 1271–1273.
Schneider, Marilyn J. et al. Proceroside, an iridoid glucoside from Pedicularis procera. *Phytochemistry* 46, 6 (1997) 1097–1098.
Schneider, Marilyn J. et al. Uptake of host plant alkaloids by root parasitic Pedicularis species. *Phytochemistry* 29, 6 (1990) 1811–1814.
Singh, K.N. and Brij Lal. Ethnomedicines used against four common ailments by the tribal communities of Lahaul–Spiti in western Himalaya. *Journal of Ethnopharmacology* 115 (2008) 147–159.

Pine

Anderson, B. et al. Monoterpenes, fatty acids, and resin acids of Pinus edulis and Pinus albicaulis. *Phytochemistry* 8 (1969) 1999–2001.
Bobalek, John F. and Morris A. Johnson. Arabinogalactan–proteins from Douglas fir and Loblolly pine. *Phytochemistry* 22, 6 (1983) 1500–1503.
Haberer, Kristine, Lutz Jaeger, and Heinz Rennenberg. Seasonal patterns of ascorbate in the needles of Scots Pine (Pinus sylvestris L.) trees Correlation analyses

with atmospheric O3 and NO2 gas mixing ratios and meteorological parameters. *Environmental Pollution* 139 (2006) 224–231.
Keeling, Christopher I. and Jorg Bohlmann. Diterpene resin acids in conifers. *Phytochemistry* 67 (2006) 2415–2423.
Snajberk, Karel and Eugene Zavarin. Composition of turpentine from Pinus edulis wood oleoresin. *Phytochemistry* 14 (1975) 2025–2028.
Stermitz, Frank et al. Piperidine alkaloid content of Picea (Spruce) and Pinus (Pine). *Phytochemistry* 35, 4 (1994) 951–953.
Süntar, Ipek et al. Appraisal on the wound healing and anti–inflammatory activities of the essential oils obtained from the cones and needles of Pinus species by in vivo and in vitro experimental models. *Journal of Ethnopharmacology* 139 (2012) 533–540.
Zavarin, Eugene and Fields W. Cobb. Oleoresin variability in Pinus ponderosa. *Phytochemistry* 9 (1970) 2509–2515.
Zavarin, Eugene et al. Variation of the Pinus ponderosa needle oil with season and needle age. *Phytochemistry* 10 (1971) 3107–3114.
Zinkel, Duane and Thomas V. Magee. Resin acids of Pinus ponderosa needles. *Phytochemistry* 30, 3 (1991) 845–848.

Pipsissewa
Galvan, Imelda J. et al. Antifungal and antioxidant activities of the phytomedicine pipsissewa, Chimaphila umbellata. *Phytochemistry* 69 (2008) 738–746.
Oka, Michiko et al. Relevance of anti–reactive oxygen species activity to anti–inflammatory activity of components of Eviprostat, a phytotherapeutic agent for benign prostatic hyperplasia. *Phytomedicine* 14 (2007) 465–472.

Plantain
Samuelsen, Anne Berit. The Traditional Uses, Chemical Constituents and Biological Activities of Plantago Major L. *Journal of Ethnopharmacology* 71 (2000) 1–21.
Samuelsen, Anne Berit et al. Characterization of a Biologically Active Arabinogalactan from the Leaves of Plantago Major L. *Carbohydrate Polymers* 35 (1998) 145–153.
Taskova, Rilka et al. Iridoid Glucosides from Plantago Cornuti, Plantago Major and Veronica Cymbalaria. *Phytochemistry* 52 (1999) 1443–1445.

Pulsatilla
Turner, Nancy J. Counter–irritant and other medicinal uses of plants in Ranunculaceae by native peoples in British Columbia and neighboring areas. *Journal of Ethnopharmacology* 11 (1984) 181–201.
Ye, Wen–Cai et al. Patensin, a saponin from Pulsatilla patens var. multifida. *Phytochemistry* 39, 4 (1995) 937–939.

Pussytoes
Bayer, Randall J. A phylogenetic reconstruction of Antennaria (Asteraceae Inuleae). *Canadian Journal of Botany* 68, (2011) 1389–1397.

Pyrola
Averett, John E. et al. Eight flavonol glycosides in Pyrola (Pyrolaceae). *Phytochemistry* 25, 8 (1986) 1995–1996.

Leonid R. Ptitsyn et al. The 1,4–naphthoquinone derivative from Pyrola rotundifolia activates AMPK phosphorylation in C2C12 myotubes. *Fitoterapia* 82 (2011) 1285–1289.

Rattlesnake Plantain
Du, Xiao–Ming. Flavonoids from Goodyera schlechtendaliana. *Phytochemistry* 53 (2000) 997–1000.

Red Osier Dogwood
Du, C.T. et al. Anthocyanins of Cornaceae, Cornus canadensis. *Phytochemistry* 13 (1974) 2002.

Graziose, Rocky et al. Antiparasitic compounds from Cornus florida L. with activities against Plasmodium falciparum and Leishmania tarentolae. *Journal of Ethnopharmacology* 142 (2012) 456–461.

Red Raspberry
Bobinaite, Ramune et al. Variation of total phenolics, anthocyanins, ellagic acid and radical scavenging capacity in various raspberry (Rubus spp.) cultivars. *Food Chemistry* 132 (2012) 1495–1501.

Okuda, Takuo et al. Hydrolysable tannins as chemotaxoncmic markers in the Rosaceae. *Phytochemistry* 31, 9 (1992) 3091–3096.

Ryan, J.J. and D.E. Coffin. Flavonol glucuronides from Red raspberry, Rubus idaeus (Rosaceae). *Phytochemistry* 10 (1971) 1675–1677.

Venskutonis, P.R. et al. Radical scavenging activity and composition of raspberry (Rubus idaeus) leaves from different locations in Lithuania. *Fitoterapia* 78 (2007) 162–165.

Red Root
Li, Xing–Cong, Cai, Lining, and Wu, D. Antimicrobial Compounds from Ceanothus Americanus against Oral Pathogens. *Phytochemistry* 40. 1 (1997) 97–102.

Baig, Mizra A. and Banthorpe, Derek V. Accumulation of Tetrapeptide Precursors of Macrocyclic Alkaloids by Callus of Ceanothus Americanus. *Phytochemistry* 34, 1 (1993) 171–174.

Ribes
Mattila, Pirjo H. et al. High variability in flavonoid contents and composition between different North–European currant (Ribes spp.) varieties. *Food Chemistry* 204 (2016) 14–20.

Tabart, Jessica et al. Antioxidant and anti–inflammatory activities of Ribes nigrum extracts. *Food Chemistry* 131 (2012) 1116–1122.

Sagebrush
Gunawardena, K., S.B. Rivera, and W.W. Epstein. The Monoterpenes of Artemisia Tridentata ssp. Vaseyana, Artemisia Cana ssp. Viscidula and Artemisia Tridentata ssp. Spiciformis. *Phytochemistry* 59 (2002) 197–203.

Kelley, B.D., J.M. Appelt, and G.D. Appelt. Artemisia Tridentata (Basin Sagebrush) in the Southwestern United States of America Medicinal Uses and Pharmacologic Implications. *International Journal of the Addictions* 27, 3 (1992) 347–366.

McCutcheon, A.R. et al. Antifungal Screening of Medicinal Plants of British

Columbian Native Peoples. *Journal of Ethnopharmacology* 44, 3 (1994) 157–169.
Smith, Bruce N. et al. Stress–Induced Metabolic Differences Between Populations and Subspecies of Artemisia Tridentata (Sagebrush) from a Single Hillside. *Thermochimica Acta* 394 (2002) 205–210.

Scarlet Pimpernel
López, Víctor et al. Pharmacological properties of Anagallis arvensis L. (scarlet pimpernel) and Anagallis foemina Mill. (blue pimpernel) traditionally used as wound healing remedies in Navarra (Spain). *Journal of Ethnopharmacology* 134 (2011) 1014–1017.
Shoji, Noboru et al. Triterpenoid glycosides from Anagallis arvensis. *Phytochemistry* 37, 5 (1994) 1397–1402.

Self Heal
Kojima, Hisashi et al. Pentacyclic triterpenoids from Prunella vulgaris. *Phytochemistry* 26, 4 (1987) 1107–1111.
Sun, Hong–Xiang et al. In vitro and in vivo immunosuppressive activity of Spica Prunellae ethanol extract on the immune responses in mice. *Journal of Ethnopharmacology* 101 (2005) 31–36.
Zhang, Yongwen et al. Chemical properties, mode of action, and in vivo anti–herpes activities of a lignin–carbohydrate complex from Prunella vulgaris. *Antiviral Research* 75 (2007) 242–249.

Shepard's Purse
Kurode, Keiko and Tenmin Kaku. Pharmacological and Chemical Studies on the Alcohol Extract of Capsella Bursa–Pastoris. *Life Sciences* 8 (1989) 151–155.
Mukherjee, Kumar D., I. Kiewitt and H. Hurka. Lipid Content and Fatty Acid Composition of Seeds of Capsella Species from Different Geographical Locations. *Phytochemistry* 23, 1 (1984) 117–119.

Silk Tassel
Cameron, Donald W. et al. Iridoids of Garrya elliptica as plant growth inhibitors. *Phytochemistry* 23, 3 (1984) 533–535.
Pelletier, S.W. and L.H. Keith. Diterpene alkaloids from Aconitum, Delphinium, and Garrya species. *Chemical Abstracts* 2 (1968) 136–206.
Roth, William B. et al. New sources of Gutta–percha in Garrya flavescens and G. wrightii. *Phytochemistry* 24, 1 (1985) 183–184.
Valenta, Z., K. Wiesner, and C.M. Wong. A total synthesis of the Garrya alkaloids. *Tetrahedron Letters* 36 (1964) 2437–2442.

Skullcap
Awad, R. et al. Phytochemical and biological analysis of Skullcap (Scutellaria lateriflora L.): A medicinal plant with anxiolytic properties. *Phytomedicine* 10 (2003) 640–649.
Li, Jing et al. Identification of phenolic compounds from Scutellaria lateriflora by liquid chromatography with ultraviolet photodiode array and electrospray ionization tandem mass spectrometry. *Journal of Pharmaceutical and Biomedical Analysis* 63 (2012) 120– 127.
Rodriguez, Beatriz et al. Neo–clerodane diterpenoids from Scutellaria galericulata.

Phytochemistry 41, 1 (1996) 247–253.
Yoon, Seo Young et al. Convulsion–related activities of Scutellaria flavones are related to the 5,7-dihydroxyl structures. *European Journal of Pharmacology* 659 (2011) 155–160.
Zhang, Zhizhen et al. Characterization of chemical ingredients and anticonvulsant activity of American skullcap (Scutellaria lateriflora). *Phytomedicine* 16 (2009) 485–493.

Sneezeweed
Fortuna, Antonio M. et al. Antimicrobial activities of sesquiterpene lactones and inositol derivatives from Hymenoxys robusta. *Phytochemistry* 72 (2011) 2413–2418.
Shemluck, Melvin. Medicinal and other uses of the Compositae by Indians. *Journal of Ethnopharmacology* 5 (1982) 303–358.
Spring, Otmar et al. Chemistry of Glandular Trichomes in Hymenoxys and Related Genera. Biochemical Systematics and Ecology 22, 1 (1994) 171–195.

Spearmint
Arumugam, P. et al. Anti–Inflammatory Activity of Four Solvent Fractions of Ethanol Extract of Mentha Spicata L. Investigated on Acute and Chronic Inflammation Induced Rats. *Environmental Toxicology and Pharmacology* 26 (2008) 92–95.
Choudhury, R. Paul, A. Kumar, and A.N. Garg. Analysis of Indian Mint (Mentha Spicata) for Essential, Trace and Toxic Elements and its Antioxidant Behaviour. *Journal of Pharmaceutical and Biomedical Analysis* 41 (2006) 825–832.
Vian, Maryline Abert et al. Microwave Hydrodiffusion and Gravity, a New Technique for Extraction of Essential Oils. *Journal of Chromatography A* 1190 (2008) 14–17.

Spruce
Keeling, Christopher I. and Jorg Bohlmann. Diterpene resin acids in conifers. *Phytochemistry* 67 (2006) 2415–2423.
Pan, Hefeng and Lennart N. Lungren. Phenolic estractives from root bark of Picea abies. *Phytochemistry* 39, 6 (1995) 1423–1428.
Stermitz, Frank et al. Piperidine alkaloid content of Picea (Spruce) and Pinus (Pine). *Phytochemistry* 35, 4 (1994) 951–953.
Tumena, Ibrahim et al. Wound repair and anti–inflammatory potential of essential oils from cones of Pinaceae Preclinical experimental research in animal models. *Journal of Ethnopharmacology* 137 (2011) 1215– 1220.

St. John's Wort
Fiebich, Bernd L. et al. Pharmacological studies in an herbal drug combination of St. John's Wort (Hypericum perforatum) and passion flower (Passiflora incarnata) In vitro and in vivo evidence of synergy between Hypericum and Passiflora in antidepressant pharmacological models. *Fitoterapia* 82 (2011) 474–480.
Fritz, Daniela et al. Herpes Virus Inhibitory Substances from Hypericum Connatum Lam., a Plant Used in Southern Brazil to Treat Oral Lesions. *Journal of Ethnopharmacology* 113 (2007) 517–520.
Linde, K. and L. Knuppel. Large–Scale Observational Studies of Hypericum Extracts in Patients with Depressive Disorders—A Systematic Review.

Phytomedicine 12 (2005) 148–157.
Piovan, Anna et al. Detection of Hypericins in the "Red Glands" of Hypericum Elodes by ESI–MS/MS. *Phytochemistry* 65 (2004) 411–414.
Sanchez, C.C. et al. Antidepressant Effects of the Methanol Extract of several Hypericum Species from the Canary Islands. *Journal of Ethnopharmacology* 79 (2002) 119–127.
Süntar, Ipek Pesin et al. Investigations on the in vivo wound healing potential of Hypericum perforatum L. *Journal of Ethnopharmacology* 127 (2010) 468–477.

Stachys
Bilusic' Vundac, Vjera et al. Content of polyphenolic constituents and antioxidant activity of some Stachys taxa. *Food Chemistry* 104 (2007) 1277–1281.
Háznagy–Radnai, E. et al. Cytotoxic activities of Stachys species. *Fitoterapia* 79 (2008) 595–597.
Tundis, Rosa et al. Phytochemical and biological studies of Stachys species in relation to chemotaxonomy A review. *Phytochemistry* 102 (2014) 7–39.

Sweet Cicely
Crowden, R.K. Chemosystematics of the Umbelliferae. *Phytochemistry* 8 (1969) 1963–1984.
Harrorne, J.B. and Christine A. Williams. Flavonoids patterns in the fruits of the Umbelliferae. *Phytochemistry* 11 (1972) 1741–1750.
Kern, John Robert. Native American medicinal plants, chemical constituents of Osmorhiza chilensis and Clematis hirsutissima. *Thesis, Montana State University* (1982).

Sweet Clover
Edwards, K.g. and J.R. Stoker. Biosynthesis of coumarin: the isomerization stage. *Phytochemistry* 6 (1961) 655–661.
Kleinhofs, A. et al. Trans–o–hydroxycinnamic acid glucosylation in cell–free extracts of Melilotus alba. *Phytochemistry* 6 (1967) 1313–1318.
Martino, Emanuela et al. Microwave–assisted extraction of coumarin and related compounds from Melilotus officinalis (L.) Pallas as an alternative to Soxhlet and ultrasound–assisted extraction. *Journal of Chromatography A*, 1125 (2006) 147–151.

Toadflax
Blanco, Armandodoriano et al. Iridoids from endemic Sardinian Linaria species. *Photochemistry* 42, 2 (1996) 89–91.
Ilieva, Emilia et al. Iridoid glucosides from Linaria vulgaris. *Phytochemistry* 31, 3 (1992) 1040–1041.
Sticher, O. Isolation of antirrinoside from Linaria vulgaris. *Phytochemistry* 10 (1970) 1974–1975.
Valdez, E. Flavonoids pigments in the flower and leaf of the genus Linaria (Scrophulariaceae). *Phytochemistry* 9 (1970) 1253–1260.

Usnea
Choudhary, Muhammad I. et al. Bioactive phenolic compounds from a medicinal lichen, Usnea longissima. *Phytochemistry* 66 (2005) 2346–2350

Honda, N.K. et al. Antimycobacterial activity of lichen substances. *Phytomedicine* 17 (2010) 328–332.
Weckesser, S. et al. Screening of plant extracts for antimicrobial activity against bacteria and yeasts with dermatological relevance. *Phytomedicine* 14 (2007) 508–516

Uva–Ursi

Dykes, Gary A., Ryszard Amarowicz, and Ronald B. Pegg. Enhancement of Nisin Antibacterial Activity by a Bearberry (Arctostaphylos Uva–ursi) Leaf Extract. *Food Microbiology* 20 (2003) 211–216.
Grases, F. et al. Urolithiasis and Phytotherapy. *International Urology and Nephrology* 26, 5 (1994) 505–511.

Valerian

Abourashed, E.A., U. Koetter, and A. Brattstrom. In Vitro Binding Experiments with a Valerian, Hops and Their Fixed Combination Extract (Ze91019) to Selected Central Nervous System Receptors. *Phytomedicine* 11 (2004) 633–638.
Bent, Stephen et al. Valerian for Sleep A Systematic Review and Meta–Analysis. *The American Journal of Medicine* 119 (2006) 1005–1012.
Fernandez, Sebastian P. et al. Synergistic Interaction Between Hesperidin, a Natural Flavonoid, and Diazepam. *European Journal of Pharmacology* 512 (2005) 189–198.
Francis, A.J.P. and R.J.W. Dempster. Effect of Valerian, Valeriana Edulis, on Sleep Difficulties in Children with Intellectual Deficits Randomized Trial. *Phytomedicine* 9 (2002) 273–279.
Lacher, Svenja K. et al. Interaction of Valerian Extracts of Different Polarity with Adenosine Receptors Identification of Isovaltrate as an Inverse Agonist at A1 Receptors. *Biochemical pharmacology* 73 (2007) 248–258.
Leathwood, Peter D. et al. Aqueous Extract of Valerian Root (Valeriana officinalis L.) Improves Sleep Quality in Man. *Pharmacology Biochemistry & Behavior* 17 (1982) 65–71.
Stevinson, Clare and E. Ernst. Valerian for Insomnia A Systematic Review of Randomized Clinical Trials. *Sleep Medicine* 1 (2000) 91–99.

Verbena

Hernández, Nancy E., M.L. Tereschuk, and L.R. Abdala. Antimicrobial Activity of Flavonoids in Medicinal Plants from Tafí del Valle (Tucumán, Argentina). *Journal of Ethnopharmacology* 73 (2000) 317–322.
Kawashty, S.A. and I.A. El-Garf. The Flavonoid Chemosystematics of Egyptian Verbena Species. *Biochemical Systematics and Ecology* 28 (2000) 919–921.

Western Mugwort

Bork, Peter M. et al. Sesquiterpene Lactone Containing Mexican Indian Medicinal Plants and Pure Sesquiterpene Lactones as Potent Inhibitors of Transcription Factor NF–B. *FEBS Letters* 402, 1 (1997) 85–90.
Fernandez, Salvador Said et al. In Vitro Antiprotozoal Activity of the Leaves of Artemisia Ludoviciana. *Fitoterapia* 76 (2005) 466–468.
Jakupovic, J. et al. Sesquiterpene Lactones from Artemisia Ludoviciana. *Phytochemistry* 30, 5 (1991) 1573–1577.
Lee, K.H. and T.A. Geissman. Sesquiterpene Lactones of Artemisia Constituents of A. Ludoviciana ssp. Mexicana. *Phytochemistry* 9, 2 (1970) 403–408.

Liu, Yong-Long and T.J. Mabry. Flavonoids from Artemisia Ludoviciana var. Ludoviciana. *Phytochemistry* 21, 1 (1982) 209-214.

Ruiz-Cancino, Alejandro, Arturo E. Cano, and Guillermo Delgado. Sesquiterpene Lactones and Flavonoids from Artemisia Ludoviciana ssp. Mexicana. *Phytochemistry* 33, 5 (1993) 1113-1115.

Wild Cherry

Horsley, Stephen and Jerrold Meinwald. Glucose-1-benzoate and prunasin from Prunus serotina. *Phytochemistry* 20, 5 (1981) 1127-11287.

Jena, Ashish Kumar et al. Amelioration of testosterone induced benign prostatic hyperplasia by Prunus species. *Journal of Ethnopharmacology* 190 (2016) 33-45.

Ordaz-Galindo, Alejandro et al. Purification and identification of Capulin (Prunus serotina Ehrh) anthocyanins. *Food Chemistry* 65 (1999) 201-206.

Santamour, Frank S. Jr. Amygdalin in Prunus leaves. *Phytochemistry* 47, 8 (1998) 1537-1538.

Wild Iris

Benoit-Vical, Francoise et al. Antiplasmodial and antifungal activities of iridal, a plant triterpenoid. *Phytochemistry* 62 (2003) 747-751.

Wong, Sui-Ming et al. Plant Anticancer Agents XXXIX Triterpenes from Iris missouriensis (Iridaceae). *Journal of Fharmaceutical Sciences* 75, 3 (1986) 320.

Wild Rose

Andersson, Staffan C. et al. Carotenoid content and composition in rose hips (Rosa spp.) during ripening, determination of suitable maturity marker and implications for health promoting food products. *Food Chemistry* 128 (2011) 689-696.

Guoa, Dejian et al. Anti-inflammatory activities and mechanisms of action of the petroleum ether fraction of Rosa multiflora Thunb. hips. *Journal of Ethnopharmacology* 138 (2011) 717- 722.

Lattanzio, Francesca et al. In vivo anti-inflammatory effect of Rosa canina L. extract. *Journal of Ethnopharmacology* 137 (2011) 880- 885.

Lee, Jin Hwan et al. Anthocyanin compositions and biological activities from the red petals of Korean edible rose (Rosa hybrida cv. Noblered). *Food Chemistry* 129 (2011) 272-278.

Nadpal, Jelena D. et al. Comparative study of biological activities and phytochemical composition of two rose hips and their preserves: Rosa canina L. and Rosa arvensis Huds. *Food Chemistry* 192 (2016) 907-914.

Zhang, Shuai et al. Effects of flavonoids from Rosa laevigata Michx fruit against high-fat diet-induced non-alcoholic fatty liver disease in rats. *Food Chemistry* 141 (2013) 2108-2116.

Wild Strawberry

Liberal, Joana et al. Bioactivity of Fragaria vesca leaves through inflammation, proteasome and autophagy modulation. *Journal of Ethnopharmacology* 158 (2014) 113-122.

Vennat, B. et al. Proanthocyanidins from the roots of Fragaria vesca. *Phytochemistry* 26, 1 (1987) 261-263.

Wild Violet

Hellinger, Roland et al. Immunosuppressive activity of an aqueous Viola tricolor herbal extract. *Journal of Ethnopharmacology* 151 (2014) 299–306.

Herrmann, Anders et al. The alpine violet, Viola biflora, is a rich source of cyclotides with potent cytotoxicity. *Phytochemistry* 69 (2008) 939–952.

Lee, Mee-Young et al. Anti–inflammatory and anti–asthmatic effects of Viola mandshurica W. Becker (VM) ethanolic (EtOH) extract on airway inflammation in a mouse model of allergic asthma. *Journal of Ethnopharmacology* 127 (2010) 159–164.

Piana, Mariana et al. Antiinflammatory effects of Viola tricolor gel in a model of sunburn in rats and the gel stability. *Journal of Ethnopharmacology* 150 (2013) 458–465.

Zeng, Hai-Rong et al. Effects of Viola yedoensis Makino anti–itching compound on degranulation and cytokine generation in RBL–2H3 mast cells. *Journal of Ethnopharmacology* 189 (2016) 132–138.

Willow

Chrubasik, Sigrun et al. Treatment of Low Back Pain Exacerbations with Willow Bark Extract A Randomized Double–Blind Study. *The American Journal of Medicine* 109 (2000) 9–14.

Orians, Colin M. et al. Phenolic Glycosides and Condensed Tannins in Salix Sericea, S. Eriocephala and their F1 Hybrids Not All Hybrids are Created Equal. *Biochemical Systematics and Ecology* 28 (2000) 619–632.

Tunón, H., C. Olavsdotter, and L. Bohlin. Evaluation of Anti–Inflammatory Activity of some Swedish Medicinal Plants. Inhibition of Prostaglandin Biosynthesis and PAF–Induced Exocytosis. *Journal of Ethnopharmacology* 48 (1995) 61–76.

Yarrow

Benedek, Birgit, B. Kopp, and M.F. Melzig. Achillea millefolium L. s.l. – Is the Anti–inflammatory Activity Mediated by Protease Inhibition? *Journal of Ethnopharmacology* 113 (2007) 312–317.

Benedek, B. et al. Choleretic Effects of Yarrow (Achillea millefolium s.l.) in the Isolated Perfused Rat Liver. *Phytomedicine* 13 (2006) 702–706.

Cavalcanti, A.M. et al. Safety and Antiulcer Efficacy Studies of Achillea Millefolium vL. After Chronic Treatment in Wistar Rats. *Journal of Ethnopharmacology* 107 (2006) 277–284.

Dalsenter, Paulo R. et al. Reproductive Evaluation of Aqueous Crude Extract of Achillea Millefolium L. (Asteraceae) in Wistar Rats. *Reproductive Toxicology* 18 (2004) 819–823.

Guedon, Didier, P. Abbe, and J.L. Lamaison. Leaf and Flower Head Flavonoids of Achillea Millefolium L. Subspecies. *Biochemical Systematics and Ecology* 21, 5 (1993) 607–611.

Innocentia, G. et al. In Vitro Estrogenic Activity of Achillea Millefolium L. *Phytomedicine* 14 (2007) 147–152.

Kelley, Bruce D., Glenn D. Appelt, and Jennifer M. Appelt. Pharmacological Aspects of Selected Herbs Employed in Hispanic Folk Medicine in the San Luis Valley of Colorado, USA II Asclepias Asperula (Inmortal) and Achillea Lanulosa (Plumajillo). *Journal of Ethnopharmacology* 22 (1988) 1–9.

Kubelka, Wolfgang et al. Chemotaxonomic Relevance of Sesquiterpenes Within

the Achillea Millefolium Group. *Biochemical Systematics and Ecology* 27 (1999) 437–444.
Kültür, A. Medicinal Plants used in Kirklareli Province (Turkey). *Journal of Ethnopharmacology* 111 (2007) 341–364.
Lans, Cheryl, N. Turner, T. Khan, and G. Brauer. Ethnoveterinary Medicines Used to Treat Endoparasites and Stomach Problems in Pigs and Pets in British Columbia, Canada. *Veterinary Parasitology* 148 (2007) 325–340.
Lietave, Jan. Medicinal Plants in a Middle Paleolithic Grave Shanidar IV? *Journal of Ethnopharmacology* 35 (1992) 263–266.
Mockute, Danute and A. Judzentiene. Variability of the Essential Oils Composition of Achillea Millefolium ssp. Millefolium Growing Wild in Lithuania. *Biochemical Systematics and Ecology* 31 (2003) 1033–1045.

Yellow Pond Lily
Bate–Smith, E.C. Chemotaxonomy of Nuphar lutea. *Phytochemistry* 7 (1968) 459.
Cybulski, Jacek and Jerzy T. Worbel. Nuphar alkaloids. *The Alkaloids* 35, 5 (1989) 215–257.
Cybulski, Jacek et al. Nuphacristine – an alkaloid form Nuphar luteum. *Phytochemistry* 27 (1988) 3339–3341.
LaLonde, R.T. and C.F. Wong. Sulfur containing alkaloids from Nuphar lutea. *Phytochemistry* 11 (1972) 3305–3306.

INDEX

A

Abies 139
  lasiocarpa 139
abscess 343
Abutilon 101
acetylcholine 54, 343
acetylcholinesterase 343
Achillea millefolium 326
acidosis 212, 214
acid reflux 50, 149
acne 360
Aconite 76, 153, 187, 328
Aconitum 187
Actaea arguta 75
  eburnea 75
  neglecta 75
  rubra 75
    forma neglecta 75
    subsp. arguta 75
    var. dissecta 75
  spicata var. rubra 75
  viridiflora 75
adaptogen 343
Addison's disease 343
adrenal cortex 343
  medulla 343
adrenaline 98, 306, 343
Africa 78
Agastache 43–45
  foeniculum 44
  glaucifolia 43
  mexicana 44
  pallidiflora 43, 44
  rugosa 44
  urticifolia 43
  wrightii 43
Agrimonia brittoniana 46
  eupatoria var. parviflora 46
  gryposepala 46
  macrocarpa 46
  parviflora var. macrocarpa 46
  striata 46
  striata var. campanulata 46
Agrimony 46, 47, 48, 65, 106
Alamo temblón 62
Alaska 67, 68, 75, 86, 97, 128, 199, 204, 298, 317, 329
albumin 343

albuminuria 235, 245
Alcea rosea 171
aldosterone 343, 344, 357
Alfalfa 48, 49, 213
allantoin 182
allergy 95, 120, 220, 318, 344, 345, 347, 363
Aloe 95, 157, 323
  vera 69, 142, 231, 279, 284
alterative 108, 220, 315, 344
Althaea rosea 171
Alumroot 50, 51, 52, 151
alveoli 344, 350
Alzheimer's disease 54, 136, 170, 344, 349
amebiasis 80, 81, 219, 220, 268, 344, 357, 365
amenorrhea 45, 76, 110, 241, 260, 309, 344
American bilberry 83
  bistort 88
  blueberry 85
  dogwood 247
  Indian 72, 130, 189, 243, 249, 253, 281
  pasqueflower 238
  red elderberry 127
  red raspberry 250
  stinging nettle 211
amoeba 309
amphoteric 197
amylase 344
Anacardiaceae 146
Anagallis arvensis 261
analgesic 68, 70, 116, 225, 259
Anaphalis 242
anaphrodisiac 175, 325, 330, 344
anaphylaxis 344
androgen 344
anemia 123
Anemone 76, 201
  occidentalis 238
    var. subpilosa 238
  patens 238
  pratensis 239
  pulsatilla 239
Anemopsis californica 189
Angelica 52–55, 118, 136, 189
  ampla 53
  archangelica 53, 54

grayi 53
officinalis 53
pinnata 53
roseana 53
sinensis 53
angina pectoris 164, 345
Animas Mountains 195
Anise 44, 288
  hyssop 44
Aniseroot 288
anodyne 64, 69, 71, 74, 189
anorexia 48, 49, 80, 93, 149, 157, 345
anovulatory cycle 345
Antennaria 242
  rosea 243
antibacterial 51, 73, 91, 104, 108, 134,
    150, 172, 175, 189, 208, 210, 216,
    222, 240, 249, 266, 277, 289, 308,
    321, 323
antibody 354
anticholinergic 168, 345, 358
antifungal 104, 150, 175, 222, 259, 289,
    308, 321, 331
antimicrobial 47, 51, 63, 64, 66, 69, 70,
    79, 83, 106, 113, 116, 140, 141, 150,
    160, 172, 175, 178, 192, 193, 196,
    197, 205, 228, 229, 244, 259, 268,
    276, 277, 287, 331
antioxidant 45, 62, 80, 84, 205, 248, 308,
    352
Antirrhinum linaria 292
antiseptic 69, 70, 74, 87, 166, 184, 197,
    209, 235, 245, 299
antiviral 73, 189, 192, 277
anxiety 45, 100, 110, 170, 175, 268, 270,
    271, 306
aortic valve 163
Apache 55, 56, 57, 189
  plume 55–57
aphthous stomatitis 345
Apiaceae 52, 114, 118, 188, 191, 288
Apocynaceae 124
Apocynum cannabinum 124
apoptosis 345
arachidonic acid 345
Arbutus arizonica 195
  menziesii 195
  procera 195
  texana 195

unedo 199
xalapensis 195
  var. arizonica 195
  var. texana 195
Archangelica officinalis 53
Arctostaphylos uva–ursi 196, 298
Arizona 44, 56, 83, 86, 94, 101, 128, 156,
    162, 173, 177, 188, 190, 196, 199,
    204, 207, 212, 215, 219, 258, 261,
    267, 281, 283, 302, 305, 310, 311,
    314
  madrone 195
Arkansas 298
Arnica 57–60
  cordifolia 58
  montana 58
aromatase 213
arrhythmia 163, 164, 170, 346
Arrowleaf balsamroot 72
Artemisia ludoviciana 307
  mexicana 307
  tridentata 258
  vulgaris 307
    var. mexicana 307
arteriosclerosis 163
arthritis 49, 58, 63, 69, 76, 95, 113, 168,
    200, 213, 214, 220, 229, 240, 241,
    259, 277, 287, 291, 318, 362. See
    also pain, arthritis
Asclepias 242
Ashy silk tassel 267
Asia 78, 83, 138, 298
Asparagus 60–62
  officinalis 60
Aspen 45, 62–64, 67, 69, 72, 112, 114, 151,
    153, 156, 188, 215, 224, 256, 272,
    276, 322
Aspergillus 290
aspirin 63, 87
Asteraceae 57, 72, 103, 119, 154, 158, 221,
    242, 258, 272, 307, 326
asthma 54, 160, 168, 178, 222, 318, 323,
    346
astringent 46, 47, 50, 51, 56, 66, 83, 87, 89,
    106, 134, 144, 146, 153, 198, 215,
    216, 217, 234, 244, 249, 251, 256,
    257, 266, 281, 282, 287, 298, 299,
    300, 301, 313, 320, 327, 331
atherosclerosis 164, 346, 355, 359, 366

INDEX

autism 101
autonomic nervous system 346
Avens 65–67, 106
Ayurveda 61, 104, 346

B

Bacillus 79
Baldhip rose 316
Balm of gilead buds 67
Balsamea 192
Balsamorhiza helianthoides 72
   sagittata 72
Balsam poplar 63, 64, 67–72, 112
Balsamroot 72–74
Baneberry 75–78, 288, 327
Barberry 51, 78–82, 120, 152, 178, 220, 255
Barberry family. *See* Berberidaceae
basophil 346, 353
Bayberry 81, 327
Bearberry 298
Bearbush 267
Bear root 188
Bebb willow 324
bedsore 59, 217, 346
Bedstraw 107
bed wetting 147, 210
Beebalm 203
Beechdrops 280
Beech family. *See* Fagaceae
Beechleaf buckthorn 94
Belladonna 71, 167
benign prostate hypertrophy 213, 346.
   See also prostatitis
Berberidaceae 78, 218
Berberis aquifolium 218
  fremontii 220
  nervosa 219
  repens 218
  trifoliolata 220
Berberis fendleri 78
  vulgaris 78
Betonica 225
Betony 225
Betula alleghaniensis
  glandulosa 85
  lenta 87
  occidentalis 85

papyrifera 85
Betulaceae 85
Bifidobacteria 120, 346
Bigbract verbena 305
Big sagebrush 258
Bilberry 83–85
bile 80, 104, 120, 157, 219, 261, 308, 328, 343, 346
biliary blockage 82, 105, 121, 309
  congestion 104
  deficiency 157
  insufficiency 262
  obstruction 96
  secretion 259
  spasm 268
  stimulant 95, 104, 120
  system 156
Bill William's giant hyssop 43
Birch 85–87
  family. *See* Betulaceae
Birchleaf buckthorn 94
Biscuit root 191
Bistort 88–90, 151
Bistorta bistortoides 88
  var. oblongifolia 88
bites 57, 74, 89, 90, 132, 134, 138, 146, 152, 182, 237. 246, 264, 287, 318, 356
Bitterbrush 91–93
Bitter dock 122
  tonic 63, 80, 93, 94, 95, 104, 120, 149, 157, 219, 293, 307, 308, 328
Black cherry 310
  chokecherry 310
  cohosh 75, 76, 77, 78
  cottonwood 67
  elderberry 127
  haw 168
  henbane 167
  nightshade 71
  willow 325
Blackfoot 73, 243
bladder 64, 69, 74, 106, 160, 169, 172, 175, 180, 197, 210, 211, 213, 235, 236, 245, 246, 266, 299, 325, 327, 349, 355, 360, 363, 366
bloating 45, 53, 120, 135, 166, 184, 189, 205, 206, 209, 259, 291, 303
blood pressure 82, 126, 163, 344, 351, 359.
  See also hypertension

sugar 93, 149, 157, 212. *See also* diabetes, hyperglycemia
Blowball 119
Blue elderberry 127
  flag 314
  spruce 275
  violet 322
Bogbean 92–93, 219
  family. *See* Menyanthaceae
Bog birch 85
Borage family. *See* Boraginaceae
Boraginaceae 182
borborygmus 53, 268
Boschniakia 280
BPH. *See* benign prostate hypertrophy
bradycardia 347
Branched solomon's seal 133
Brassicaceae 265
Brickellia 212
  californica 351
British Columbia 43, 68, 83, 196, 207, 258, 270, 317
Broadleaf arnica 57
  dock 122
  plantain 236
bronchial inflammation. *See also* inflammation, bronchial
bronchitis 54, 73, 74, 91, 92, 102, 110, 115, 116, 134, 141, 159, 160, 169, 172, 189, 192, 193, 222, 229, 243, 259, 260, 277, 311, 312, 347
Bronchorrhoea 160
Brook mint 135
Broomrape family. *See* Orobanchaceae
bruises 58, 59, 168, 200
Buckbean 92
Buckbrush 252
Buckthorn 94–96, 157, 218, 323
  family. *See* Rhamnaceae
Buckwheat 88, 89, 122
  family. *See* Polygonaceae
Bugleweed 97–101
burns 51, 64, 71, 113, 138, 147, 152, 183, 193, 216, 217, 237, 246, 247, 264, 284, 291, 292, 323
bursitis 69
Bush cinquefoil 107
  mint 274
Butcher's broom 291

Butter and eggs 292
Buttercup family. *See* Ranunculaceae

C

Cactus 99
caffeine 102, 104, 255
California 43, 52, 56, 68, 72, 88, 94, 101, 128, 148, 156, 159, 161, 165, 177, 185, 192, 196, 204, 207, 212, 218, 234, 238, 253, 258, 261, 263, 267, 298, 310, 317, 324, 329
  buckthorn 94
  figwort 137
Caltha bicolor 199
  leptosepala 199
  palustris 200
Camellia sinensis 145
Camphor 229
Campylobacter spp. 51
Canada 43, 52, 68, 75, 86, 88, 115, 148, 159, 177, 191, 212, 236, 239, 246, 248, 263, 283, 290, 293, 302, 314
Canadian fleabane 145, 268
  violet 322
cancer 78, 108, 281, 345, 353, 358
Cancer root 280
Candida albicans 79, 80, 81, 140, 175, 205, 262, 300
Canker lettuce 244
canker sores 89, 245
Cannabaceae 173
Canoe birch 85
Canutillo 180
Capsella bursa–pastoris 265
carcinoma 347
cardiac glycosides 347
  sphincter 150
cardiomyopathy 163
cardiovascular 44, 45, 59, 98, 99, 100, 125, 126, 162, 163, 164, 187, 311, 312, 356, 358, 365
carminative 44, 53, 63, 115, 116, 135, 156, 178, 179, 184, 189, 205, 208, 219, 274, 288, 323, 347
Carpenter's square 137
Carpenter weed 263
Carrot family. *See* Apiaceae
Cascades 72, 128, 199, 267

Cascara sagrada 95, 218
Cashew family. *See* Anacardiaceae
Castela 222
cataracts 84
Catch weed 107
Catspaw 242
Catstoes 242
Ceanothus 252
  americanus 253
  fendleri 252
  greggii 252
  integerrimus 255
Cebadilla 156
Celery 118
central nervous system 110, 143, 169, 174, 225, 270, 279, 303, 343, 347, 350, 352, 358
Cerro hawthorn 161
cervical dysplasia 347, 348, 353
cervicitis 251, 317, 321, 347
chai 145
Chamaenerion angustifolium 144
Chamerion angustifolium 144
Chamisso arnica 57
Chamomile 44, 101, 222
Chamomilla 222
Checkerbloom 101
Checker mallow 80, 101–103, 140, 277
Chelidonium 268
chemotherapy 108, 286
Cheyenne 73
chicken pox 284, 347, 362
Chicken toe 109
Chicoria 103, 119
Chicory 103–105
childbirth 282
Chimaphila menziesii 233
  umbellata 233
China 171, 224
Chisos Mountains 196
Chokecherry 250
cholecystokinin 347
cholera 140, 229, 277
choleretic 80, 308, 328, 348
cholesterol 45, 346, 348, 356
cholinergic 169, 348
cholinesterase 54, 55, 136
chologogue 80, 158, 348
chronic fatigue syndrome 193

venous insufficiency 291, 318
Chrysanthemum cinerariaefolium 223
  leucanthemum 221
Chuchupate 188
Cichorium intybus 103
Cinquefoil 65, 105–107, 321
circulation 44, 45, 76, 110, 193, 205, 208, 216, 239, 240, 302, 306
cirrhosis 104, 158, 220, 318
Citronella 179
Citrus geranium 153
Cleavers 107–108
Clematis 76, 201
Clusiaceae 283
Coccidioides immitis 348
coccidioidomycosis 348
Coffee 102, 104, 240, 299, 304
  weed 103
Coffeeberry 94
colic 53, 54, 189, 274, 275
colitis 87, 145, 268, 308, 327, 328
collagen 348
Collinsonia 266
Colorado 43, 44, 56, 68, 72, 78, 86, 128, 148, 161. 162, 188, 215, 302
  barberry 78
  cough root 188
Common agrimony 46
  barberry 78
  dogbane 124
  henbane 167
  hollyhock 171
  horsetail 180
  mullein 209
Condyloma acuminatum 348, 352
Conioselinum scopulorum 188
conjunctivitis 81, 240, 241, 348
Conopholis alpina 280
  americana 280
  mexicana 280
  panamensis 280
  sylvatica 280
constipation 95, 124, 125, 157, 218, 261, 262, 323
Continental Divide 91, 97
contusions 58, 59, 64, 113, 168, 200, 225, 259, 260, 273, 291
Convallaria 133. 163
convulsions 115, 170

Coptis 178
Coralbells 50
Corallorhiza 109
   maculata 109
   odontorhiza 110
   striata 109
Coral root 45, 109–111, 244, 246
Cornaceae 247
Corn mint 135
   silk 197, 229
Cornus florida 248
   sericea 247
   stolonifera 247
coronary artery 162
corpus luteum 348, 361
cortisol 343, 348
Cottonwood 63, 64, 67, 69, 112–114, 145, 205, 325
cough 73, 91, 110, 125, 140, 141, 159, 160, 169, 172, 180, 189, 200, 210, 227, 228, 229, 242, 243, 277, 311
Cough root 191
coumadin 291
coumarin 63, 290
counter–irritant 200
Cow parsnip 55, 114–119, 194
cowper's gland 240
Cowslip 199
Coyote mint 207
   willow 324
Cramp bark 44, 54, 168
Cranberry 74, 197, 299
Crataegus erythropoda 161
   rivularis 161
Crawley 109
Creek dogwood 247
Creeping holly grape 218
Creosote bush 95, 308
crones disease 145
Crucifixion thorn 66, 80, 268
Culpepper 261
Culver's root 293
Cupressaceae 183
Curlycup gumweed 158
Currant 256
   family. *See* Grossulariaceae
cuts 51, 74, 91, 134, 146, 175, 182, 193, 201, 206, 216, 217, 219, 230, 249, 257, 264, 278, 281, 284, 287, 289, 318, 323
CVI. *See* chronic venous insufficiency
cyanosis 125
Cylindropuntia 102
Cynoglossum officinale 182
Cypress 51, 66, 102, 106, 206, 281, 318, 330
cystitis 47, 74, 106, 108, 172, 184, 198, 210, 211, 214, 234, 235, 245, 251, 300, 318, 321, 349, 355
cytokines 323

D

Dalmatian daisy 223
   toadflax 292
Dandelion 103, 105, 119–121, 212, 261, 326
Dasiphora 105
Datura 59, 71, 167, 168
Davis Mountains 196
Deerbrush 252
Deer's ears 156
dehydroepiandrosterone 349
Delphinium ajacis 186
   staphisagria 186
dementia 54, 170, 344, 349
demulcent 349
depression 77, 163, 169, 170, 239, 241, 284, 303, 304
dermatitis 55, 80, 81, 118, 285, 306, 363
Desert parley 191
detoxification 344, 352
DHEA. *See* Dehydroepiandrosterone
DHT. *See* dihydrotestosterone
diabetes 93, 149, 157, 358. *See also* hyperglycemia
diabetic neuropathy 84
diaphoresis 54, 63, 130, 137, 205, 208, 306, 328, 349
diaphoretic 44, 45, 54, 110, 116, 128, 129, 136, 137, 155, 166, 189, 192, 204, 208, 259, 271, 288, 308, 328, 329, 349, 364
diarrhea 51, 54, 56, 57, 80, 83, 84, 87, 89, 90, 94, 144, 145, 146, 147, 150, 152, 168, 169, 178, 205, 216, 217, 229, 237, 241, 243, 249, 257, 259, 260, 264, 268, 277, 281, 282, 287, 308,

309, 316, 330, 331, 344, 352, 363, 365
dicumarol 290
Digitalis 125
dihydrotestosterone 349
Dioscorides 114, 261
disinfectant 56, 66, 74, 175, 206, 266, 277
Disporum trachycarpum 134
diuretic 61, 63, 70, 87, 105, 113, 120, 129, 145, 180, 213, 237, 259, 308, 349
Dock 122–124
Doctrine of Signatures 281
Dogbane 124–126, 163
  family. *See* Apocynaceae
Dog violet 322
Dogwood family. *See* Cornaceae
Dong quai 53
dopamine 350
Douglas fir 75, 128, 139, 276
Dragonhead 286
Dragon's claw 109
Dugaldia hoopesii 272
dust cell 350
Dwarf birch 85
dysentery 89, 140, 229, 264, 277, 287, 363
dysmenorrhea 45, 76, 241, 328, 331, 350, 357
dyspepsia 44, 45, 93, 149, 150, 156, 157, 178, 184, 206, 309, 315, 350
dysuria 66, 69. *See also* urinary, pain

E

earache 210, 211
Echinacea 73, 79, 129, 220, 254, 281, 354
Eclectics 239, 248, 315, 350
ectomorph 239
eczema 80, 81, 87, 108, 116, 160, 184, 315, 318, 363
edema 84, 125, 163, 235, 291, 350
  pulmonary 163
Edwards Plateau 196
Elder 113, 127–130
Elderberry syrup 129
Elephanthead lousewort 224
Elkslip 199
Elkweed 156
emetic 91, 249
emmenagogue 166, 208, 350

emphysema 160
endometriosis 350
endometrium 350
Engelmann spruce 275
Entamoeba histolytica 152, 308, 344, 350
enteric fever 140, 277
eosinophil 323, 351, 353
epididymitis 240, 330
Epifagus 280
epilepsy 115, 271
Epilobium angustifolium 144
epinephrine 343
Epstein–Barr virus 193
Equisetaceae 180
Equisetum arvense 180
  boreale 180
  calderi 180
  saxicola 180
Ericaceae 83, 195, 233, 244, 298
Eriogonum 89
erythrocyte 351
Escherichia coli 79, 197, 234, 244, 259, 262, 299, 351
Espeletia helianthoides 72
  sagittata 72
Estafiate 307
estrogen 47, 56, 66, 76, 174, 175, 255, 327, 351
Eucalyptus 172, 206, 229, 259
Eupatorium britonianum 46
  gryposepalum 46
  purpureum 102
Eupatory tribe 351
Eurasian buckthorn 95
Europe 46, 61, 68, 71, 78, 83, 98, 108, 119, 132, 145, 173, 174, 182, 186, 210, 215, 233, 236, 239, 250, 283, 298
European barberry 78
  bilberry 83
  pasqueflower 239
  red raspberry 250
  white waterlily 330
Evening primrose family. *See* Onagraceae
Everlasting 242
expectorant 54, 69, 70, 73, 91, 192, 193, 259, 289
Explorer's gentian 148

F

Fabaceae 48, 290
Fagaceae 215
Fairy bells 134
Fallopia multiflora 89
Fallugia micrantha 55
  paradoxa 55
  var. acuminata 55
False lily of the valley 133
  pennyroyal 165
  solomon's seal 133–135
  wintergreen 244
Feather duster bush 55
  rose 55
Fendler barberry 78
Fennel 44
Ferula dissecta 191
fever 44, 45, 54, 64, 69, 70, 99, 108, 110, 113, 116, 128, 129, 136, 140, 155, 166, 170, 189, 192, 193, 204, 206, 208, 209, 220, 222, 235, 245, 248, 249, 260, 271, 275, 277, 306, 309, 311, 328, 348, 361, 362
Feverfew 222
fibroids 255, 351
fibromyalgia 63, 76, 95
Field mint 80, 93, 120, 135–137, 136, 149, 152, 157, 250, 270, 286, 293
  primrose 131
Figwort 137–138, 293
  family. *See* Scrophulariaceae
Fingergrass 105
Fir 83, 139–144, 275, 276, 278, 279, 331
Fireweed 144–146
Fivefingers 105
flatulence 53
Florida 177, 204
Flowering dogwood 248
flu 63, 69, 73, 76, 115, 116, 129, 141, 172, 189, 192, 229, 271, 277. *See also* influenza
follicle stimulating hormone 100, 351
food poisoning 50, 51, 79, 80, 81, 129, 168, 178, 205, 219, 220, 259, 260, 331, 352, 362
Foothill arnica 57
Fo-ti 89
Four Corners 159, 204

Fragaria vesca 320
  virginiana 320
Fragrant sumac 146–148
France 61
Frangula betulifolia 94
  californica 94
Frasera speciosa 156
Fremont's cottonwood 112
FSH. *See* follicle stimulating hormone
fungus 79, 80, 81, 116, 129, 166, 175, 184, 193, 205, 206, 219, 220, 222, 259, 260, 262, 289, 295, 309, 331
Fusarium 175, 351

G

G6PD. *See* glucose phosphate dehydrogenase deficiency
GABA 270, 303
Galium aparine 107
gallbladder 104, 120, 121, 157, 158, 221, 260, 262, 268, 314, 347, 348. *See also* biliary
gallstones 104
Gamble oak 215
gamma linolenic acid 132
Garden valerian 301
Garlic 162, 210, 300
Garryaceae 267
Garrya flavescens 267
  fremontii 267
  wrightii 267
gastritis 44, 45, 53, 54, 89, 90, 92, 105, 149, 150, 152, 175, 308, 309, 311, 327, 352, 353. *See also* heartburn
gastroenteritis 129, 170, 316, 352
gastrointestinal 48, 50, 51, 52, 53, 54, 57, 60, 63, 75, 80, 83, 85, 88, 90, 91, 92, 93, 94, 95, 96, 104, 117, 134, 135, 137, 140, 147, 149, 153, 157, 177, 178, 180, 181, 192, 198, 200, 201, 205, 206, 207, 217, 219, 229, 231, 247, 257, 260, 263, 266, 277, 279, 282, 288, 289, 293, 294, 300, 307, 308, 314, 315, 316, 320, 323, 327, 328, 329
  cramps 54
  irritation 52
  spasm 54

INDEX

Gelsemium 328
Gentian 63, 91, 93, 148–150, 156, 219
   family. *See* Gentianaceae
Gentiana affinis 148
   calycosa 148
   parryi 148
Gentianaceae 148, 156
Georgia 298
Geraniaceae 151
Geranium 151–153, 265
   caespitosum 151
   family. *See* Geraniaceae
   richardsonii 151
Gerard 261
Germany 215, 294
Geum 65
Giant creek nettle 211
   goldenrod 154
   hyssop 43
   lousewort 224
   rattlesnake plantain 246
Giardia lamblia 352
giardiasis 80, 81, 152, 219, 220, 268, 308
gingivitis 352, 359
glaucoma 352, 355
Globemallow 101
glomerulonephritis 352
glucose–6–phosphate–dehydrogenase 82, 221
glutathione 352
Gnaphalium 242
Goldenrod 154–155
Goldenseal 81, 216, 327
Golden smoke 220
Goodyera oblongifolia 246
Gooseberry 256
Goosegrass 105, 107
Gordolobo 209
gout 61, 120, 121, 212, 352, 366
Grand fir 139
granulocyte 353
Gravel root 47, 66, 102
Graves' disease 98
Gray's angelica 52
Great Basin 72, 91
   Lakes 75
   ox–eye 221
   Plains 97, 204, 234, 244, 253
   willow herb 144

Greater periwinkle 99
Green gentian 91, 149, 156–158
   leaved rattlesnake plantain 246
   tea 145
Greenland 86
Grindelia 73, 74, 158–161
   nuda 158
   robusta 159
   squarrosa 158
Grossulariaceae 256
Groundcone 280
Ground holly 233
Guadalupe Mountains 196
gums, bleeding 50, 51, 89, 147
Gumweed 158
Gypsyflower 132

H

Hairy arnica 57
   hedgenettle 286
   henbane 167
hallucinations 171
hangover 205
Hawaii 97, 204
Hawthorn 59, 99, 161–165, 318
hayfever 240, 309, 362. *See also* rhinitis
HCL. *See* Hydrochloric acid
headache 64, 69, 76, 77, 80, 113, 136, 168, 170, 240, 241, 249, 260, 287, 293, 303, 306, 308, 314
Heal all 263
heart 59, 76, 98, 99, 116, 125, 133, 162, 163, 164, 170, 187, 306, 311, 322, 345, 347, 349, 350, 365, 366
heartburn 53, 94, 137, 150, 271. *See also* gastritis
Heartleaf arnica 57
Heath family. *See* Ericaceae
Hedeoma 165–167, 208
   oblongifolia 166
Hedgenettle 285
Helenium 226
   hoopesii 272
Helicobacter pylori 175, 308, 353
hematuria 66, 69, 266, 327, 328, 353
Hemlock parsley 188
hemolysis 353
hemorrhage 51, 89, 99, 100, 152, 180, 181,

198, 265, 266, 282, 300, 327
hemorrhoids 69, 84, 168, 266, 291, 353
hemostatic 66, 265, 266, 353
Hemp family. *See* Cannabaceae
Henbane 59, 69, 71, 160, 167–170, 216
hepatic antioxidant 80
   congestion 262
   deficiency 81, 157
   detoxification 80
   enzymes 80
   inflammation 81, 104, 220, 309. *See also* hepatitis
   irritation 52
   obstruction 96
   rhythm 95
   secretions 149, 259, 314
   sluggishness 81
   stimulant 80, 82, 120, 255, 261
   toxins 80
hepatitis 80, 104, 120, 158, 220, 254, 255, 293, 308, 318, 353
hepatocyte 308, 353, 362
hepatoprotective 80, 149, 220, 308
Heracleum lanatum 114
   maximum 114
   persicum 115
   sphondylium 115
herpes 115, 262, 264, 284, 308, 309
Heuchera 50
Hill Country 196
histamine 356
HIV 193
Hoary nettle 211
Hogweed 114
Holly grape 218
Hollyhock 140, 171–173, 229, 277
homeopathic 60
Honeysuckle family. *See* Caprifoliaceae
Hooker's evening primrose 131
Hopi 189
Hops 173–176, 179
Hoptree 177–179
Horehound 98
Horse chestnut 291
Horsemint 43, 203
Horsetail 48, 65, 180–181, 251
   family. *See* Equisetaceae
Ho shu wu 89
hot flashes 49, 99, 100, 174

Hound's tongue 182–183
human papillomavirus 348, 353
Humulus lupulus var. lupuloides 174
   var. lupulus 174
   var. neomexicanus 173
   var. pubescens 174
hydrochloric acid 93, 149, 219, 259, 354, 359
Hymenoxys 226
   hoopesii 272
Hyoscyamus niger 167
hyperglycemia 93, 149, 150, 157, 213, 354, 355, 358. *See also* diabetes
Hypericum perforatum 283
   scouleri 283
hyperlipidemic 213
hyperplasia 78
hypertension 45, 99, 100, 163, 164, 213, 351, 354
hyperthyroidism 98, 100
hypoglycemia 354
hypotension 343, 359
hypothyroidism 81, 100, 284, 303, 315
Hyssop 43
Hyssopus 43
hysteria 239, 240, 304

I

Idaho 68, 72, 86, 97, 101, 128, 165, 167, 207, 212, 234, 238, 270, 317
Illinois 204
immunity 73, 84, 87, 89, 95, 102, 110, 115, 128, 129, 154, 155, 172, 193, 227, 228, 235, 245, 254, 314
immunoglobulin 345, 354
incontinence 47, 66, 106, 170, 210
Indiana 75
Indian balsam 191
   hemp 124
   wickopy 144
indigestion 44, 53, 63, 64, 70, 80, 81, 91, 93, 104, 113, 120, 121, 125, 149, 156, 163, 166, 175, 178, 205, 209, 219, 220, 240, 241, 259, 262, 274, 275, 293, 294, 303, 304, 306, 307, 328
infection, bacterial 51
   fungal 362, 363, 366

intestinal 141, 229, 277
urinary 61, 87
inflammation, bronchial 54, 222
  chronic 58
  gums 51
  intestinal 50, 145, 213, 237
  oral 51
  subacute 58
  urinary 57
  vascular 59
influenza 110, 189, 193, 277, 311, 354. See also flu
insecticide 168, 186, 187
insect repellent 179
insomnia 99, 100, 110, 116, 169, 174, 175, 225, 239, 241, 270, 271, 284, 304, 354
interleukin 355
interstitial cystitis 172
intraocular pressure 352, 355
Iridaceae 313
Iris arizonica 313
  family. See Iridaceae
  longipetala var. montana 313
  missouriensis 313
  montana 313
  pariensis 313
  pelogonus 313
  tolmieana 313
  versicolor 314
irritable bowel syndrome, 168
ischemia 345, 355, 359

J

Jack-in-the-pulpit 189
Jesuit Priests 159
Jumping cholla 102
Juniper 51, 66, 102, 106, 172, 196, 330
Juniperus canadensis 183
  communis 183

K

Kansas 159, 204
Kaporie tea 145
Kava 270, 289
Kentucky 204
keratinocyte 355

kidney 51, 52, 61, 63, 70, 72, 75, 102, 113, 120, 121, 143, 154, 155, 160, 167, 169, 180, 181, 185, 197, 202, 207, 232, 235, 236, 245, 279, 282, 299, 350, 352, 358, 366
  infection 51 See also nephritis
  inflammation 83
  irritation 52. 90
  stones 51, 61, 66, 102, 181
Kinnikinnick 243, 250, 298
Klamath 91
Klamathweed 283
Klebsiella pneumoniae 210
Knight's spur 185
Kola nut 240
Korean mint 44
Koumaro 199
Krameria 99
kupffer cell 355

L

lactation 49, 306, 361
Lactobacillus 355
Lady slipper 110
Lamiaceae 43, 97, 135, 165, 203, 207, 263, 269, 274, 286
Lanceleaf figwort 137
Larch 227
large intestine 95, 140. See also gastrointestinal
Large-leaved avens 65
Larix 227
Lark's claw 185
Larkspur 153, 185–187
Larrea 284
laryngitis 69, 70, 192, 193
laxative 91, 96, 124, 130, 157, 158, 220, 294, 323
LDL. See Low density lipoprotein
leaky gut syndrome 120
Lemonade berry 146
Lemon balm 45
  beebalm 203
  horsemint 203
  mint 203
Leontodon taraxacum 119
Leptandra 293
Leptotaenia dissecta 191

Leucanthemum vulgare 221
leukocyte 346, 351, 356, 365, 367
leukotriene 356
LH. *See* luteinizing hormone
libido 240, 241, 344
lice 186, 187
Licorice 44, 77
Ligusticum 59, 73, 116, 160, 188–191, 192, 210, 242, 288, 289
 porteri 188
Liliaceae 60, 133
Lily family. *See* Liliaceae
 of the valley 133
Limber pine 226
Linaria dalmatica 292
 vulgaris 292
Lion's teeth 119
Listerine 206
lithiasis 47, 356
lithotropic 47, 66, 180, 266
Littleleaf alumroot 50
Little prince's pine 233
 wild rose 316
liver 77, 80, 81, 95, 104, 120, 121, 149, 150, 157, 158, 202, 205, 213, 220, 232, 254, 260, 262, 279, 286, 287, 293, 294, 308, 309, 314, 315, 344, 346, 348, 350, 352, 353, 355, 356, 361, 362, 366
 inflammation 362. *See also* hepatitis
Lobelia 47, 59, 66, 160
Lodgepole pine 83, 226
Lomatium 73, 116, 191–194, 210, 242
 dissectum 191
 nevadense 194
 suksdorfii 193
Louisiana sagewort 307
low density lipoprotein 356, 366
Lucerne 48
lungs 54, 55, 73, 74, 99, 110, 115, 129, 140, 159, 172, 192, 193, 200, 228, 242, 243, 259, 277, 311
Lupinus 226
lupulin 175
lupulinum 175
lupus 318
Lupus erythematosus 254
luteinizing hormone 77, 100, 356
Lyall's angelica 52

Lycopus americanus 97
 asper 97
 europaeus 98
 parviflorus 97
 uniflorus 97
 virginicus 98
  var. parviflorus 97
Lyme's disease 193
lymph 123, 192, 253, 254, 255, 315, 363, 365
lymphocyte 356

M

MacDougal verbena 305
macrophage 355, 356, 357, 360
macular degeneration 84
Madder family. *See* Rubiaceae
Madrone 74, 102, 195–199, 234, 281, 299
Madrono 195
Mahonia aquifolium 218
 repens 218
Maianthemum racemosum 133
 stellatum 134
Maine 177, 248
malabsorption 123, 214, 315
malaria 248, 253, 356, 360
Mallow 101
 family. *See* Malvaceae
malnourishment 48, 49
Malvaceae 101, 171
Malva neglecta 101
Manzanita 74, 102, 195, 196, 198, 199, 299
Marguerite 221
Marrubium vulgare 98
Marsh betony 286
 marigold 199–202, 240
 mint 135
 skullcap 269
 trefoil 92
Massachusetts 97
mast cell 356
Masterwort 114
mastitis 254, 255, 291, 292
Matricaria 222
Maudlin daisy 221
Medicago sativa 48
 tunetana 48
melanocyte 356

Melilotus alba 290
  albus 290
  graveolens 290
  leucanthus 290
  officinalis 290
    fo. suaveolens 290
memory 349
menopause 357, 359. *See* perimenopause
menorrhagia 56, 106, 327, 328, 357
menorrhalgia 357. *See also* dysmenorrhea
menses 44, 47, 56, 66, 76, 110, 111, 116, 166, 174, 189, 193, 208, 240, 251, 259, 266, 275, 308, 321, 344
menstrual 56, 99, 116, 168, 193, 208, 240, 259, 260, 268, 291, 330
  spotting 45, 106, 251, 266, 318, 321, 327
Mentha aquatica
  arvensis 135
  pulegium 165
  spicata 274
Menyanthaceae 92
Menyanthes trifoliata 92
mesomorph 213, 239, 241
Mexican agastache 44
  squawroot 280
  valerian 301
Micrococcus 175, 357
Microsporum 79, 357
migraine 76, 77, 240
Milfoil 326
Milk thistle 80, 104, 120, 149, 294, 318
mineralocorticoid 343, 348, 357
Minnesota 148, 177, 314
Mint 274
  family. *See* Lamiaceae
miscarriage 251, 266
Mississippi River 204
Missouri 159
Mock pennyroyal 165
Monarda 80, 93, 120, 149, 152, 157, 172, 178, 203–207, 250, 293, 331
  austromontana 203
  citriodora 203
  fistulosa 203
  menthifolia 203
  pectinata 203
Monardella 165, 207–209
  crispa 208

  glauca 207
  odoratissima 207
monoamine oxidase 284, 357
monocyte 357
Montana 43, 68, 72, 86, 88, 97, 128, 131, 148, 156, 161, 162, 167, 173, 191, 207, 234, 238, 239, 302, 317, 324
Monument plant 156
motion sickness 168
Mountain arnica 57
  birch 85
  bog gentian 148
  figwort 137
  lovage 188
  nettle 211
  pennyroyal 207
  rose 316
  sagebrush 258
  sidalcea 101
mucilaginous 101, 323
Mucor 175
Mugwort 307
Mullein 243
multiple sclerosis 358
muscle pulls 58, 136, 225
Mustard family. *See* Brassicaceae
myasthenia gravis 358
Mycobacterium 116, 175, 358
Myrrh 79, 216
Myrtle blueberry 83

N

Nana–pennyroyal 166
Narrowleaf cottonwood 112
  fireweed 144
  skullcap 269
natural killer cells 358
nausea 44, 53, 54, 80, 89, 90, 94, 126, 135, 136, 150, 152, 168, 169, 178, 189, 205, 245, 249, 250, 260, 273, 274, 275, 288, 289, 293, 314, 352
Navajo 91, 249
Nebraska 204
nephritis 47, 102, 106, 113, 154, 184, 235, 245, 358
nervousness 45, 175, 240, 306
Nettle 65, 211–214, 251, 286
  family. *See* Urticaceae

Nettleleaf hyssop 43
neuralgia 69, 115, 168, 304
Nevada 43, 56, 68, 72, 94, 97, 128, 161, 165, 188, 192, 204, 208, 212, 234, 267, 270
New Jersey tea 253
  Mexican figwort 137
  Mexican verbena 305
  Mexico 44, 56, 83, 86, 88, 94, 101, 128, 156, 162, 165, 173, 188, 190, 191, 195, 196, 199, 204, 207, 212, 215, 219, 234, 239, 258, 267, 281, 283, 302, 305, 310, 314, 317, 329
  York 75, 97
Nightshade family. See Solanaceae
night vision 84
nocturnal emission 364
Nootka rose 316
norepinephrine 343, 357, 358
North Dakota 161
Northern bugleweed 97
  water horehound 97
Northern Hemisphere 83, 86, 144, 183, 242, 270
nose bleeds 100
Nuphar lutea subsp. polysepala 329
  polysepala 329
nursing 60, 92, 96, 101, 118, 126, 143, 161, 167, 176, 190, 194, 202, 209, 215, 232, 236, 246, 250, 260, 262, 269, 280, 294, 304, 316, 332
Nymphaea alba 330
  odorata 330
  polysepala 329
Nymphaeaceae 329

O

Oak 51, 63, 87, 128, 196, 215–217, 265, 281
Ocotillo 254
Oenothera biennis 131
  elata 131
  hookeri 131
Ohio 75
Oklahoma 159, 204, 324
Old man's whiskers 65
oleoresin 69, 139, 140, 141, 142, 143, 227, 228, 229, 230, 231, 232, 233, 276, 277, 278, 279, 280

Onagraceae 131, 144
Ongra biennis 131
  hookeri 131
Orange Sneezeweed 272
Orchidaceae 109, 246
Orchid family. See Orchidaceae
orchitis 240
Oregano 205
Oregon 52, 68, 72, 94, 97, 128, 131, 148, 165, 196, 204, 207, 212, 238, 261, 263, 267, 270, 317, 324, 329
Oregongrape 79, 80, 218–221, 255, 315
Orobanchaceae 224, 280
Orobanche 280
orthorexia 93, 149, 157
Oshá 188
ovulation 345, 356
Owl's claws 272
Ox–eye daisy 221–223

P

Pacific madrone 195
  red elderberry 127
pain 63, 69, 87, 112, 291, 325
  acute 95
  arthritis 76, 95, 115, 213, 229, 259, 277. See also arthritis
  bronchial 110, 242
  chronic 69
  ear 210
  flu 189
  gas 116, 135, 189, 274, 328
  genital 266
  headache 64, 113, 136, 168
  heart 163
  intestinal 327, 331
  kidney 51, 235, 245
  mastitis 291
  menstrual 44, 168, 205, 268, 291, 327, 330
  migraine 76
  muscular 63, 69, 76, 115, 225
  nerve 115, 284. See also neuralgia
  ovarian 168, 240, 330
  rheumatic 69
  subacute 69
  throat 189, 317
  toothache 328

topical 58, 113, 117, 168, 200, 259, 273
urinary 69, 102, 106, 108, 155, 169, 180, 184, 234, 237, 244, 266, 327. *See also* dysuria
Paiute 73, 91, 189
palpitations 76, 99, 100, 163, 303, 304, 311
pancreas 96, 314
pancreatic juice 344
Paper birch 85
paralysis 115, 170, 171
parasites 56, 219, 222, 226, 254, 259, 309, 351, 352, 362, 366
parasympathetic nervous system 169, 343, 345, 346, 359, 366
parathyroid 213
Parry's gentian 148
Parsnip 118
Pasqueflower 238
Passionflower 101, 284, 303, 364
Peachleaf willow 324
Pea family. *See* Fabaceae
Pediacus Dioscorides 114
Pedicularis 45, 224–226
 grayi 224
 groenlandica 224
 procera 224
 racemosa 224
Pelargonium 153
Penicillium 290
Pennyroyal 165, 208, 232
Penstemon 138, 293
Peppermint 135, 274, 289
pepsin 93, 149
pepsinogen 219, 259, 359
perimenopause 47, 49, 66, 76, 77, 99, 100, 174, 255, 318, 359
period cramps. *See* dysmenorrhea
periodontitis 359, 362
peripheral vascular disease 359
peristalsis 360
Periwinkle 240
permethrin 186, 187
Persicaria bistortoides 88
pertussis 169
phagocytosis 360
pharmaceuticals 345, 352
pharyngitis 51, 59, 70, 74, 79, 81, 89, 102, 134, 152, 189, 192, 193, 217, 254, 255, 287, 289, 319, 331, 360

phosphaturia 266
photosensitivity 55
Picea 275
Pickpocket 265
Pinaceae 139, 226, 275
Pine 139, 142, 196, 226–233, 276, 278, 331
 family. *See* Pinaceae
Pineland figwort 137
Pineywoods geranium 151
Pink alumroot 50
 elephants 224
Pinus edulis 226
 flexilis 228
 monophylla 233
 ponderosa 226
 strobus 227
 sylvestris 233
pinworms 178, 259, 260, 308, 360
Pinyon pine 226
Pipsissewa 233–236, 244
pituitary 98, 99, 100
placenta 361
Plains beebalm 203
Plantaginaceae 236, 292
Plantago borysthenica 236
 dregeana 236
 latifolia 236
 major 236
 ovata 237
 psyllium 237
Plantain 236–237, 326
 Family. *See* Plantaginaceae
Plasmodium falciparum 360
platelet aggregation 360, 365
Pleated gentian 148
pleurisy 311, 361
Pleurisy root 228, 277
Pliny 261
Plumajillo 326
pneumonia 311
Poison hemlock 188
 ivy 123, 146, 160
Poke root 254, 255, 315
Poléo 135
 chino 166
Poliomintha 165, 208
polycystic ovarian syndrome 330
Polygonaceae 88, 122
Polygonatum multiflorum 134

Polygonum bistortoides 88
  multiflorum 89
  var. linearifolium 88
  var. oblongifolium 88
Ponderosa pine 134, 226
Poñil 55
Poplar buds 67
Populus angustifolia 63, 112
  aurea 62
  balsamifera 63, 67, 112
    ssp. balsamifera 67
    ssp. trichocarpa 67
    var. candicans 67
    var. subcordata 67
  candicans 67
  fremontii 112
  nigra 68
  tacamahacca 67
  tremula subsp. tremuloides 62
  tremuloides 62, 112
    var. aurea 62
    var. magnifica 62
    var. vancouveriana 62
  trichocarpa 63, 67
  x hastata 67
Porter's lovage 188
postpartum 47, 51, 66, 89, 90, 106, 152, 198, 243, 251, 266, 282, 300, 321
Potentilla 65, 105
  arguta 105
  diversifolia 105
  fruticosa 105, 106
Prairie crocus 238
  dogbane 124
  gentian 148
  grub 177
  sagewort 307
  smoke 65
pregnancy 45, 52, 55, 60, 72, 75, 77, 90, 92, 96, 101, 111, 118, 124, 126, 137, 143, 147, 153, 158, 161, 167, 170, 176, 185, 187, 190, 194, 199, 202, 207, 215, 218, 232, 236, 241, 246, 250, 251, 260, 262, 266, 269, 273, 275, 280, 285, 289, 294, 300, 304, 306, 309, 316, 329, 332, 348, 351, 361
Prickly ash 314
  pear 212

Primrose family. *See* Primulaceae
Primulaceae 261
Prince's pine 233
progesterone 47, 56, 66, 255, 348, 356, 361
prolactin 306, 361
prostate 64, 70, 145, 213, 214, 234, 235, 245, 346
prostatitis 70, 113, 145, 214, 234, 325, 330, 361
Prostrate verbena 305
Prunella vulgaris 263
Prunus serotina 310
  virginiana 310
Pseudognaphalium 242
Pseudotsuga 139
psoriasis 81, 87, 108, 116, 184, 220, 361
psychotic behavior 171
psyllium 142, 231, 237, 279
Ptelea crenulata 177
  trifoliata 177
Puccinia graminis 82
pulegone 45, 135, 137, 165, 208, 209
Pulsatilla 45, 76, 201, 238–241
  hirsutissima 238
  ludoviciana 238
  occidentali 238
  vulgaris 239
Purple horsemint 43
  hyssop 43
Purshia tridentata 90
Pussytoes 242–243
pycnogenol 228
pyelitis 235, 245
pyrethrins 223
Pyrola 244–246
pyrrolizidine alkaloids 58, 182, 202, 351

Q

Quaking aspen 62
Quercus gambelii 215

R

Raíz de cochino 188
  del lobo 272
Ranunculaceae 75, 185, 199, 202, 238
rashes 90, 132, 138, 152, 237, 282, 319
Rattlesnake orchid 246

INDEX

plantain 246–247
rattlesnakes 191
Raynaud's syndrome 84, 362
Red baneberry 75
  birds in a tree 137
  chickweed 261
  dogwood 247
  elderberry 127
  osier dogwood 86, 247–250
  raspberry 48, 250–252, 317, 321
  root 252–256
  twig dogwood 247
reproductive 53, 54, 55, 77, 100, 118, 165, 190, 199, 207, 208, 243, 300, 320, 321, 327, 329, 330, 331, 332
Resin birch 85
Reye's syndrome 65, 114, 326, 362
Rhamnaceae 94, 252
Rhamnus betulifolia 94
  californica 94
  cathartica 95
  purshiana 95
rhinitis 213, 214, 317, 319, 362. *See also* hayfever
Rhode Island 75
Rhus aromatica 146
  trilobata 146
Ribbed melilot 290
Ribes 256, 256–257
Ribwort 236
Richardson's geranium 151
ringworm 357, 362
River birch 85
  hawthorn 161
Roadside agrimony 46
Rocky mountain elder 127
  mountain goldenrod 154
  mountain iris 313
  mountain pond lily 329
  mountain white oak 215
Rocky Mountains 53, 67, 68, 75, 78, 86, 128, 131, 148, 183, 190, 199, 212, 222, 248, 258, 272, 286, 302, 310, 311, 314, 329
Rosaceae 46, 55, 65, 90, 105, 161, 250, 310, 316, 320
Rosa gymnocarpa 316
  nutkana 316
  woodsii 316

Rose angelica 52
  family. *See* Rosaceae
  geranium 153
  hips 318
Rosebay 144
rosin 227, 232, 276, 279
Ross's avens 65
Rosy pussytoes 243
Roundleaf alumroot 50
roundworms 178, 259, 260, 362
rubefacient 200, 240, 362
Rubiaceae 107
Rubus idaeus 250
Rue family. *See* Rutaceae
Rumex 122
  hymenosepalus 122
Russia 145, 182
Ruta 179
Rutaceae 177

S

Sage 206, 258, 260, 307, 311
Sagebrush 91, 178, 307, 308, 318
Salicaceae 62, 67, 112, 324
Salix amygdaloides 324
  bebbiana 324
  exigua 324
  nigra 325
Salmonella 51, 79, 129, 259, 362
Salt spring checkerbloom 101
Sambucus cerulea 127
  glauca 127
  melanocarpa 127
  mexicana 127
  microbotrys 127
  neomexicana 127
  nigra 127
  racemosa var. melanocarpa 127
  velutina 127
San Juan Mountains 78
Saxifragaceae 50
Saxifrage 151
Scarlet pimpernel 261–263, 323
Scented geranium 153
Scotch pine 233
Scouler's St. John's wort 283
scrapes 51, 56, 57, 64, 74, 91, 113, 134, 146, 147, 175, 193, 206, 216, 217, 246,

247, 257, 264, 281, 282, 287, 318, 319, 323
Scrophularia 137
  macrantha 137
Scrophulariaceae 137, 209
scurvy 141
Scutellaria angustifolia 269
  galericulata 269
sea sickness 168
sedative 44, 45, 76, 98, 99, 101, 110, 115, 169, 170, 174, 175, 176, 222, 225, 259, 271, 284, 302, 303, 304, 305, 306, 311, 327
seizures 115, 270, 271
Selenicereus 59, 99
Self heal 263–265, 286
seminal vesicle 240, 266
Senecio 226, 264
Senna 95, 157
Seriphidium tridentatum 258
serotonin 357
Serviceberry 250
Shepherd's heart 265
  purse 265–267
shingles 115, 284, 353, 363
Shinleaf 244
Shoshoni 91
Shrubby trefoil 177
sialagogue 314, 315
Sickletop lousewort 224
Sidalcea neomexicana 101
Sierra Nevada 72, 196, 199
Sieversia paradoxa 55
Silk tassel 178, 205, 216, 243, 267–269
  family. *See* Garryaceae
Simaruba family 51, 66, 80, 152
sinuses 363
sinusitis 79, 81, 89, 90, 141, 152, 217, 220, 259, 277, 317, 319, 363
Skullcap 269–272, 284, 286
Skunk bush 146
Slippery elm 80
Small leaf angelica 52
  pasqueflower 239
Smilacina racemosa 133
Smokeweed 88
Snakeberry 75
snakebite 354
Sneezeweed 272–273

Solidago 154
  canadensis 154
Solomon's plume 133
  seal 133
Sonoran hyssop 43
sore throat 50, 56, 57, 141, 152, 172, 189, 216, 245, 256, 257, 282, 289, 317. *See also* pharyngitis
South Dakota 156, 258
  Carolina 204
Southwestern black cherry 310
Spanish Flu 192
spasmolytic 44, 53, 168, 327
Spearleaf arnica 57
Spearmint 274–275
sperm 365
spermatorrhea 325, 358, 364
Spikenard 332
splenitis 253, 254, 255
Spotted beebalm 203
  horsemint 203
sprains 58, 64, 113, 136, 225, 259
Spruce 83, 139, 142, 275–280, 331
Squaw bush 146
Squawroot 280–282
Stachys 225, 270, 286–287
  palustris subsp. pilosa 286
  pilosa 286
Staphylococcus 79, 175, 210, 259, 331, 364
Star solomon's seal 134
Stavesacre 186
Stillingia 189, 220, 254
stings 56, 89, 90, 138, 146, 152, 182, 213, 237, 246, 264, 286, 287
Stinking roger 167
  sumac 146
St. John's wort 69, 270, 283–286, 286
  family. *See* Clusiaceae
stomach 44, 48, 50, 63, 72, 89, 93, 107, 116, 143, 149, 150, 166, 184, 208, 216, 219, 232, 236, 240, 247, 259, 271, 279, 288, 308, 322
stomachic 135, 175
Strawberry 321
  tree 199
Stream orchid 110
strep throat 364
Streptococcus 79, 259, 364
Streptomycetes 175

stroke 349
Subalpine fir 139
sudorific 44, 110
Sumac 146
sunburn 56, 57, 132, 146, 281, 282
Sunflower family. *See* Asteraceae
Swamp hedgenettle 286
Sweet cicely 288–289
 clover 168, 254, 290–292
Sweetroot 288
swelling 348, 362
Swertia radiata 156

T

T3. *See* triiodothyronine
T4. *See* thyroxine
Tacamahac 67
tachycardia 99, 100, 164, 170, 364
takotsubo cardiomyopathy 163
Tanacetum parthenium 222
Tarahumara 189
Taraxacum dens–leonis 119
 officinale 119
 retroflexum 119
 sylvanicum 119
TCM. *See* Traditional Chinese Medicine
Tea tree 232
tendinitis 69
Tennessee 204
testosterone 344, 364
Texas 44, 56, 94, 148, 156, 159, 162, 165, 173, 179, 196, 204, 251, 261, 267, 281, 293, 305, 310, 317, 324, 326
 madrone 195
 Trans–Pecos 44
Thermopsis 226
Three leaf sumac 146
thrush 81, 365. *See also* Candida albicans
Thuja 51, 66, 102, 232, 300, 318
Thyme 205
thyroid 98, 100, 101, 125, 314, 365
 stimulating hormone 98, 100, 365
thyroxin 81
thyroxine 81, 98, 100, 314, 365
Tigarea tridentata 90
Toadflax 292–294, 294
Tobacco 59, 243, 292, 365
tonsillitis 255, 365

Towering lousewort 224
Toxicodendron 146
Traditional Chinese Medicine 53, 346
traveler's diarrhea 344, 365
Tree of heaven 56, 66, 80, 268
 primrose 131
Trefoil 92
Tremble 62
Trichomonas vaginalis 152
trichomoniasis 66, 222
Trichophyton 79, 175, 365
Trifolium officirale 290
triiodothyronine 81, 98, 100, 314, 365
TSH. *See* thyroid stimulating hormone
tuberculosis 116
Turmeric 95, 149, 294, 318, 323
turpentine 227, 229, 231

U

ulcerative colitis 87, 145, 268, 308, 327, 365
ulcers 87, 89, 92, 123, 150, 160, 175, 182, 183, 216, 217, 222, 245, 246, 249, 259, 264, 266, 277, 281, 284, 291, 308, 323, 327
Unani 104
ureter 327
ureteritis 235, 245
urethra 69, 106, 160, 169, 197, 210, 266, 299, 327
urethritis 47, 74, 106, 108, 198, 234, 235, 245, 251, 300, 318, 321, 366
uric acid 61, 120, 212, 266, 366
urinary tract 46, 47, 51, 52, 56, 66, 69, 70, 74, 79, 87, 106, 108, 113, 140, 141, 169, 172, 180, 184, 196, 197, 198, 210, 213, 229, 234, 237, 244, 245, 257, 265, 266, 277, 299, 319, 321, 325, 327, 330
Urticaceae 211
Urtica dioica subsp. gracilis 211
 gracilis 211
 holosericea 211
Utah 43, 68, 72, 78, 86, 128, 148, 162, 177, 188, 204, 212, 215, 234, 267, 270
uterine 45, 47, 54, 66, 76, 77, 78, 96, 106, 169, 185, 199, 208, 241, 255, 259, 268, 285, 300, 309, 321, 361

Uva–ursi 74, 83, 102, 172, 196, 198, 234, 244, 298–300

V

Vaccinium corymbosum 85
  myrtillus 83
  oreophilum 83
vaginitis 47, 51, 56, 57, 66, 90, 106, 107, 152, 193, 222, 251, 300, 317, 319, 321, 327, 328, 331, 366. *See also* inflammation, vaginal
vagus nerve 242, 366
Valerian 45, 174, 225, 301–304
  family. *See* Valerianaceae
Valeriana acutiloba 301
  arizonica 302
  edulis 301
  occidentalis 302
  officinalis 301
Valerianaceae 301
valium 305
valley fever 348
varicella zoster virus 284, 363. *See also* shingles
varicoceles 240
varicosities 164, 291
venous insufficiency 291, 318
Veratrum 328
Verbascum thapsus 209
Verbena 305–306
  bracteata 305
  macdougalii 305
Verbenaceae 305
vermifuge 366
Verruca vulgaris 366
vertigo 366
Vervain family. *See* Verbenaceae
Very low density lipoprotein 366
Vinca major 99, 240
Viola 322
  adunca 322
  canadensis 322
  nephrophylla 322
Violaceae 322
Violet dock 122
  family. *See* Violaceae
Virginia strawberry 320
vitamin C 141, 152, 199, 228, 229, 277

vitiligo 366
VLDL. *See* Very low density lipoprotein
vocal cords 59
vomiting 44, 135, 168, 205, 289
vulnerary 104, 138, 182, 264, 287, 291, 323, 367
VZV. *See* varicella zoster virus

W

Wafer ash 177
warfarin 291
warts 348, 352, 353, 366
  genital 348, 353
Washington 52, 68, 72, 86, 97, 128, 131, 148, 156, 165, 212, 238, 239, 248, 263, 267, 270, 311, 317, 324, 329
Washoe Indians 192
Water avens 65
  birch 85
  hemlock 188
  lily family. *See* Nymphaeaceae
Weatherglass 261
Western balsam poplar 67
  barberry 78
  bistort 88
  blue flag 313
  chokecherry 310
  dock 122
  elder 127
  goldenrod 154
  hops 173
  mugwort 44, 149, 294, 307–309, 318
  pasqueflower 238
  pennyroyal 165, 207
  peony 44, 54, 168, 216, 327, 330
  rattlesnake plantain 246
  valerian 301
  yarrow 326
White avens 65
  fir 139
  marsh marigold 199
  melilot 290
  pasqueflower 238
  pine 227
  sage 172, 189
  sagewort 307
  spruce 275
  sweet clover 290

waterlily 330
white blood cell 356, 360, 367
whooping cough 169
Whortleberry 83
Wickup 144
Wight's silk tassel 267
Wild bergamot 203
  cherry 169, 228, 277, 310–312
  crocus 238
  geranium 151
  iris 261, 313–315
  lilac 252
  mint 135
  oregano 203
  parsnip 114
  rhubarb 122
  rose 65, 106, 282, 316–318
  strawberry 317, 320–321
  violet 323–324
Willow 69, 113, 205, 324–326
  dock 122
  family. *See* Salicaceae
Wingseed 177
Wintergreen 87
Woodland agrimony 46
  strawberry 320
Woods' rose 316
Woolly mullein 209
wounds 58, 59, 84, 87, 116, 129, 138, 181, 182, 183, 201, 206, 219, 259, 264, 278, 281, 284, 291, 292, 327, 328
Woundwort 286
Wyoming 67, 68, 101, 128, 148, 159, 162, 167, 188, 302, 305

Y

Yarrow 223, 326–329
yeast infections. *See* Candida albicans
Yellow avens 65
  melilot 290
  pond lily 54, 168, 216, 329–333
  sweet clover 290
  water lily 329
Yellowdock 122, 213
Yerba buena 274
  del lobo 272
  mansa 59, 81, 189, 327
  santa 73, 74, 91

Z

Zea mays 197
Ziziphus 253